T0259169

Pediatric Critical Care

Editors

MARY W. LIEH-LAI
KATHERINE CASHEN

PEDIATRIC CLINICS
OF NORTH AMERICA

www.pediatric.theclinics.com

Consulting Editor
BONITA F. STANTON

June 2022 • Volume 69 • Number 3

ELSEVIER

1600 John F. Kennedy Boulevard • Suite 1800 • Philadelphia, Pennsylvania, 19103-2899

http://www.theclinics.com

THE PEDIATRIC CLINICS OF NORTH AMERICA Volume 69, Number 3
June 2022 ISSN 0031-3955, ISBN-13: 978-0-323-98675-5

Editor: Kerry Holland
Developmental Editor: Axell Ivan Jade M. Purificacion

© **2022 Elsevier Inc. All rights reserved.**

This periodical and the individual contributions contained in it are protected under copyright by Elsevier, and the following terms and conditions apply to their use:

Photocopying
Single photocopies of single articles may be made for personal use as allowed by national copyright laws. Permission of the Publisher and payment of a fee is required for all other photocopying, including multiple or systematic copying, copying for advertising or promotional purposes, resale, and all forms of document delivery. Special rates are available for educational institutions that wish to make photocopies for non-profit educational classroom use. For information on how to seek permission visit www.elsevier.com/permissions or call: (+44) 1865 843830 (UK)/(+1) 215 239 3804 (USA).

Derivative Works
Subscribers may reproduce tables of contents or prepare lists of articles including abstracts for internal circulation within their institutions. Permission of the Publisher is required for resale or distribution outside the institution. Permission of the Publisher is required for all other derivative works, including compilations and translations (please consult www.elsevier.com/permissions).

Electronic Storage or Usage
Permission of the Publisher is required to store or use electronically any material contained in this periodical, including any article or part of an article (please consult www.elsevier.com/permissions). Except as outlined above, no part of this publication may be reproduced, stored in a retrieval system or transmitted in any form or by any means, electronic, mechanical, photocopying, recording or otherwise, without prior written permission of the Publisher.

Notice
No responsibility is assumed by the Publisher for any injury and/or damage to persons or property as a matter of products liability, negligence or otherwise, or from any use or operation of any methods, products, instructions or ideas contained in the material herein. Because of rapid advances in the medical sciences, in particular, independent verification of diagnoses and drug dosages should be made.

Although all advertising material is expected to conform to ethical (medical) standards, inclusion in this publication does not constitute a guarantee or endorsement of the quality or value of such product or of the claims made of it by its manufacturer.

The Pediatric Clinics of North America (ISSN 0031-3955) is published bimonthly by Elsevier Inc., 360 Park Avenue South, New York, NY 10010-1710. Months of issue are February, April, June, August, October, and December. Periodicals postage paid at New York, NY and additional mailing offices. Subscription prices are $263.00 per year (US individuals), $1028.00 per year (US institutions), $331.00 per year (Canadian individuals), $1074.00 per year (Canadian institutions), $395.00 per year (international individuals), $1074.00 per year (international institutions), $100.00 per year (US students and residents), $100.00 per year (Canadian students and residents), and $165.00 per year (international residents and students). To receive students/resident rare, orders must be accompanied by name of affiliated institution, date of term, and the signature of program/residency coordinator on institution letterhead. Orders will be billed at individual rate until proof of status is received. Foreign air speed delivery is included in all *Clinics* subscription prices. All prices are subject to change without notice. **POSTMASTER:** Send address changes to *The Pediatric Clinics of North America*, Elsevier Health Sciences Division, Subscription Customer Service, 3251 Riverport Lane, Maryland Heights, MO 63043. **Customer Service: 1-800-654-2452 (US and Canada). From outside of the US and Canada: 1-314-447-8871. Fax: 1-314-447-8029. For print support, E-mail: JournalsCustomerService-usa@elsevier.com. For online support, E-mail: JournalsOnlineSupport-usa@elsevier.com.**

Reprints. For copies of 100 or more, of articles in this publication, please contact the Commercial Reprints Department, Elsevier Inc., 360 Park Avenue South, New York, NY 10010-1710. Tel.: 212-633-3874; Fax: 212-633-3820; E-mail: reprints@elsevier.com.

The Pediatric Clinics of North America is also published in Spanish by McGraw-Hill Inter-americana Editores S.A., Mexico City, Mexico; in Portuguese by Riechmann and Affonso Editores, Rua Comandante Coelho 1085, CEP 21250, Rio de Janeiro, Brazil; and in Greek by Althayia SA, Athens, Greece.

The Pediatric Clinics of North America is covered in *MEDLINE/PubMed (Index Medicus), Excerpta Medica, Current Contents, Current Contents/Clinical Medicine, Science Citation Index, ASCA, ISI/BIOMED,* and *BIOSIS.*

PROGRAM OBJECTIVE
The goal of the *Pediatric Clinics of North America* is to keep practicing physicians and residents up to date with current clinical practice in pediatrics by providing timely articles reviewing the state-of-the-art in patient care.

TARGET AUDIENCE
All practicing pediatricians, physicians, and healthcare professionals who provide patient care to pediatric patients.

LEARNING OBJECTIVES
Upon completion of this activity, participants will be able to:
1. Review the appropriate use of evidence-based clinical guidelines, interventions, medications, and supportive therapies to promote safe, quality care and positive outcomes in critically ill children.
2. Discuss education in the pediatric critical care setting using traditional and novel teaching strategies and technology to improve diagnostic abilities and clinical decision-making skills.
3. Recognize the significance and impact of multidisciplinary collaboration in pediatric intensive care planning, decision making, coordination of care, and serving the needs of patients and families.

ACCREDITATIONS
Physician Credit

The Elsevier Office of Continuing Medical Education (EOCME) is accredited by the Accreditation Council for Continuing Medical Education (ACCME) to provide continuing medical education for physicians.

The EOCME designates this journal-based activity for a maximum of 13 *AMA PRA Category 1 Credit*(s)™. Physicians should claim only the credit commensurate with the extent of their participation in the activity.

All other healthcare professionals requesting continuing education credit for this journal-based activity will be issued a certificate of participation.

ABP Maintenance of Certification Credit

Successful completion of this CME activity, which includes participation in the activity and individual assessment of and feedback to the learner, enables the learner to earn up to 13 MOC points in the American Board of Pediatrics' (ABP) Maintenance of Certification (MOC) program. It is the CME activity provider's responsibility to submit learner completion information to ACCME for the purpose of granting ABP MOC credit.

DISCLOSURE OF CONFLICTS OF INTEREST
The EOCME assesses conflict of interest with its instructors, faculty, planners, and other individuals who are in a position to control the content of CME activities. All relevant conflicts of interest that are identified are thoroughly vetted by EOCME for fair balance, scientific objectivity, and patient care recommendations. EOCME is committed to providing its learners with CME activities that promote improvements or quality in healthcare and not a specific proprietary business or a commercial interest.

The planning committee, staff, authors, and editors listed below have identified no financial relationships or relationships to products or devices they or their spouse/life partner have with commercial interest related to the content of this CME activity:
Omar Alibrahim, MD; Michael R. Anderson, MD, MBA; Orkun Baloglu, MD; Rukhmi Bhat, MD, MS; Katherine Cashen, DO; Meera Chitlur, MD; Jeff A. Clark, MD; Kshama Daphtary, MD, MBI; Moreshwar Desai, MBBS; Meena Kalyanaraman, MD; Janelle Kummick, PharmD, BCPPS; Mary W. Lieh-Lai, MD; Amarilis A. Martin, MD; Marvin B. Mata, MD, MSHS-HCQ, CPHQ, CPPS, FAAP; Rajkumar Mayakrishnan, BSc, MBA; Kathleen L. Meert, MD; Andrew G. Miller, MSc, RRT; Andrew Prout, MD; Katherine Regling, DO; Kyle J. Rehder, MD, FCCM; Divya Sabapathy, MD; Raya Safa, MD; Arun Saini, MD, MS; Alexander Santos, MD, FAAP; Ajit Ashok Sarnaik, MD; Doreen Thomas-Payne, MSN, BSN, RN, PMHNP-BC; Judith Ugale-Wilson, MD, FAAP; Kevin Valentine, MD

The planning committee, staff, authors and editors listed below have identified financial relationships or relationships to products or devices they or their spouse/life partner have with commercial interest related to the content of this CME activity:
Alexandre T. Rotta, MD, FCCM: *Speaker*: Breas Medical, Inc, Vapotherm

UNAPPROVED/OFF-LABEL USE DISCLOSURE

The EOCME requires CME faculty to disclose to the participants:

1. When products or procedures being discussed are off-label, unlabelled, experimental, and/or investigational (not US Food and Drug Administration [FDA] approved); and
2. Any limitations on the information presented, such as data that are preliminary or that represent ongoing research, interim analyses, and/or unsupported opinions. Faculty may discuss information about pharmaceutical agents that is outside of FDA-approved labelling. This information is intended solely for CME and is not intended to promote off-label use of these medications. If you have any questions, contact the medical affairs department of the manufacturer for the most recent prescribing information.

TO ENROLL

To enroll in the *Pediatric Clinics of North America* Continuing Medical Education program, call customer service at 1-800-654-2452 or sign up online at http://www.theclinics.com/home/cme. The CME program is available to subscribers for an additional annual fee of USD 324.00.

METHOD OF PARTICIPATION

In order to claim credit, participants must complete the following:

1. Complete enrolment as indicated above.
2. Read the activity.
3. Complete the CME Test and Evaluation. Participants must achieve a score of 70% on the test. All CME Tests and Evaluations must be completed online.

In order to claim MOC points, participants must complete the following:

1. Complete steps listed above for claiming CME credit
2. Provide your specialty board ID#, birth date (MM/DD), and attestation.
3. Online MOC submission is only available for the American Board of pediatrics' (ABP) Maintenance of Certification (MOC) program

CME INQUIRIES/SPECIAL NEEDS

For all CME inquiries or special needs, please contact elsevierCME@elsevier.com

Contributors

CONSULTING EDITOR

BONITA F. STANTON, MD
Professor of Pediatrics and Founding Dean, Robert C. and Laura C. Garrett Endowed Chair, Hackensack Meridian School of Medicine, President, Academic Enterprise, Hackensack Meridian Health, Nutley, New Jersey

EDITORS

MARY W. LIEH-LAI, MD
Professor of Pediatrics (Vol), Wayne State University School of Medicine, Detroit, Michigan, USA

KATHERINE CASHEN, DO
Associate Professor of Pediatrics, Division of Pediatric Critical Care Medicine, Department of Pediatrics, Duke Children's Hospital, Duke University Medical Center, Duke University School of Medicine, Durham, North Carolina

AUTHORS

OMAR ALIBRAHIM, MD
Associate Professor of Pediatrics and PICU Medical Director, Division of Pediatric Critical Care Medicine, Department of Pediatrics, Duke University School of Medicine, Durham, North Carolina

MICHAEL R. ANDERSON, MD MBA
Senior Advisor, Children's National Hospital, Adjunct Professor of Leadership and Clinical Research, George Washington University School of Medicine and Health Sciences

ORKUN BALOGLU, MD
Staff Physician, Department of Pediatric Critical Care Medicine, Clinical Assistant Professor of Pediatrics, Cleveland Clinic Lerner College of Medicine, Case Western Reserve University, Cleveland, Ohio

RUKHMI BHAT, MD, MS
Division of Hematology, Oncology and Stem Cell Transplantation, Associate Professor of Pediatrics, Northwestern University Feinberg School of Medicine, Ann & Robert H. Lurie Children's Hospital of Chicago, Chicago, Illinois

KATHERINE CASHEN, DO
Associate Professor of Pediatrics, Division of Pediatric Critical Care Medicine, Department of Pediatrics, Duke Children's Hospital, Duke University Medical Center, Duke University School of Medicine, Durham, North Carolina

MEERA CHITLUR, MD
Barnhart-Lusher Hemostasis Research Endowed Chair, Wayne State University, Professor of Pediatrics, Central Michigan University, Director, Hemophilia Treatment

Center and Hemostasis Program, Special Coagulation Laboratory, Division of Hematology/Oncology, Children's Hospital of Michigan, Detroit, Michigan

JEFF A. CLARK, MD
Staff Intensivist, Division of Pediatric Critical Care Medicine, Vice Chair of Pediatrics, Ascension St. John Children's Hospital, Detroit, Michigan

KSHAMA DAPHTARY, MD, MBI
Staff Physician, Department of Pediatric Critical Care Medicine, Clinical Assistant Professor of Pediatrics, Cleveland Clinic Lerner College of Medicine, Case Western Reserve University, Cleveland, Ohio

MORESHWAR S. DESAI, MBBS
Director of Pediatric Liver ICU, Associate Professor, Department of Pediatrics, Division of Critical Care Medicine, Baylor College of Medicine, Houston, Texas

MEENA KALYANARAMAN, MD
Associate Director, Pediatric Critical Care Medicine, Children's Hospital of New Jersey at Newark, Beth Israel Medical Center, Newark, New Jersey

JANELLE KUMMICK, PharmD, BCPPS
Indianapolis, Indiana

AMARILIS A. MARTIN, MD
Division of Pediatric Critical Care Medicine, Assistant Professor of Pediatrics, Central Michigan University College of Medicine, Children's Hospital of Michigan, Detroit, Michigan

MARVIN B. MATA, MD, MSHS-HCQ, CPHQ, CPPS, FAAP
Medical Director, Department of Pediatrics, PICU and Pediatric Hospital Medicine, Rapides Regional Medical Center, Alexandria, Louisiana

KATHLEEN L. MEERT, MD
Professor of Pediatrics, Chair, Discipline of Pediatrics, Children's Hospital of Michigan, Detroit, Michigan; Central Michigan University, Mt. Pleasant, Michigan

ANDREW G. MILLER, MSc, RRT
Respiratory Care Services, Duke University Medical Center, Durham, North Carolina

ANDREW PROUT, MD
Assistant Professor of Pediatrics, Division of Pediatric Critical Care Medicine, Discipline of Pediatrics, Children's Hospital of Michigan, Detroit, Michigan; Central Michigan University, Mt. Pleasant, Michigan

KATHERINE REGLING, DO
Assistant Professor of Pediatrics, Division of Pediatric Hematology Oncology, Children's Hospital of Michigan, Detroit, Michigan; Central Michigan University, Mt. Pleasant, Michigan

KYLE J. REHDER, MD, FCCM
Associate Professor of Pediatrics and Vice-Chair of Education, Department of Pediatrics, Duke University School of Medicine, Durham, North Carolina

ALEXANDRE T. ROTTA, MD, FCCM
Professor of Pediatrics and Chief, Division of Pediatric Critical Care Medicine, Department of Pediatrics, Duke University School of Medicine, Durham, North Carolina

DIVYA G. SABAPATHY, MD
Department of Pediatrics, Division of Pediatric Critical Care Medicine and Liver ICU,
Baylor College of Medicine, Houston, Texas

RAYA SAFA, MD
Assistant Professor of Pediatrics, Divisions of Cardiology and Critical Care, Children's
Hospital of Michigan, Detroit, Michigan; Central Michigan University, Mt. Pleasant,
Michigan

ARUN SAINI, MD, MS
Assistant Professor of Pediatrics, Division of Pediatric Critical Care Medicine, Texas
Children's Hospital, Baylor University, Houston, Texas

ALEXANDER SANTOS, MD, FAAP
Pediatric Intensivist, Pediatric Critical Care, Children's Healthcare of Atlanta – Scottish
Rite, Neonatology Associates of Atlanta, Atlanta, Georgia

AJIT A. SARNAIK, MD
Associate Professor of Pediatrics, Central Michigan University College of Medicine, Carls
Building, Pediatric Critical Care, Children's Hospital of Michigan, Detroit, Michigan

JUDITH UGALE-WILSON, MD
Clinical Associate Professor, Department of Pediatrics, Pediatric Critical Care Medicine,
East Carolina University Greenville, ECU Brody School of Medicine, Greenville,
North Carolina

KEVIN VALENTINE, MD
Associate Professor of Clinical Pediatrics, Indiana University School of Medicine,
Riley Hospital for Children, Indianapolis, Indiana

Contents

> Pediatric cardiac critical care has evolved with advances in congenital heart surgery, interventional cardiac catheterization, and diagnostic advances. Debate remains over the optimal location of care and training background despite data showing that systems established in collaboration with multidisciplinary experts in the care of children with congenital heart disease are associated with the best outcomes. Operative mortality is low, and preventing morbidity is the new focus of the future. Advances in screening and fetal diagnosis, mechanical circulatory support, and collaborative research and quality improvement initiatives are reviewed in this article.

> Brain injury in children is a major public health problem, causing substantial morbidity and mortality. Cause of pediatric brain injury varies widely and can be from a primary neurologic cause or as a sequela of multisystem illness. This review discusses the emerging field of pediatric neurocritical care (PNCC), including current techniques of imaging, treatment, and monitoring. Future directions of PNCC include further expansion of evidence-based practice guidelines and establishment of multidisciplinary PNCC services within institutions.

> Neonatal and pediatric extracorporeal membrane oxygenation (ECMO) has evolved over the past 50 years. Advances in technology, expertise, and application have increased the number of centers providing ECMO with expanded indications for use. However, increasing the use of ECMO in recent years to more medically complex critically ill children has not changed overall survival despite increased experience and improvements in technology. This review focuses on ECMO history, circuits, indications and contraindications, management, complications, and outcome data. The authors highlight important areas of progress, including unintubated and awake patients on ECMO, application during the COVID-19 pandemic, and future directions.

> Extracorporeal membrane oxygenation (ECMO) and ventricular assist devices (VADs) are increasingly used in critically ill children. Despite improvements in

mechanical design and clinical management, thromboembolic and hemorrhagic events remain significant causes of morbidity and mortality related to the use of both devices. Choice of anticoagulant agents and assays for monitoring continue to present challenges in management. In this review, we describe the incidence and risk factors for thrombosis and hemorrhage, the different types of anticoagulants currently in use, the assays available for monitoring anticoagulation, and management of thromboembolic and bleeding complications in children on mechanical circulatory support (MCS). We conclude by emphasizing the areas that need further study to minimize the risk for thrombosis and hemorrhage in the use of ECMO and VAD in children.

Divya G. Sabapathy and Moreshwar S. Desai

Acute liver failure (ALF) in children, irrespective of cause, is a rapidly evolving catastrophic clinical condition that results in high mortality and morbidity without prompt identification and intervention. Massive hepatocyte necrosis impairs the synthetic, excretory, and detoxification abilities of the liver, with resultant coagulopathy, jaundice, metabolic disturbance, and encephalopathy. Extrahepatic organ damage, multiorgan failure, and death result from circulating inflammatory mediators released by the hepatocytes undergoing necrosis. There are yet no treatment options available for reversing or halting hepatocellular necrosis, thus current therapy focuses on supporting failing organs and preventing life threatening complications pending either spontaneous liver recovery or transplantation. The aims of this review are to define pediatric acute liver failure (PALF), understand the pathophysiologic processes that lead to multiorgan failure, to describe the consequences of a failing liver on extrahepatic organs, to enumerate the critical care challenges encountered during PALF management, and to describe pharmacologic and extracorporeal options available to support a critically ill child with ALF in the intensive care unit.

Marvin B. Mata, Alexander Santos, and Judith Ugale-Wilson

Community pediatric intensive care units (PICUs) play a crucial role in providing high-quality care to critically ill children in the rural setting. Setting one up requires meticulous planning and allocation of limited resources. The design and layout of PICUs vary widely but need to meet the required minimum standards and follow local and federal policies and regulatory standards. The building block is investing in the education and training of health care providers. Collaboration with tertiary facilities and community organizations helps provide care closer to home. Care coordination necessitates partnering with the families and the community and including telemedicine to increase accessibility.

Kevin Valentine and Janelle Kummick

The care of the critically-ill child often includes medications used to optimize organ function, treat infections, and provide comfort. Pediatric pharmacology has some key differences that should be leveraged for safe pharmacologic management.

Kevin Valentine and Janelle Kummick

The care of the critically ill child often includes medications used for the relief of pain and anxiety. Children have key differences in pharmacokinetics and pharmacodynamics compared with adults that should always be considered to achieve safe medication use in this population. Pain must be addressed, and sedative use should be minimized when possible. Our understanding of sedation safety is evolving, and studies have shown that minimizing exposure to multiple medications can reduce the burden of delirium and iatrogenic withdrawal.

Meena Kalyanaraman and Michael R. Anderson

Coronavirus disease 2019 (COVID-19) is an ongoing pandemic caused by the severe acute respiratory syndrome coronavirus-2 (SARS-CoV-2) virus. More than 5 million children have been infected in the United States. Risk factors for more severe disease progression include obesity, pulmonary disease, gastrointestinal disorders, and neurologic comorbidities. Children with COVID-19 are admitted to the pediatric intensive care unit because of severe acute COVID-19 illness or COVID-19-associated multisystem inflammatory syndrome in children. The delta surge of 2021 was responsible for an increased disease burden in children and points to the key role of vaccinating children against this sometimes-deadly disease.

Kshama Daphtary and Orkun Baloglu

Clinical informatics can support quality improvement and patient safety in the pediatric intensive care unit (PICU) in several ways including data extraction, analysis, and decision support enabled by electronic health records (EHRs), and databases and registries. Clinical decision support (CDS), embedded in EHRs, now an integral part of the workflow in the PICU, includes several tools and is increasingly leveraging artificial intelligence (AI). Understanding the opportunities and challenges can improve the engagement of clinicians with the design, validation, and implementation of CDS, improve satisfaction with CDS, and improve patient safety, care quality, and value.

Omar Alibrahim, Kyle J. Rehder, Andrew G. Miller, and Alexandre T. Rotta

Children admitted to the pediatric intensive care unit often require respiratory support for the treatment of respiratory distress and failure. Respiratory support comprises both noninvasive modalities (ie, heated humidified high-flow nasal cannula, continuous positive airway pressure, bilevel positive airway pressure, negative pressure ventilation) and invasive mechanical ventilation. In this article, we review the various essential elements and considerations involved in the planning and application of respiratory support in the treatment of the critically ill children.

Andrew Prout and Kathleen L. Meert

Many important clinical questions remain unanswered in the practice of pediatric intensive care due to the lack of high-quality evidence. Although challenges exist in conducting research in pediatric intensive care units, identification of research priorities, interdisciplinary collaborations, innovative trial designs, and the use of common datasets and outcome measures helps to bring new knowledge to our field. The topic of "Research in PICUs" is extremely broad; therefore, this review focuses on a few common themes receiving increased attention in the literature, including research agendas, core outcome sets, precision medicine, and novel clinical trial strategies.

Jeff A. Clark

This article addresses the latest data and ideas related to education in the pediatric intensive care unit, including traditional education methods with newer and technology-based methods. A review of adult learning theory is included with discussions regarding medical decision making and error prevention, bedside teaching, medical simulation, and electronic methods of education.

PEDIATRIC CLINICS OF NORTH AMERICA

SERIES OF RELATED INTEREST

Critical Care Clinics of North America
www.criticalcare.theclinics.com

THE CLINICS ARE AVAILABLE ONLINE!
Access your subscription at:
www.theclinics.com

Preface

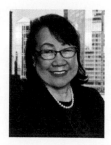 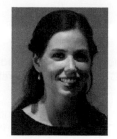

Mary W. Lieh-Lai, MD   Katherine Cashen, DO
Editors

The very first pediatric intensive care units were established in the late 1960s with one attending physician who was always on call, and a couple of fellows who usually were on call every other night. One-hundred-hour work weeks and forty-eight hours without sleep were common, and the ability to brag about this was a badge of honor. Despite the fatigue and sleep deprivation, we were taught, and we learned. Along the way, we saw evidence that the lack of sleep caused harm in many ways, so long work hours and bleary eyes, missing meals, living in the call room, and not seeing our families for days on end are no more. While these are steps in the right direction, we hope that education does not disappear with the constraints on our time.

Technology has evolved in the aspects of respiratory and cardiovascular support, medications, smart pumps, renal replacement therapy, neurointensive care, treatment for hepatic failure, cardiopulmonary resuscitation, and biological therapeutics. What remains central to the evolution and success in all we do in pediatrics and pediatric critical care medicine is education. As Yoda said in *The Last Jedi*, "We are what they grow beyond." Our students learn and grow and go out into the world and practice pediatrics and pediatric critical care and teach others in turn, and our greatest honor and hope is that they surpass us in all that they do.

Amid technological advances, the demands on our time, and the limits placed by rules and regulations, one must make time to continue to share knowledge and teach, whether it is at the bedside, in the hallway, in writing, or by example in our words and actions.

In this issue, we have the honor of inviting former students to be contributors to share their knowledge and experience. They have come far and embody the vision of why teachers teach. What they do, and what they have become is a reward that teachers dream of. On behalf of all the children and the families that they have taken care of and will continue to take care of, our humblest thanks and gratitude to all our students for serving as an inspiration to their teachers and for carrying on the tradition of teaching others.

Pediatr Clin N Am 69 (2022) xv–xvi
https://doi.org/10.1016/j.pcl.2022.03.001
0031-3955/22/© 2022 Published by Elsevier Inc.

Just as importantly, we are grateful to all our teachers and mentors, particularly those who taught us compassion and the importance of selflessly serving our patients. With that in mind, we dedicate this issue to Dr Bonita F. Stanton, our mentor and friend.

Mary W. Lieh-Lai, MD
Wayne State University School of Medicine

Katherine Cashen, DO
Division of Pediatric Critical Care Medicine, Department of Pediatrics, Duke Children's Hospital, Durham, NC, USA Duke University School of Medicine.

E-mail addresses:
mary.liehlai@svinpa.com (M.W. Lieh-Lai)
katherine.cashen@duke.edu (K. Cashen)

Cardiovascular Critical Care in Children

Katherine Cashen, DO[a,b,*], Raya Safa, MD[c,d]

KEYWORDS

- Pediatric • Congenital heart disease • Cardiac surgery • Acquired heart disease
- Outcomes • Infants • Children

KEY POINTS

- Children with congenital or acquired heart disease require complex multidisciplinary care.
- Outcomes for children with cardiovascular disease have improved significantly, with low operative mortality but the burden of morbidity remains high.
- The ideal location of cardiac critical care and training requirements for cardiac intensivists is controversial.
- Advances in congenital heart disease screening and fetal diagnosis, interventional cardiac catheterization, mechanical circulatory support, and collaborative research and quality improvement allow earlier detection and data for focused initiatives to decrease morbidity.

INTRODUCTION

Pediatric cardiac critical care has developed as a collaborative field with cardiac surgery, anesthesiology, critical care, cardiology, and other subspecialties working together. The need for pediatric specific complex postoperative management evolved with advances in surgical technique and life-support technology. Many early pediatric intensive care units were developed and staffed by pediatric anesthesiologists.[1] As pediatric critical care medicine became a distinct subspecialty, cardiac surgical technique, cardiac catheterization, and medical treatments for children with cardiovascular disease also progressed. In this review, the authors provide current data about the care environment/location of care for children with cardiac disease in the United States, provide an overview of training pathways and care models, review outcome data and advances in the field, and discuss future directions.

[a] Division of Pediatric Critical Care Medicine, Department of Pediatrics, Duke Children's Hospital, Durham, NC 27710, USA; [b] Duke University Medical Center, 2301 Erwin Road, Suite 5260Y, DUMC 3046, Durham, NC 27710, USA; [c] Divisions of Cardiology and Critical Care, Children's Hospital of Michigan 3901 Beaubien Boulevard, Detroit, MI 48201, USA; [d] Central Michigan University, Mt. Pleasant, MI, USA
* Corresponding author.
E-mail address: katherine.cashen@duke.edu

Pediatr Clin N Am 69 (2022) 403–413
https://doi.org/10.1016/j.pcl.2022.02.002
0031-3955/22/© 2022 Elsevier Inc. All rights reserved.

CARE ENVIRONMENT/LOCATION OF CARE

In the current era, many children's hospitals have either distinct cardiac intensive care units (CICU) or dedicated cardiac beds in the general pediatric intensive care unit (PICU.) There is ongoing debate about the optimal environment of care for children with cardiovascular disease.[2] Substantial variability in the care environment and location of care exists between centers in the United States (US). Much of the focus has surrounded care of neonates with congenital heart disease (CHD) in the preoperative period and the postoperative care of children with CHD or acquired heart disease. Importantly, the spectrum of cardiovascular critical care also includes children with arrhythmias (with or without CHD), acquired heart disease such as myocarditis, cardiomyopathies, Kawasaki disease, infectious endocarditis, and systemic diseases with cardiac insufficiency or failure. Cardiac insufficiency in multisystem inflammatory syndrome in children with COVID-19 infections is an important example. In some centers these children are preferentially cared for in CICUs, whereas others provide care for these children in PICUs, reserving dedicated cardiac beds or CICU beds for postoperative patients.

Neonates

Critically ill neonates with CHD have a long history of receiving care in the neonatal intensive care unit (NICU). However, many centers have moved preoperative care of neonates born with CHD to CICUs or PICUs with dedicated cardiac beds. A recent study using data from the Pediatric Health Information Systems (PHIS) database suggests that neonates with CHD who were initially admitted to a CICU versus the NICU had a reduction in total hospital cost, shorter hospital and ICU length of stay, and fewer days of mechanical ventilation but no difference in mortality.[3] Another study using PHIS data reported lower mortality for neonates cared for in CICUs compared with NICUs. In this study, preoperative and total length of stay and total length of mechanical ventilation were significantly greater in patients cared for in NICUs compared with CICUs. There was no difference in mortality for "low" complexity operations or patients undergoing treatment at high-volume hospitals.[4] Unfortunately, both these studies use PHIS data, which are from an administrative database that lacks the clinical detail needed to determine why a patient is first admitted to the NICU instead of the CICU and the rationale for transfer between the units. These studies suggest that despite trying to account for all variables, location of care could be a surrogate for other factors that drive outcome in different health systems. Thus, optimal location for preoperative neonates remains unclear.

Perioperative Care

Even more debate exists over the optimal care location for children in the perioperative period. Burstein and colleagues linked survey data to the Society of Thoracic Surgeons Congenital Heart Surgery Database to report a multivariable analysis of outcomes for children undergoing cardiac surgery in dedicated CICUs compared with general PICUs.[5] In this study, there was no difference in overall mortality, length of stay, or complications. In stratified analysis, CICUs were associated with lower mortality among STS-European Association for Cardiothoracic Surgery risk category 3 (primarily related to atrioventricular canal repair and arterial switch operation).[5] Experience of nurses, physicians, and surgeons were not evaluated in this study. Another recent study used data from the Virtual Pediatric Systems Database (VPS, LLC) and showed no difference in outcomes for children undergoing cardiac surgery based on unit type.[6] This study suggested that in centers with a large volume of cases, a dedicated CICU may have survival benefit. Other studies have shown significant hospital variation in morbidity and mortality after congenital heart surgery, including in lower risk surgical procedures.[7]

High-performance programs have an organized infrastructure, a critical mass of specialized providers, focused provider training, and adequate ancillary personnel.[8] Thus, in the perioperative period, location of care is likely less important than the structure of care. Many centers have adopted a Heart Center model with clear service lines and organization, which may include fetal, perioperative, and postoperative long-term care (**Fig. 1**). These high performing programs have standardization of management protocols, efficient resource utilization, and focused quality improvement initiatives.

TRAINING PATHWAYS/STAFFING MODELS

Current training pathways for pediatric cardiac intensive care physicians have substantial variability with unique strengths and weaknesses. These pathways have historically included pediatric critical care medicine (PCCM), pediatric cardiology, pediatric anesthesiology, and neonatology. The 3 predominant training pathways in the US include Accreditation Council for Graduate Medical Education (ACGME)

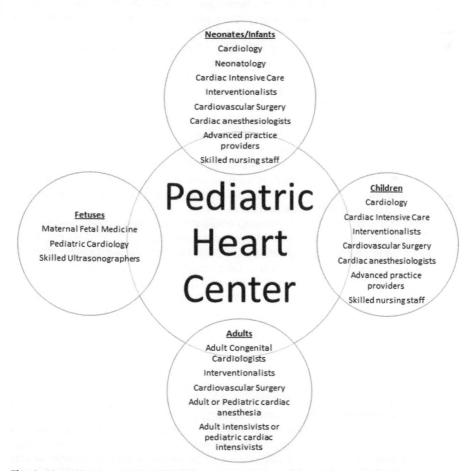

Neonates/Infants
Cardiology
Neonatology
Cardiac Intensive Care
Interventionalists
Cardiovascular Surgery
Cardiac anesthesiologists
Advanced practice providers
Skilled nursing staff

Fetuses
Maternal Fetal Medicine
Pediatric Cardiology
Skilled Ultrasonographers

Pediatric Heart Center

Children
Cardiology
Cardiac Intensive Care
Interventionalists
Cardiovascular Surgery
Cardiac anesthesiologists
Advanced practice providers
Skilled nursing staff

Adults
Adult Congenital Cardiologists
Interventionalists
Cardiovascular Surgery
Adult or Pediatric cardiac anesthesia
Adult intensivists or pediatric cardiac intensivists

Fig. 1. Heart Center model with different key personnel based on age of patient.

accredited, American Board of Pediatrics (ABP) categorical postdoctoral training in PCCM, pediatric cardiology, or both (dual PCCM/pediatric cardiology). In addition, an unaccredited fourth year of training in pediatric cardiac critical care is currently offered by 23 programs in North America. There is no standardization of training or oversight for the fourth year fellowship but a recent initiative endorsed by the Pediatric Cardiac Intensive Care Society developed a standardized curriculum.[9] Attempts to standardize training and certification are focused on optimizing care.

In a 2018 national survey, Horak and colleagues report a detailed evaluation of the landscape of 120 US and Canadian centers providing pediatric cardiac intensive care.[10] Respondents were from mixed ICUs (N = 61, 51%) and separate CICUs (N = 59, 49%). All centers reported use of extracorporeal membrane oxygenation and the majority reported caring for patients older than 18 years. The most common training background for practicing cardiac intensivists in this study was pediatric critical care (98% of attendings in mixed ICUs and 63% of attendings in CICUs). In separate CICUs, dual PCCM/cardiology fellowship (80%) or critical care with 1 year of cardiac critical care training (77%) was more common in the physician group when compared with mixed ICUs. Advanced practice providers were consistent frontline providers in CICUs and mixed ICUs. Separate CICUs had more access to electrophysiology, heart failure, and cardiac anesthesiology consultation than mixed ICUs.[10] These separate CICUs were located in higher volume centers and may explain the increased subspecialty access.

Additional subspecialty training of attending physicians has not been associated with improved outcome in pediatric cardiac intensive care.[11] Cardiac intensivists must have a thorough understanding of cardiac physiology, the breadth of critical care, leadership skills, and the technical skills needed to care for critically ill cardiac patients. The training pathways and the learning objectives for PCCM or board-certified pediatric cardiology subspecialists pursuing a fourth year of training in pediatric cardiac critical care are variable. Recently, a taskforce including content experts and program directors of these fellowships developed and published learning objectives and minimum rotational requirements for dual PCCM/pediatric cardiology fellowship programs and fourth year pediatric cardiac critical care fellowships.[9] Regardless of subspecialty training pathway, all stakeholders agree that the goal of standardizing education is to provide optimal patient care.

Controversy surrounds efforts to develop additional subspecialty board certification and maintenance of certification (MOC) to practice as a cardiac intensive care physician. Proponents of additional certification argue that variation in training leads to some strengths but many limitations. Defined standards for education should decrease this variability. In addition, they suggest that regulators may use board certification as a quality metric and subspecialization should therefore be recognized.[12] Opponents to additional subspecialty certification point out that the collaboration between different subspecialties likely contributes to optimal care. However, there is lack of clarity regarding which training pathway should lead to board certification. For many pediatric cardiac intensivists, a third (Pediatrics/PCCM + Pediatric Cardiac Critical Care) or even fourth subspecialty certification (Pediatrics/PCCM/Pediatric Cardiology + Pediatric Cardiac Critical Care) and related MOC would add substantial and unnecessary costs to the certification process. Additional concerns exist about burnout and staffing shortages and unintentionally limiting the pediatric cardiac critical care workforce by creating restrictive standards.[12] The true benefits and challenges associated with subspecialty board certification are unclear. In a recent survey study, most of the medical directors of pediatric cardiac intensive care units and faculty favored accreditation of pediatric critical care fellowships by the ACGME and respondents supported development of specific ABP certification.[13] Contrary to concerns about a workforce shortage, predictive modeling suggests that faculty will fill current and projected open positions over the next 5 years, leading to an increasingly competitive job market.[14]

Many children with CHD have comorbidities. At least 15% have associated genetic conditions, and critically ill children with acquired heart disease often have multiorgan involvement.[15,16] Therefore, physicians providing care for these patients need training and experience in a wide spectrum of anomalies and organ dysfunction or failure, instead of a narrow focus on cardiovascular physiology or pathophysiology. In addition, there is a growing population of older children and adults with palliative surgery or full correction of CHD. The ongoing care of these children and young adults is frequently outside of a specialized CICU. With the increasing subspecialization in the field, many of the frontline providers in distinct CICUs are now composed of advanced practice providers.[10] Although having a dedicated team streamlines care and provides more continuity, this has led to a reduced exposure for trainees (medical students, residents, and fellows) to pediatric patients with CHD. The balance between increased specialization with the need for experience and education for trainees who may eventually provide care for these patients in a community or medically underserved population is an important consideration.

OUTCOMES

Advances in the care of children with cardiovascular disease have led to low operative mortality with reports of 2.5% to 8.1% depending on the age of the patient at surgery.[17] This evolution in care has been attributed to improved intraoperative and postoperative assessment and imaging, surgical technique, cardiovascular pharmacology, mechanical ventilation, interventional cardiac catheterization, anesthesiology and cardiopulmonary bypass, and mechanical circulatory support.[18] Although physicians have been focused on ways to reduce mortality, future practice is focused on decreasing morbidity. The authors provide a review of the progress in fetal and neonatal detection of critical congenital heart disease (CCHD), fetal and pediatric interventional cardiac catheterization, mechanical circulatory support, and collaborative research and quality improvement networks.

Advances in Fetal and Neonatal Diagnosis

Prenatal detection of fetal CHD has been associated with improved neonatal survival and decreased morbidity.[19–21] Improved ultrasound technology, standardization of cardiac screening during routine ultrasound, and increased multidisciplinary collaboration in the management of patients with maternal risk factors have led to increased prenatal detection.[22] This allows coordinated care for fetal intervention and risk assessment for anticipated complications in the delivery room and planning for delivery in the appropriate setting.

The Secretary of Health and Human Services recommended uniform screening for CCHD in 2011. Standard pulse oximetry screening in the newborn period is highly specific and moderately sensitive for detection of CCHD with very low false-positive rates.[23] CCHD screening has been shown to decrease infant mortality from CCHD in states with mandatory screening policies.[24]

Advances in Interventional Cardiac Catheterization

Fetal cardiac interventions include percutaneous ultrasound-guided and catheter-based fetal cardiac interventions. These interventions are performed in fetal centers with specialists in maternal fetal medicine, anesthesiology, radiology or pediatric cardiology, and interventional cardiac catheterization. Most data are from fetal cardiac interventions for fetuses with severe aortic stenosis (AS), pulmonary atresia with intact ventricular septum (PA/IVS), and hypoplastic left heart syndrome (HLHS) with restrictive atrial septum.[25] These fetuses carry a high risk of death in utero and postnatally. Currently, the American Heart Association recommendation is to consider fetal catheter intervention for fetuses with AS with antegrade flow and evolving HLHS; with AS, severe mitral regurgitation, and restrictive atrial septum; with HLHS and a severely restrictive or intact atrial septum; or those with PA/IVS.[22] Immediate postnatal data so far are promising but optimal timing of intervention and additional longitudinal data are needed.[25]

Advances in pediatric cardiac catheter interventions have led to less invasive options. Persistent patent ductus arteriosus in preterm and low-birth-weight infants have historically been limited to surgical options because percutaneous approaches have been hampered by sheath size and size of occlusion devices. Recent literature supports the use percutaneous closure with ductal occlusion devices.[26] Right ventricular outflow tract (RVOT) stenting in symptomatic neonates with tetralogy of Fallot (TOF) and adverse risk factors have been reported. There are no studies comparing outcome of early repair of TOF with Blalock-Taussig-Thomas shunt or RVOT stent. Despite limitations, the latter provides options for patients who may not be surgical candidates. Ductal stenting in patients with ductal-dependent pulmonary blood flow has also advanced with the use of drug-eluting stents in neonates without significant adverse outcomes. Finally, in the current era, advances in bioprosthetic pulmonary valves or homografts and transcatheter tricuspid and mitral valve replacement have become viable options in small children and adults with CHD. With appropriate application, transcatheter valves have longevity and help avoid open heart surgery. Long-term data are needed to determine whether catheter or surgical interventions have the best outcome.[26]

Advances in Mechanical Circulatory Support

Recent substantial improvements in device technology and clinical management have led to more options for short- and long-term support for children with heart failure. **Table 1** shows different devices used for mechanical circulatory support in children. For many unstable patients with severe heart failure or cardiogenic shock, extracorporeal membrane oxygenation (ECMO) is used as a bridge to recovery, heart transplant, or ventricular assist device (VAD) placement. A detailed review of ECMO is provided in Cashen and colleagues' article, "Extracorporeal Membrane Oxygenation in Critically Ill Children," in this issue. In this section, the authors focus on VADs. Depending on the size of the child, short-term VAD support may be provided by central or peripheral cannulation. The TandemHeart and Impella can be placed by peripheral/percutaneous cannulation and have been used in children but experience is limited.[27,28] Other approaches for short-term support have included placement of Berlin Heart cannulas but attached to a temporary continuous flow device such as the Pedimag. Long-term VAD support became an option for children with widespread application of the pulsatile paracorporeal device known as the Berlin Heart EXCOR. Newer devices include implantable continuous-flow VADs. These intracorporeal devices were developed for adults and include the HeartMate II and 3 and HeartWare (HVAD). However, Medtronic has recently stopped the distribution of the HeartWare (HVAD) system due to a growing number of reports of adverse neurologic events and increased mortality compared with other commercially available LVAD systems. Another option for mechanical circulatory support is the SynCardia total artificial heart (TAH). This device

Table 1
Features of commonly used mechanical circulatory support devices in children

Name	Location/Route of Insertion	Type of Flow/Mechanism	Challenges in Pediatrics
Venoarterial extracorporeal membrane oxygenation	Extracorporeal/peripheral or central cannulation	Nonpulsatile/centrifugal	Temporary support Complications: anticoagulation risk of bleeding and thrombosis
PediMag (Thoratec Corp)	Paracorporeal/sternotomy	Nonpulsatile/centrifugal	Temporary support CE mark approved for short-term use
Impella 2.5, 5.0 (Abiomed)	Intracorporeal/percutaneous femoral access	Non-pulsatile/Microaxial continuous	Approved for short-term support up to 6 h Smallest size: 12 F
TandemHeart (Kardia)	Extracorporeal/percutaneous femoral access OR transthoracic	Continuous, centrifugal	Temporary support Few hours to up to 14 d of support; 21 F transseptal cannula
Berlin Heart EXCOR (Berlin Heart GmbH)	Paracorporeal/sternotomy	Pulsatile/pneumatic	Anticoagulation risk of bleeding and thrombosis For weight>3 kg
Total Artificial Heart (Syncardia)	Intracorporeal/sternotomy	Pulsatile/pneumatic	70 cc: Approved for BTT and humanitarian status for DT/sizes: 50, 70 cc BSA >1.2
HeartMate II and 3 (Thoratec Corp)	Intracorporeal/sternotomy	Continuous flow/axial	Weight>30 kg, but reports of >19 kg patient with HeartMate 3
HeartWare (Medtronic)	Intracorporeal/sternotomy	Continuous flow/centrifugal	Recalled/no longer available due to increased complications compared with other LVADs

Abbreviations: BSA, body surface area; BTT, bridge to transplant; DT, destination therapy; F, French; Kg, kilogram; LVAD, left ventricular assist device.

provides pulsatile flow replacing the ventricular contraction and has served as a bridge for children to heart transplant.[29]

Timing of implantation, optimal anticoagulation, and indications for explant are all determined by risk benefit assessment according to institutions. A recent study using data from children enrolled in the International Society for Heart and Lung Transplantation registry (n = 5095) found that 26% of patients received MCS before transplant. Of these patients, children supported with ECMO before or after heart transplant had the highest mortality, and patients supported with VADS had similar short- and long-term survival compared with patients who were not supported with VADs.[30]

Collaborative Networks and Quality Improvement Initiatives

The development of national and international registries to standardize nomenclature, develop risk adjustment tools, and collect case and outcome data for benchmarking has been an integral part of the CHD community.[31] The Society of Thoracic Surgeons (STS) National Database was established in 1989 with public reporting since 2010. The STS database is useful for benchmarking and research but lacks the level of granularity that is needed for many questions related to critical care of children with CHD. Growth and development of specific registries related to the care of children with CHD have increased significantly. In the pediatric cardiac critical care community, the Pediatric Cardiac Critical Care Consortium (PC4) was developed to improve the quality of care for patients with cardiovascular disease cared for in an intensive care unit. The advantage of PC4 over surgical registries is that it includes all critically ill children cared for in the CICU, and internal institutional quality improvement metrics can be reviewed in a timely manner via a dashboard that are available to designated site personnel. In addition, collaboration is available and encouraged to allow lower performing centers in certain areas to work with higher performing centers for ideas and guidelines to improve care.

The development of multiple networks and registries that include children with cardiac disease (PC4, Pediatric Acute Care Cardiology Collaborative, Cardiac Neurodevelopmental Outcome Collaborative, Advanced Cardiac Therapies Improving Outcomes Network, National Pediatric Cardiology Quality Improvement Collaborative) led to the development of Cardiac Networks United. The goal of this "super" network is to unite and align similar networks for research and quality improvement to create the infrastructure to share data and encourage collaboration, with the important addition of parent advocates as key stakeholders.

Participation in pediatric cardiac network allows for benchmarking results, quality improvement, internal review of data, and encourages collaboration between centers. The current era seems more focused on attempts to improve outcome based on processes used at high performing centers rather than a punitive focus on lower performance. It is hoped that collaboration over competition will lead to improved outcomes targeted at modifiable risk factors for morbidity and mortality. Finally, precision care tailored to specific patients is only achievable with prognostic and predictive enrichment from data based on the biological responses to illness and treatment.[31] The hope is that precision care will be achievable in the not-too-distant future in large part due to robust databases.

SUMMARY

In conclusion, pediatric cardiac critical care has evolved with advances in diagnosis, congenital heart surgery, interventional cardiac catheterization, and mechanical circulatory support, which have all contributed to improved outcomes. Debate continues over the optimal location of care and training requirements. Operative mortality is low, and preventing morbidity is the new focus of the future. Ongoing collaboration facilitated by pediatric cardiac research and quality improvement networks makes the future of pediatric cardiac critical care promising.

CLINICS CARE POINTS

- Cardiac intensive care physicians have variable training backgrounds.
- The location of care and training of physicians is likely less important than the structure of care.
- High performing centers encourage multidisciplinary collaboration and standardized approaches to care.
- Mortality has declined for postoperative congenital heart disease, and the focus is now on decreasing morbidity.
- Advances in fetal diagnosis and CCHD screening have led to earlier detection.
- Advances in interventional cardiac catheterization have led to less invasive treatment approaches for children who are not ideal surgical candidates and children who meet select criteria.
- Advances in collaborative research and quality improvement initiatives allow for ongoing collaboration between centers and use of high-quality data for focused initiatives to decrease morbidity.

DISCLOSURE

The authors have nothing to disclose.

REFERENCES

1. Epstein D, Brill JE. A history of pediatric critical care medicine. Pediatr Res 2005; 58:987–96.
2. Hickey P, Gauvreau K, Curley MAQ, et al. The effect of critical care nursing and organizational characteristics on pediatric cardiac surgery mortality in the United States. J Nurs Adm 2014;44(10 Suppl):S19–26.
3. Johnson JT, Wilkes JF, Menon SC, et al. Admission to dedicated pediatric cardiac intensive care units is associated with decreased resource use in neonatal cardiac surgery. J Thorac Cardiovasc Surg 2018;155(6):2606–14.
4. Gupta P, Beam BW, Noel TR, et al. Impact of preoperative location on outcomes in congenital heart surgery. Ann Thorac Surg 2014;98(3):896–903.
5. Burstein DS, Jacobs JP, Li JS, et al. Care models and associated outcomes in congenital heart surgery. Pediatrics 2011;127(6):e1482–9.
6. Bagdure DN, Custer JW, Foster CB, et al. The impact of dedicated cardiac intensive care units on outcomes in pediatric cardiac surgery: a virtual pediatric systems database analysis. J Pediatr Intensive Care 2021;10(3):174–9.
7. Pasquali SK, Thibault D, O'Brien SM, et al. National variation in congenital heart surgery outcomes. Circulation 2020;142(14):1351–60.
8. Backer CL, Pasquali SK, Dearani JA. Improving national outcomes in congenital heart surgery: the time has come for regionalization of care. Circulation 2020; 141(12):943–5.

9. Tabbutt S, Krawczeski C, McBride M, et al. Standardized training for physicians practicing pediatric cardiac critical care. Ped Crit Care Med 2021. https://doi.org/10.1097/PCC.0000000000002815.

10. Horak RV, Alexander PM, Amirnovin R, et al. Pediatric cardiac intensive care distribution, service delivery, and staffing in the United States in 2018. Pediatr Crit Care Med 2020;21:797–803.

11. Bhaskar P, Rettiganti M, Gossett JM, et al. Impact of intensive care unit attending physician training background on outcomes in children undergoing heart operations. Ann Pediatr Cardiol 2018;11:48–55.

12. Anand V, Kwiatkowski DM, Ghanayem NS, et al. Training pathways in pediatric cardiac intensive care: proceedings from the 10th international conference of the Pediatric Cardiac Intensive Care Society. World J Pediatr Congenit Heart Surg 2016;7:81–8.

13. Horak RV, Bai S, Marino BS, et al. Workforce demographics and unit structure in paediatric cardiac critical care in the United States. Cardiol Young 2021;1–5. https://doi.org/10.1017/S1047951121004753.

14. Horak R, Marino B, Werho D, et al. Assessment of physician training and prediction of workforce needs in paediatric cardiac intensive care in the United States. Cardiol Young 2021;1–6.

15. Oyen N, Poulsen G, Boyd HA, et al. Recurrence of congenital heart defects in families. Circulation 2009;120:295–301.

16. Hartman RJ, Rasmussen SA, Botto LD, et al. The contribution of chromosomal abnormalities to congenital heart defects: a population-based study. Pediatr Cardiol 2011;32:1147–57.

17. Society of Thoracic Surgeons Congenital Heart Surgery Database Executive Summaries. Available: https://www.sts.org/sites/default/files/Congenital-STSExec Summary_Neonates.pdf. Accessed November 25, 2021.

18. Checchia PA, Brown KL, Wernovsky G, et al. The evolution of pediatric cardiac critical care. Crit Care Med 2021;49:545–57.

19. Bonnet D, Coltri A, Butera G, et al. Detection of transposition of the great arteries in fetuses reduces neonatal morbidity and mortality. Circulation 1999;99:916–8.

20. Franklin O, Burch M, Manning N, et al. Prenatal diagnosis of the aorta improves survival and reduces morbidity. Heart 2002;87:67–9.

21. Kaguelidou F, Fermont L, Boudjemline Y, et al. Foetal echocardiographic assessment of tetralogy of Fallot and post-natal outcome. Eur Heart J 2008;29:1432–8.

22. Donofrio MT, Moon-Grady AJ, Hornberger LK, et al. Diagnosis and treatment of fetal cardiac disease. A scientific statement from the American Heart Association. Circulation 2014;129:183–2242.

23. Plana MN, Zamora J, Suresh G, et al. Pulse oximetry screening for critical congenital heart defects. Cochrane Database Syst Rev 2018;3(3):CD011912.

24. Abouk R, Grosse SD, Ailes EC, et al. Association of US state implementation of newborn screening policies for critical congenital heart disease with early infant cardiac death. JAMA 2017;318:2111–8.

25. Schidlow DN, Freud L, Friedman K, et al. Fetal interventions for structural heart disease. Echocardiography 2017;34:1834–41.

26. Kang SL, Benson L. Recent advances in cardiac catheterization for congenital heart disease. F1000Res 2018;7:370.

27. Dimas VV, Murthy R, Guleserian KJ. Utilization of the Impella 2.5 micro-axial pump in children for acute circulatory support. Catheter Cardiovasc Interv 2014;83:261–2.

28. Kulat BT, Russell HM, Sarwark AE, et al. Modified TandemHeart ventricular assist device for infant and pediatric circulatory support. Ann Thorac Surg 2014;98: 1437–41.
29. Park SS, Sanders DB, Smith BP, et al. Total artificial heart in the pediatric patient with biventricular heart failure. Perfusion 2014;29:82–8.
30. Edelson JB, Huang Y, Griffis H, et al. The influence of mechanical circulatory support on post-transplant outcomes in pediatric patietns: A multicenter study from the International Society for Heart and Lung Transplant (ISHTL) registry. J Heart Lung Transplant 2021;40:1443–53.
31. Laussen PC. Sharing and learning through the pediatric cardiac critical care consortium: moving toward precision care. J Thorac Cardiovasc Surg 2020. https:// doi.org/10.1016/j.jtcvs.2020.05.092.

Pediatric Neurocritical Care

Ajit A. Sarnaik, MD

KEYWORDS

- Pediatric traumatic brain injury • Pediatric neurocritical care • Pediatric stroke
- Neuroimaging • Neurologic monitoring

KEY POINTS

- Pediatric brain injury can occur from a primary neurologic cause or as a sequela of multisystem illness.
- Pediatric neurocritical care (PNCC) is an expanding multidisciplinary field incorporating brain-specific imaging, monitoring, and treatment modalities along with focused efforts in education, quality improvement, and collaboration.
- Although PNCC is emerging as a specialty, services are not universally available. Thus, all pediatric practitioners should develop an approach to diagnosis, monitoring, and management for children with brain injuries.

INTRODUCTION

Whether the disease process originates from the neurologic system or manifests as a neurologic complication of a systemic critical illness, pediatric brain injury is a major health problem, accounting for 20% to 25% of all admissions and 65% of all deaths in pediatric intensive care units (PICUs).[1] Au and colleagues[2] reported that more than half of all patients in a large tertiary care PICU who died had an acute neurologic injury, and in 90% of those, brain injury was the proximate cause of death. There are numerous causes of primary pediatric brain injury. Traumatic brain injury (TBI) is the leading cause of death and disability related to trauma in children. In the United States, pediatric TBI caused 7440 deaths, 60,000 inpatient stays, and 600,000 visits to the emergency department.[3] Although the Brain Trauma Foundation has released guidelines for the management of severe pediatric TBI,[4,5] significant variability exists in management among practitioners.[6] Status epilepticus is another common neurologic emergency, with an annual incidence of approximately 20 cases per 100,000 children, with a 3% mortality.[7] Stroke in children carries an annual incidence of 1–2 cases per 100,000.[8] In contrast to adult stroke, which is primarily caused by atherosclerotic disease, the causes of stroke in children range widely and include sickle cell disease, inherited or acquired hypercoagulability, congenital heart disease, and arterial

Central Michigan University College of Medicine, Carls Building, Pediatric Critical Care, Children's Hospital of Michigan, 3901 Beaubien Avenue, Detroit, MI 48201, USA
E-mail address: sarna1aa@cmich.edu

Pediatr Clin N Am 69 (2022) 415–424
https://doi.org/10.1016/j.pcl.2022.01.007
0031-3955/22/© 2022 Elsevier Inc. All rights reserved.

dissection. The field of pediatric neurocritical care (PNCC) has been ushered in recent years by the recognition of this vast heterogeneity in causes, natural history, pathophysiology, and treatment. Several large pediatric centers have instituted neurocritical care services, consisting of specialists from several disciplines including critical care, neurosurgery, and neurology. Because these services are not universal, all pediatric practitioners should develop an approach to diagnosis, monitoring, and management for pediatric brain injuries. The purpose of this review is to discuss the emerging subspecialty of PNCC, to review the pathophysiology of primary and secondary brain injuries, and to highlight contemporary imaging and monitoring modalities.

DISCUSSION
PNCC Subspecialty Service

Pediatric critical care as a subspecialty is only several decades old.[9] Unlike ICUs for adults, most PICUs are general and not designated based on a specific organ system. However, this has changed in pediatric cardiac critical care, which has been increasingly recognized as a field requiring specific resources and teams with a highly specialized skill set.[10] PNCC is an expanding field directed toward the mitigation of secondary brain injury caused by systemic illness, stroke, cardiac arrest, trauma, infection/inflammation, postneurosurgical conditions, and seizures. Although the development of guidelines in adult neurocritical care may be several years ahead than that of its pediatric counterpart, developmental differences between adults and children prevent drawing undue parallels between the natural history of neurologic disease and treatments across the age groups. A comprehensive, multidisciplinary approach to care, including current techniques of imaging, neuromonitoring, and neuroprotective strategies, augmented by focus on patient safety, quality, and education can improve outcomes in children with brain injury.[11] Recent data indicate that the development of a PNCC service within an institution that includes experts from neurosurgery, neurology, and critical care medicine may improve patient outcomes.[12,13] Potential benefits of neurocritical care services include facilitation of communication among the numerous services involved in the care of patients who often have complicated needs, focused efforts on patient safety, quality improvement and education among diverse groups of practitioners, as well as coordination of limited resources in imaging and monitoring. In addition, the involvement of neurology and neurosurgery services facilitates long-term follow-up after ICU and hospital discharge. A recent survey of PICU medical directors and program directors of pediatric neurosurgery and child neurology fellowships reported the existence of 45 neurocritical care services in the United States, 80% of which were consultant services to the PICU/CICU.[14] Respondents had an overall positive opinion on the value of PNCC as a specialty service. The few negative opinions pointed out that developing a PNCC service would be "redundant." Recent studies have shown that a PNCC service can add diagnostic considerations,[15] and that it can be associated with a reduction in mortality and an improvement in the favorable outcome.[12] However, an important limitation in studies exploring outcomes in specialized services in any discipline is uncertainty regarding generalizability across different institutions, and whether it is the service itself conferring benefit, or if it is due to increased resources and attention. Overall, the impact on outcome of dedicated PNCC services warrants more study.

Pathophysiology of Brain Injury

Brain injury can be classified as either primary or secondary. Primary injury results from the inciting event. In TBI, this consists of direct disruption of neurons and vascular structures that occurs at the moment of impact or acceleration/deceleration force. Practitioners are relatively powerless against primary TBI, outside of physical prevention measures and anticipatory guidance. In hypoxia/ischemia, stroke, infection, and seizures, the primary event leading to brain injury can often be treated or prevented. If possible, every measure should be considered to reverse the primary cause of brain injury. Secondary brain injury begins the instant following the inciting event and is therefore the target of therapeutic interventions from the prehospital stage through the entire hospitalization and rehabilitation phases. There are many ways a brain cell can die from secondary injury, including inadequate supply of oxygen and substrates to meet the metabolic demands of the vulnerable brain, inflammation, apoptosis, and excitotoxicity. Mitigating imbalances in the supply and demand of oxygen and nutrients following brain injury begins with supportive care of other organ systems. Establishing and maintaining adequate airway, breathing, and circulation is essential in ensuring cerebral oxygen delivery. This can be achieved using pediatric critical care principles of airway management, ventilator strategies, fluid resuscitation, and inotropic or vasopressor therapies.

Cerebral oxygen delivery = cerebral blood flow × arterial oxygen content.

Arterial oxygen content (mL/dL) = 1.36 × S_aO_2/100 × Hb (g/dL) + 0.003 × P_aO_2 (mm Hg).

Considering the determinants of cerebral oxygen delivery, it is important to ensure adequate cardiac output, hemoglobin concentration, hemoglobin oxygen saturation, and partial pressure of arterial oxygen. In children, there exist age-related differences in cerebral blood flow, which range from 60 mL/100 g/min at 3 years, to 70 mL/100 g/min at age 6 years, to 50 mL/100 g/min in adulthood.[16] In addition, prevention of hypoglycemia is also essential in maintaining adequate cellular respiration.

Local oxygen delivery in the injured brain also depends on cerebral perfusion. Cerebral perfusion pressure is equal to the difference between the mean arterial pressure (MAP) and the intracranial pressure (ICP).

CPP = MAP–ICP.

Ensuring an adequate MAP and limiting ICP are important in maintaining cerebral perfusion. Strategies to increase MAP include optimizing intravascular volume, use of inotropes, and vasopressors if needed. ICP is influenced by the Monro–Kellie principle, which states that the volume of the contents of the intracranial vault, that is, the brain, cerebrospinal fluid, and blood, is constant. Therefore, if the volume of one of the components increases, the volume of the other components must decrease to compensate. When the compensatory mechanisms are exhausted, ICP rapidly increases. Brain volume can increase with cytotoxic, vasogenic, osmotic, and interstitial cerebral edema. An increase in the blood component can occur with cerebral hyperemia or hemorrhage. Finally, the CSF volume can be increased due to disorders of CSF drainage or resorption. Relative to the magnitude of increase in the volume of intracranial contents, ICP can be lower in children with an open fontanelle or in those who have undergone decompressive craniectomy. However, it is important to note that ICP can still be high in such circumstances, and that injury can still be severe in the absence of ICP elevation. Given the developmental differences in norms of systemic blood pressure and cerebral blood flow, there is likely an age-related continuum for optimal cerebral perfusion pressure. In a recent report, Allen and colleagues[17] studied 317 adults and children with severe TBI using specific CPP targets more than 50–60 mm Hg in adults, more than 50 mm Hg in the 6–17-year age group, and more than 40 mm Hg in the 0–5-year age group. Regardless of the likely existence of a similar age-related continuum, the 2019 Brain Trauma Foundation guidelines for severe pediatric TBI support a CPP threshold of greater than 40 mm Hg irrespective of age.[18]

In addition to ensuring an adequate supply of blood and energy substrate, limiting cerebral oxygen demand is also important to prevent secondary brain injury. Studies on the effects of different classes of sedatives and anesthetics on cerebrovascular response and compensatory reserve in TBI are conflicting,[19,20] and studies in children are even more limited. However, sedatives can reduce the cerebral metabolic rate of oxygen, an effect that is possibly coupled with a global reduction in cerebral blood flow. Thus, in the brain-injured child requiring mechanical ventilation, analgesia and sedation are mainstays of treatment to prevent pain, agitation, and ventilator desynchrony, all of which can increase cerebral blood volume and ICP.[21–23] Preventing fever through targeted temperature management and management of seizures with the antiepileptic therapy with electroencephalography (EEG) monitoring can also reduce the cerebral metabolic demand.

Neurologic Examination

Evaluation of neurologic injury in a child begins with the pupillary examination and measurement of vital signs. Any combination of bradycardia, systemic hypertension, disordered regulation of respiration, and abnormal pupillary reflex could indicate an acute herniation syndrome, requiring immediate medical or surgical treatment. Another early step in assessment is the Glasgow Coma Score (GCS). The GCS was initially developed in 1974 to assess the altered consciousness after TBI.[24] The GCS ranges from 3 to 15, with a score between 1 and 6 assigned for motor function, between 1 and 5 for verbal function, and between 1 and 4 for eye opening. The initial 1974 scale did not include children younger than 5 but modified scales are available and can be applied to children,[25] although they have not been widely validated for the younger age groups.[26] Initial GCS in children correlates with outcome,[27,28] and it is often used to stratify severity of TBI among mild (GCS 13–15), moderate (GCS 9–12), and severe (GCS 3–8) both in clinical practice and in research. A recent study showed that further stratifying the group of children with severe TBI with GCS between 3 and 8 is associated with mortality.[29] Although the GCS has not been rigorously validated outside of trauma, its ease, reproducibility, and quantitative nature have resulted in wide acceptance to represent the degree of impairment across various neurologic conditions. Indeed, it is often used by practitioners to communicate the severity of injury to each other for several different disease states causing encephalopathy.[26] It can also be applied serially to determine improvement or deterioration. Limitations of the GCS in the assessment of severe brain injury includes lack of inclusion of other important neurologic examination parameters such as pupillary and brainstem reflexes, focality/laterality, and airway protective reflexes.[30] Therefore, a more comprehensive neurologic examination assessing consciousness, airway protection, cranial nerves, motor function, reflexes, and sensory function should be performed along with the GCS.

Imaging

Indications for imaging of a child with brain injury are based on the mechanism of injury, findings from the clinical neurologic examination and GCS, likelihood of imaging findings to affect management decisions, and the stability of the patient for transport. Computed tomography (CT) continues to be widely used to detect and stage various neurologic injuries because it is usually readily available, expeditious, and does not always require sedation of the patient. Noncontrast head CT is a good first-line test to detect bony abnormalities in the skull and upper cervical spine, acute intracranial hemorrhage, hydrocephalus, mass effect, cerebral edema, and extraaxial fluid collections. Because the detection of these abnormalities can change the medical or surgical management following head trauma, CT is the preferred modality for the initial evaluation and staging of adults and children with severe TBI.[31–33] One drawback of CT is the risk of acquired malignancy due to radiation.[34] A study of CT scans in the US children from 1996 to 2011 projected that 4 million pediatric CT scans per year would cause about 5000 future cancers, and reducing the highest radiation doses given might prevent cancers.[35] Other important limitations of noncontrast head CT include failure to detect important neurologic abnormalities such as ischemia, inflammation, subacute hemorrhage, axonal injury, ligamentous high cervical spine injury, subtle cerebral edema, thrombosis, vascular abnormalities, and abnormalities of posterior fossa contents. If any of these conditions are suspected, magnetic resonance imaging (MRI) should be performed. Limitations of MRI include availability, duration, requirement of sedation in young children, and challenges of monitoring during the procedure. It is therefore not routinely performed in children during the acute stage of TBI because patients are often unstable in the first several days following injury, and most of the information necessary to guide therapy can be obtained from CT. However, it is superior to CT in the evaluation of ischemic stroke, and rapid sequence MRI protocols confer the added benefits of shorter duration, more widespread availability, and the dispensing with the need for sedation. A recent study showed that the rapid sequence MRI can be used in the evaluation of both ischemic and nonischemic brain attacks in children.[36] In that study, diffusion-weighted imaging was shown to be more sensitive and specific in detecting ischemic strokes compared with fluid-attenuated inversion recovery techniques, as the latter was useful in the identification of inflammatory and metabolic disorders.

Other Monitoring Modalities

Nonconvulsive seizures (NCS) and nonconvulsive status epilepticus (NCSE) are increasingly recognized conditions in pediatrics. The gold standard for diagnosis of NCS, and for monitoring of children with neurologic injuries at risk for NCS, is continuous EEG (cEEG). In the past, limitations of cEEG included inadequate equipment, lack of technologists and personnel to interpret the study at regular intervals, and lack of data on its benefit on outcome. In adults, studies have shown that the mental status changes out of proportion to the degree of the primary neurologic illnesses of TBI, stroke, or intracerebral hemorrhages can be due to NCS.[37] A growing body of pediatric literature recognizes NCS as a common primary diagnosis or a common harmful sequela of other neurologic conditions.[1,38,39] Prompt recognition and treatment of seizures is essential, as NCSE has been shown to be an independent predictor of mortality in children.[40,41] Various studies have shown that delayed initiation of treatment of seizures is associated with refractoriness of status epilepticus.[42] In addition, failure to treat seizures according to a protocol is associated with the development of status epilepticus,[43] and a proportion of seizure-related deaths are preventable.[44] Specific disease states in pediatrics warrant heightened index of suspicion for NCS, as it can occur frequently in children on extracorporeal membrane oxygenation,[45] following neonatal cardiac surgery on bypass,[46] and following TBI.[47] cEEG monitoring should be considered for children at high risk for NCS in whom a neurologic examination cannot be used for sequential evaluation, such as children on sedation or neuromuscular blockade. cEEG should also be used to monitor response to intensive therapies for known status epilepticus, for example, high-dose benzodiazepines or barbiturates.

Cerebral oximetry is an additional modality useful for monitoring a child with brain injury. It can be used to assess imbalances between the supply and demand of oxygen delivery to titrate therapies intended to mitigate secondary brain injury. Analogous to the use of central venous oxygen saturation to monitor oxygen delivery, cardiac output, and oxygen extraction in shock, jugular bulb oximetry ($S_{jv}O_2$) can be used to assess the cerebral blood flow, oxygen delivery, and extraction. Although it has been used in pediatric neurosurgery,[48,49] and there are reports of correlation between $S_{jv}O_2$ and outcome after brain injury in adults and children,[50–52] it is not currently widely used in pediatric critical care. Another tool used to monitor cerebral oxygenation is the brain tissue oxygen monitoring ($P_{br}O_2$), where a catheter is inserted directly into the brain tissue. Therapeutic measures to improve $P_{br}O_2$ include pulmonary and hemodynamic strategies to increase the cerebral oxygen delivery and arterial PO_2 to facilitate oxygen diffusion to brain tissue, and neuroprotective measures such as limiting cerebral metabolic demand and raised ICP. Studies in both adult and pediatric neurotrauma showed an association between unfavorable outcome and $P_{br}O_2$ less than 10 mm Hg.[53–56] An important limitation of the goal-directed $P_{br}O_2$ therapy is related to the placement of the $P_{br}O_2$ catheters. In one of the largest pediatric studies, the monitors were placed either in normal appearing right frontal white matter if there were no focal lesions or in the hemisphere with the greater swelling or more localized lesions.[53,54] If the monitor is placed in healthy brain tissue, the impact of therapy may not reflect effects on at-risk brain tissue. Conversely, if the monitor is placed in dead brain tissue with minimal local cerebral blood flow, therapy may not change measured $P_{br}O_2$. Because there was variability and subjectivity even in a single center series which is considered a landmark study in this area, this modality may have limited generalizability. The 2019 Brain Trauma Foundation Guidelines for Management of Severe TBI state that while there is insufficient data to make a recommendation regarding $P_{br}O_2$ monitoring, therapy should aim for a threshold of greater than 10 mm Hg if it is used.[18] Transcranial near-infrared spectroscopy (NIRS) is a noninvasive modality of cerebral oximetry, which uses a probe attached to the skin of the forehead to measure the absorption of light in the near-infrared spectrum. Because oxyhemoglobin and deoxyhemoglobin absorb light at different wavelengths, the proportion of absorption can represent the oxygenation of brain tissue deep to the probe. Using the goal-directed therapy for cerebral hypoxia monitored by NIRS to decrease the risk of death or improved survival with severe brain injury in preterm infants has shown promise in a phase II study.[57,58] Cerebral NIRS has been extensively used intraoperatively in cardiac surgery in children and adults[59] and has been used as a marker of hemodynamics in pediatric critical care.[60] Specifics of the NIRS signal and the duration of desaturation have been shown in the pediatric cardiac ICU setting to be associated with longer time on mechanical ventilation, and longer duration of PICU and hospital stay.[61] One important limitation of NIRS, similar to that of $P_{br}O_2$ monitoring, is the uncertainty of using a local problem as a representation of global cerebral oxygenation, and whether the probe placement limits the assessment of oxygenation locally where brain is at risk. Overall, studies evaluating the use of NIRS to provide the goal-directed therapy in PNCC are lacking.

SUMMARY

The greatest advances in medicine are generalizable across institutions regardless of resources and are based on universal fundamentals of assessment, pathophysiology, and natural history of disease, and applied through continuous processes of education, safety, and quality improvement. Recently, there have been tremendous improvements in the field of PNCC, including the development and implementation of monitoring and imaging techniques, evidence-based practice guidelines for stroke and TBI, and the organization of multidisciplinary PNCC programs. Because the cause of pediatric brain injury is at once diverse and relatively infrequent, a specialized model similar to adult neurocritical care and high-volume pediatric areas such as cardiac critical care may not be feasible. To further advance the field, the PNCC community must continue to foster a culture of brain-oriented critical care through a focus on education, quality improvement, and multidisciplinary collaboration within and across institutions.

CLINICS CARE POINTS

- A comprehensive, multidisciplinary approach to care, including current techniques of imaging, neuromonitoring, and neuroprotective strategies augmented by a focus on patient safety, quality, and education can improve outcomes in children with brain injury.

- The overarching goal of PNCC in mitigating secondary brain injury can be achieved by balancing the supply and demand of blood, oxygen, and nutrients of vulnerable brain tissue. Ensuring adequate cerebral oxygen delivery begins with applying pediatric critical care principles of airway management, ventilator strategies, fluid resuscitation, and inotropic or vasopressor therapies, and continues with brain-specific therapies of ICP control, improvement of CPP, and limiting cerebral metabolic demand.

- Evaluating and assessing illness severity in a child with brain injury begins with the interpretation of vital signs and pupillary examination, as well as determining the GCS. Indications for CT or MRI to evaluate injury depend on the mechanism of injury, initial clinical examination, and patient stability.

- cEEG can be used to evaluate for NCS or NCSE, monitor intensive therapies for seizures such as barbiturates or high-dose benzodiazepines, or if neurologic examination is limited, such as in the setting of neuromuscular blockade or ECMO. Cerebral oximetry via NIRS, jugular venous oximetry, or brain tissue oximetry can be used to assess imbalances between the supply and demand of oxygen delivery to guide therapy intended to mitigate secondary brain injury.

DISCLOSURE

Author has nothing to disclose.

REFERENCES

1. Moreau JF, Fink EL, Hartman ME, et al. Hospitalizations of children with neurologic disorders in the United States. Pediatr Crit Care Med 2013;14(8):801–10.
2. Au AK, Carcillo JA, Clark RS, et al. Brain injuries and neurological system failure are the most common proximate causes of death in children admitted to a pediatric intensive care unit. Pediatr Crit Care Med 2011;12(5):566–71.
3. Stanley RM, Bonsu BK, Zhao W, et al. US estimates of hospitalized children with severe traumatic brain injury: implications for clinical trials. Pediatrics 2012; 129(1):e24–30.
4. Carney NA, Chesnut R, Kochanek PM, et al. Guidelines for the acute medical management of severe traumatic brain injury in infants, children, and adolescents. Pediatr Crit Care Med 2003;4(3 Suppl):S1.
5. Kochanek PM, Carney N, Adelson PD, et al. Guidelines for the acute medical management of severe traumatic brain injury in infants, children, and adolescents–second edition. Pediatr Crit Care Med 2012;13(Suppl 1):S1–82.
6. Dean NP, Boslaugh S, Adelson PD, et al. Physician agreement with evidence-based recommendations for the treatment of severe traumatic brain injury in children. J Neurosurg 2007;107(5 Suppl):387–91.

7. Gurcharran K, Grinspan ZM. The burden of pediatric status epilepticus: epidemiology, morbidity, mortality, and costs. Seizure 2019;68:3–8.
8. Mallick AA, Ganesan V, Kirkham FJ, et al. Childhood arterial ischaemic stroke incidence, presenting features, and risk factors: a prospective population-based study. Lancet Neurol 2014;13(1):35–43.
9. Epstein D, Brill JE. A history of pediatric critical care medicine. Pediatr Res 2005; 58(5):987–96.
10. Johnson JT, Wilkes JF, Menon SC, et al. Admission to dedicated pediatric cardiac intensive care units is associated with decreased resource use in neonatal cardiac surgery. J Thorac Cardiovasc Surg 2018;155(6):2606–2614 e5.
11. Murphy S. Pediatric neurocritical care. Neurotherapeutics 2012;9(1):3–16.
12. Pineda JA, Leonard JR, Mazotas IG, et al. Effect of implementation of a paediatric neurocritical care programme on outcomes after severe traumatic brain injury: a retrospective cohort study. Lancet Neurol 2013;12(1):45–52.
13. O'Lynnger TM, Shannon CN, Le TM, et al. Standardizing ICU management of pediatric traumatic brain injury is associated with improved outcomes at discharge. J Neurosurg Pediatr 2016;17(1):19–26.
14. LaRovere KL, Murphy SA, Horak R, et al. Pediatric neurocritical care: evolution of a new clinical service in PICUs across the United States. Pediatr Crit Care Med 2018;19(11):1039–45.
15. Bell MJ, Carpenter J, Au AK, et al. Development of a pediatric neurocritical care service. Neurocrit Care 2009;10(1):4–10.
16. Schoning M, Hartig B. Age dependence of total cerebral blood flow volume from childhood to adulthood. J Cereb Blood Flow Metab 1996;16(5):827–33.
17. Allen BB, Chiu YL, Gerber LM, et al. Age-specific cerebral perfusion pressure thresholds and survival in children and adolescents with severe traumatic brain injury*. Pediatr Crit Care Med 2014;15(1):62–70.
18. Kochanek PM, Tasker RC, Carney N, et al. Guidelines for the management of pediatric severe traumatic brain injury, third edition: update of the brain trauma foundation guidelines. Pediatr Crit Care Med 2019;20(3S Suppl 1):S1–82.
19. Froese L, Dian J, Batson C, et al. The Impact of vasopressor and sedative agents on cerebrovascular reactivity and compensatory reserve in traumatic brain injury: an exploratory analysis. Neurotrauma Rep 2020;1(1):157–68.
20. Froese L, Dian J, Gomez A, et al. Cerebrovascular response to phenylephrine in traumatic brain injury: a scoping systematic review of the human and animal literature. Neurotrauma Rep 2020;1(1):46–62.
21. Minardi C, Sahillioglu E, Astuto M, et al. Sedation and analgesia in pediatric intensive care. Curr Drug Targets 2012;13(7):936–43.
22. Tume LN, Baines PB, Lisboa PJ. The effect of nursing interventions on the intracranial pressure in paediatric traumatic brain injury. Nurs Crit Care 2011;16(2): 77–84.
23. Kerr ME, Weber BB, Sereika SM, et al. Effect of endotracheal suctioning on cerebral oxygenation in traumatic brain-injured patients. Crit Care Med 1999;27(12): 2776–81.
24. Teasdale G, Jennett B. Assessment of coma and impaired consciousness. A practical scale. Lancet 1974;2(7872):81–4.
25. Reilly PL, Simpson DA, Sprod R, et al. Assessing the conscious level in infants and young children: a paediatric version of the Glasgow Coma Scale. Childs Nerv Syst 1988;4(1):30–3.
26. Teasdale G, Maas A, Lecky F, et al. The glasgow coma scale at 40 years: standing the test of time. Lancet Neurol 2014;13(8):844–54.

27. Fulkerson DH, White IK, Rees JM, et al. Analysis of long-term (median 10.5 years) outcomes in children presenting with traumatic brain injury and an initial Glasgow Coma Scale score of 3 or 4. J Neurosurg Pediatr 2015;16(4):410–9.
28. Morray JP, Tyler DC, Jones TK, et al. Coma scale for use in brain-injured children. Crit Care Med 1984;12(12):1018–20.
29. Murphy S, Thomas NJ, Gertz SJ, et al. Tripartite stratification of the glasgow coma scale in children with severe traumatic brain injury and mortality: an analysis from a multi-center comparative effectiveness study. J Neurotrauma 2017;34(14): 2220–9.
30. Moulton C, Pennycook A, Makower R. Relation between Glasgow coma scale and the gag reflex. BMJ 1991;303(6812):1240–1.
31. Liesemer K, Riva-Cambrin J, Bennett KS, et al. Use of Rotterdam CT scores for mortality risk stratification in children with traumatic brain injury. Pediatr Crit Care Med 2014;15(6):554–62.
32. Maas AI, Hukkelhoven CW, Marshall LF, et al. Prediction of outcome in traumatic brain injury with computed tomographic characteristics: a comparison between the computed tomographic classification and combinations of computed tomographic predictors. Neurosurgery 2005;57(6):1173–82 [discussion: 1173-82].
33. Levi L, Guilburd JN, Linn S, et al. The association between skull fracture, intracranial pathology and outcome in pediatric head injury. Br J Neurosurg 1991;5(6): 617–25.
34. Hennelly KE, Mannix R, Nigrovic LE, et al. Pediatric traumatic brain injury and radiation risks: a clinical decision analysis. J Pediatr 2013;162(2):392–7.
35. Miglioretti DL, Johnson E, Williams A, et al. The use of computed tomography in pediatrics and the associated radiation exposure and estimated cancer risk. JAMA Pediatr 2013;167(8):700–7.
36. De Jong G, Kannikeswaran N, DeLaroche A, et al. Rapid sequence MRI protocol in the evaluation of pediatric brain attacks. Pediatr Neurol 2020;107:77–83.
37. Friedman D, Claassen J, Hirsch LJ. Continuous electroencephalogram monitoring in the intensive care unit. Anesth Analg 2009;109(2):506–23.
38. Abend NS. Electrographic status epilepticus in children with critical illness: Epidemiology and outcome. Epilepsy Behav 2015;49:223–7.
39. O'Neill BR, Handler MH, Tong S, et al. Incidence of seizures on continuous EEG monitoring following traumatic brain injury in children. J Neurosurg Pediatr 2015; 16(2):167–76.
40. Abend NS, Arndt DH, Carpenter JL, et al. Electrographic seizures in pediatric ICU patients: cohort study of risk factors and mortality. Neurology 2013;81(4): 383–91.
41. Shah S, Shah N, Johnson R, et al. Single center outcomes of status epilepticus at a paediatric intensive care unit. Can J Neurol Sci 2016;43(1):105–12.
42. Brophy GM, Bell R, Claassen J, et al. Guidelines for the evaluation and management of status epilepticus. Neurocrit Care 2012;17(1):3–23.
43. Tirupathi S, McMenamin JB, Webb DW. Analysis of factors influencing admission to intensive care following convulsive status epilepticus in children. Seizure 2009; 18(9):630–3.
44. Sidebotham P, Hunter L, Appleton R, et al. Deaths in children with epilepsies: a UK-wide study. Seizure 2015;30:113–9.
45. Piantino JA, Wainwright MS, Grimason M, et al. Nonconvulsive seizures are common in children treated with extracorporeal cardiac life support. Pediatr Crit Care Med 2013;14(6):601–9.

46. Naim MY, Gaynor JW, Chen J, et al. Subclinical seizures identified by postoperative electroencephalographic monitoring are common after neonatal cardiac surgery. J Thorac Cardiovasc Surg 2015;150(1):169–78 [discussion: 178-80].
47. Arndt DH, Lerner JT, Matsumoto JH, et al. Subclinical early posttraumatic seizures detected by continuous EEG monitoring in a consecutive pediatric cohort. Epilepsia 2013;54(10):1780–8.
48. Sharma D, Ellenbogen RG, Vavilala MS. Use of transcranial Doppler ultrasonography and jugular oximetry to optimize hemodynamics during pediatric posterior fossa craniotomy. J Clin Neurosci 2010;17(12):1583–4.
49. Sharma D, Siriussawakul A, Dooney N, et al. Clinical experience with intraoperative jugular venous oximetry during pediatric intracranial neurosurgery. Paediatr Anaesth 2013;23(1):84–90.
50. Cormio M, Valadka AB, Robertson CS. Elevated jugular venous oxygen saturation after severe head injury. J Neurosurg 1999;90(1):9–15.
51. Perez A, Minces PG, Schnitzler EJ, et al. Jugular venous oxygen saturation or arteriovenous difference of lactate content and outcome in children with severe traumatic brain injury. Pediatr Crit Care Med 2003;4(1):33–8.
52. Sheinberg M, Kanter MJ, Robertson CS, et al. Continuous monitoring of jugular venous oxygen saturation in head-injured patients. J Neurosurg 1992;76(2):212–7.
53. Figaji AA, Zwane E, Thompson C, et al. Brain tissue oxygen tension monitoring in pediatric severe traumatic brain injury. Part 2: relationship with clinical, physiological, and treatment factors. Childs Nerv Syst 2009;25(10):1335–43.
54. Figaji AA, Zwane E, Thompson C, et al. Brain tissue oxygen tension monitoring in pediatric severe traumatic brain injury. Part 1: Relationship with outcome. Childs Nerv Syst 2009;25(10):1325–33.
55. Narotam PK, Burjonrappa SC, Raynor SC, et al. Cerebral oxygenation in major pediatric trauma: its relevance to trauma severity and outcome. J Pediatr Surg 2006;41(3):505–13.
56. Figaji AA, Zwane E, Graham Fieggen A, et al. The effect of increased inspired fraction of oxygen on brain tissue oxygen tension in children with severe traumatic brain injury. Neurocrit Care 2010;12(3):430–7.
57. Hansen ML, Pellicer A, Gluud C, et al. Cerebral near-infrared spectroscopy monitoring versus treatment as usual for extremely preterm infants: a protocol for the SafeBoosC randomised clinical phase III trial. Trials 2019;20(1):811.
58. Hyttel-Sorensen S, Austin T, van Bel F, et al. A phase II randomized clinical trial on cerebral near-infrared spectroscopy plus a treatment guideline versus treatment as usual for extremely preterm infants during the first three days of life (SafeBoosC): study protocol for a randomized controlled trial. Trials 2013;14:120.
59. Zaleski KL, Kussman BD. Near-infrared spectroscopy in pediatric congenital heart disease. J Cardiothorac Vasc Anesth 2020;34(2):489–500.
60. Ghanayem NS, Hoffman GM. Near Infrared Spectroscopy as a Hemodynamic Monitor in Critical Illness. Pediatr Crit Care Med 2016;17(8 Suppl 1):S201–6.
61. Flechet M, Guiza F, Vlasselaers D, et al. Near-infrared cerebral oximetry to predict outcome after pediatric cardiac surgery: a prospective observational study. Pediatr Crit Care Med 2018;19(5):433–41.

Extracorporeal Membrane Oxygenation in Critically Ill Children

Katherine Cashen, DO[a,b,*], Katherine Regling, DO[c,d],
Arun Saini, MD, MS[e,f]

KEYWORDS

- Pediatric intensive care unit • Infants • Children
- Extracorporeal membrane oxygenation

KEY POINTS

- In children, extracorporeal membrane oxygenation (ECMO) is a well-established technology to support refractory respiratory and/or cardiac failure with the largest growth in the cardiac population.
- Survival is highest in neonates and children with respiratory failure.
- The number of centers providing ECMO internationally continues to grow.
- Modes of support include venovenous ECMO for respiratory indications and venoarterial ECMO for cardiac support.

INTRODUCTION

Extracorporeal membrane oxygenation (ECMO) is a mode of life support evolved from cardiopulmonary bypass used to treat children and adults with cardiorespiratory failure refractory to conventional therapy. Gibbon[1] in 1953 used artificial oxygenation and perfusion for the first tIme to support a patient undergoing open heart surgery. In 1965, Rashkind and colleagues[2] reported the use of a bubble oxygenator to support an infant with refractory respiratory failure. The development of silicon-based capillary channels in oxygenator membranes prolonged the circuit life and allowed for a longer ECMO run.[3] In 1972, Dr Robert Bartlett and associates successfully supported a

[a] Division of Pediatric Critical Care Medicine, Department of Pediatrics, Duke Children's Hospital, Durham, NC, USA; [b] Duke University Medical Center, 2301 Erwin Road, Suite 5260Y, DUMC 3046, Durham, NC 27710, USA; [c] Division of Pediatric Hematology Oncology, Children's Hospital of Michigan, 3901 Beaubien Boulevard, Detroit, MI 48201, USA; [d] Central Michigan University, Mt. Pleasant, MI, USA; [e] Division of Pediatric Critical Care Medicine, Texas Children's Hospital, 6651 Main Street, Suite 1411, Houston, TX 77030, USA; [f] Baylor University School of Medicine, Houston, TX, USA
* Corresponding author. Duke University Medical Center, 2301 Erwin Road, Suite 5260Y, DUMC 3046, Durham, NC 27710.
E-mail address: katherine.cashen@duke.edu

Pediatr Clin N Am 69 (2022) 425–440
https://doi.org/10.1016/j.pcl.2022.01.008
0031-3955/22/© 2022 Elsevier Inc. All rights reserved.
pediatric.theclinics.com

2-year-old child with cardiac failure after a Mustard procedure for transposition of the great vessels. They followed this by providing support for a neonate with persistent pulmonary hypertension of the newborn for 72 hours.[4] These early successes helped drive expansion of use in neonates worldwide. **Fig. 1** illustrates key milestones in the evolution of ECMO use.

Most information regarding the use and application of ECMO comes from the Extracorporeal Life Support Organization (ELSO), an international nonprofit consortium group, founded by Dr Bartlett in 1989, that provides support to institutions and researchers and maintains a comprehensive registry of ECMO patient data. The most recent registry report includes data from outcomes from 76,348 ECMO runs in children from 1989 to 2021.[20] The registry separates children into 2 groups: neonates (0–28 days) and pediatric patients (29 days–17 years of age.) Overall, survival for neonatal respiratory ECMO is highest. **Table 1** shows survival data based on indication for ECMO.[20] Most recent pediatric growth has occurred in the cardiac population, but improvements in technology and experience have led to even broader indications. Current public attention has focused on the application of ECMO during the severe acute respiratory syndrome coronavirus 2 (SARS-CoV-2) pandemic.

Although ECMO is lifesaving, it is an invasive, expensive therapy with known complications and morbidity in survivors. This review provides an overview of the ECMO circuit, cannulation strategies, indications, contraindications, management considerations, complications, and outcome data. Areas of recent progress, including extracorporeal cardiopulmonary resuscitation (ECPR), awake ECMO, early mobility, and mobile ECMO, are highlighted, and use of ECMO during the SARS-CoV-2 pandemic is described. Future directions and research are discussed.

EXTRACORPOREAL MEMBRANE OXYGENATION CIRCUITRY

ECMO involves removing a patient's blood from the venous circulation via cannula and using a pump to advance the blood through a membrane lung, heating, and returning the blood to the patient (**Fig. 2**). For venovenous (VV) ECMO, the blood is returned to the venous circulation via a second venous cannula or via a dual-lumen VV cannula. For venoarterial (VA) ECMO, the blood is returned to the arterial circulation via an arterial cannula. Circuit variation is significant and based on center needs, patients supported, and experience.

Key milestones in the past 50 y of ECMO use

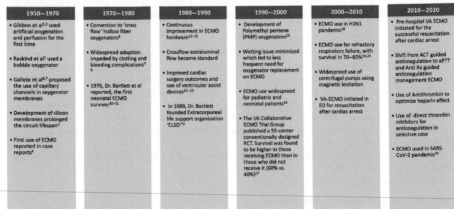

Fig. 1. Key milestones in the past 50 years of extracorporeal membrane oxygenation use[5–19]

	ECMO	Total	Survived to
Age	Indication	Runs	Discharge
Neonatal	Respiratory	33,484	24,457 (73%)
	Cardiac	9620	4218 (43%)
	ECPR	2261	961 (42%)
Pediatric	Respiratory	11,223	6775 (60%)
	Cardiac	14,078	7594 (53%)
	ECPR	5682	2417 (42%)
Total		76,348	46,422 (61%)

Table 1
Extracorporeal membrane oxygenation outcome by age and indication

Blood Pump

The blood pump needs to provide adequate flow appropriate for the patient within a safe range of pressure to prevent hemolysis. Roller pumps were the standard for

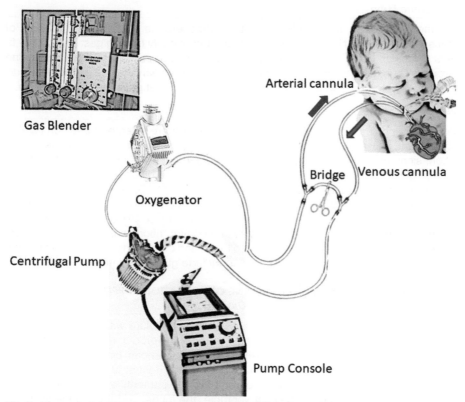

Fig. 2. Venoarterial ECMO circuit. Venous blood drains from the patient's internal jugular vein/right atrium and is pumped via the centrifugal pump through the oxygenator. The oxygenated, warmed blood then passes back into the carotid artery of the baby. There are multiple infusion and access ports as well as pressure and flow monitors not shown in this figure. (*Reprinted from* Maslach-Hubbard A, Bratton SL. Extracorporeal membrane oxygenation for pediatric respiratory failure: History, development and current status. *World J Crit Care Med* 2013; 2(4): 29-39 Creative Common Attribution Non Commercial (CC BY-NC 4.0) http://creativecommons.org/licenses/by-nc/4.0/).

decades, but now centrifugal pumps are most common.[21] Roller pumps are positive displacement pumps that generate flow via sequential compression of the circuit tubing as a function of tubing size and pump speed. The venous drainage inlet is gravity dependent and requires constant monitoring to prevent rupture of tubing with prolonged use.[22,23] Centrifugal pumps deliver flow using centrifugal force generated by a spinning rotor, which applies suction to the blood inlet and propels the blood outward from a pump by generating positive pressure. The flow on the centrifugal pump can vary based on the venous pressure (inlet) and the return pressure (outlet) on the same rotation per minute. Benefits of centrifugal pumps include smaller and more mobile circuits and elimination of circuit compression. A recent propensity-score matched study of ECMO recipients less than 10 kg found those supported with centrifugal pumps compared with roller pumps were associated with increased mortality and ECMO complications.[22] Others have reported increased hemolysis, circuit thrombosis, or inadequate support in neonates maintained with centrifugal pumps.[22,24] Although most adult and pediatric ECMO programs have transitioned from roller pumps to centrifugal pumps, many neonatal ECMO programs continue to use roller pumps.[25-27]

Membrane Lung

The membrane lung, sometimes called the oxygenator, is made up of a network of thousands of hollow fibers that are filled with continuously flowing gas. The hollow fibers allow gas to diffuse across the membrane wall but prevent liquid from passing through. Thus, oxygen and carbon dioxide diffuse between the gas and countercurrent flowing blood owing to a gradient between the partial pressures on each side.

Vascular Cannula

Vascular cannulas are available in different sizes and are selected based on level of support and vessel size. For patients receiving VV ECMO with multisite venous cannulation, single-lumen cannulas are used. Dual-lumen cannulas are used for VV ECMO via a single jugular access site where one lumen removes blood and the second lumen returns blood to the patient. For patients receiving VA ECMO, venous and arterial cannulas are used. Most cannulas are made from biocompatible polyurethane coated with heparin or nonheparin polymers designed to decrease platelet activation and inflammatory response.[21,28] Different cannula tip configurations are available, and most are wire-reinforced to prevent collapse and occlusion of the lumen. Other cannulas are designed for percutaneous cannulation and include guidewire introducer sets.

MODES OF EXTRACORPOREAL MEMBRANE OXYGENATION SUPPORT
Venovenous Extracorporeal Membrane Oxygenation

VV ECMO is used for children with primary respiratory failure without cardiovascular compromise. In general, VV ECMO has a more favorable risk profile than VA ECMO.[29-31] In VV ECMO, blood is returned to the venous circulation and mixes with venous blood coming from systemic organs to the right atrium. This mixed blood (higher in oxygen content and lower in carbon dioxide content) is pumped via the patient's own cardiac output to the right ventricle, the lungs, and then to the systemic circulation. Patients with respiratory failure requiring inotropes/vasopressors are often placed on VA ECMO, but newer data suggest cannulation type is not independently associated with survival in this population.[32]

Venoarterial Extracorporeal Membrane Oxygenation

VA ECMO is used for children with significant cardiovascular compromise. For peripheral cannulation, the internal jugular vein and carotid artery are used. For a larger patient with adequate vessel size, the femoral vein and artery may be used, but there are risks for ischemic injury to the leg. For central (transthoracic) cannulation, the aorta and right atrium are directly cannulated to transition from cardiopulmonary bypass or in a child with recent sternotomy. Benefits of central cannulation include insertion of larger cannula with potentially better flow and that the carotid artery is spared. Risks of central cannulation include the need for an open chest, infection, and bleeding. Centers have reported improved outcomes with central cannulation in pediatric refractory septic shock.[33,34] Other meta-analyses suggest no difference in outcome for patients with central versus peripheral cannulation for non-postcardiotomy shock.[35] If the metabolic demand is higher than flows achieved that can be achieved through peripheral cannulation, central cannulation should be considered.

In patients requiring VA ECMO for cardiogenic shock, left heart decompression is necessary to provide optimal cardiac support, decrease left ventricular (LV) wall stress, and prevent hemorrhagic pulmonary edema. Centers vary in approach to decompress the LV, but when indicated, early LV decompression is associated with improved outcome.[36]

CANNULATION

Cannulation for VV ECMO is achieved by a dual-lumen cannula in the internal jugular vein, or by draining blood from the inferior vena cava via the femoral vein and returning blood to the right atrium via the internal jugular vein. Pediatric cannulation is performed by direct cutdown and cannulation of the vessel, or by percutaneous access. It is limited by vessel size. Dual-lumen cannulas require adequate positioning, which can be challenging in neonates and small children. Placement with fluoroscopic or echo-cardiographic guidance decreases risks of complication.[37] Percutaneous cannulation performed by intensivists on adult patients have been shown to have good outcome and low rate of complications.[38–40] One report details high success and low complica-tion rates for percutaneous cannulation by pediatric and adult intensivists of 100 pa-tients, including 23 children.[40] In a recent survey by the American Pediatric Surgical Association, most pediatric patients had ECMO cannulation performed by pediatric general surgeons and cardiac surgeons. The same study showed that pediatric inten-sivists performed ECMO cannulation 1.6% of the time, with 83% of cannulations per-formed in the intensive care unit.[41]

INDICATIONS

This review focuses on indications for ECMO in pediatric (>28 days to <18 years) res-piratory failure, neonatal (<28 days) and pediatric cardiac failure, and ECPR. ECMO in neonatal respiratory support has been reported in a recent publication and will not be covered here.[42] Before ECMO cannulation for any indication, intensivists should consider whether the pathologic condition is potentially reversible; if the condition is considered irreversible, considerations should be made whether ECMO is a reason-able bridge to a destination therapy (ie, transplant, more permanent support device, or other therapeutics), and whether the risk of providing ECMO is less than not providing ECMO. In general, decisions should focus on the patient's disease, institu-tional experience, and expert consensus and consultation.[43]

Respiratory

ECMO should be considered in children with respiratory failure in patients with progres-sive and persistent failure despite optimized conventional therapies.[43] Intensivists should consider ECMO when the risk of mortality approached 50% and definitely in situations when mortality approaches 80%.[43] ELSO specifically recommends strong consideration for ECMO in the following: (1) patients with oxygenation index greater than 40; (2) a lack of response to conventional ventilation; and (3) elevated ventilator pressures (mean airway pressures >20–25 cm H_2O on conventional ventilation or >30 on high-frequency oscillating ventilator or evidence of barotrauma).[44] The use of ECMO has been reported in patients with anterior mediastinal masses causing extrinsic airway compression, in those with pulmonary hemorrhage, for perioperative support of patients with airway anomalies, and as a bridge to lung transplant and preoperative rehabilitation.

Neonatal and Pediatric Cardiac Failure

Indications for cardiac ECMO include respiratory failure and impaired cardiac output, septic shock, cardiogenic shock from toxidrome, myocarditis, cardiomyopathy, intractable arrhythmias, pulmonary hypertension, and during cardiac arrest (ECPR). In patients with congenital heart disease, ECMO can be used preoperatively to stabilize a patient for surgery, for high-risk cardiac catheterization procedures, for failure to wean from cardiopulmonary bypass, and for low cardiac output in the postoperative period or ECPR.

ELSO defines ECPR as the use of ECMO during cardiopulmonary resuscitation (CPR) or the application of rapid deployment VA ECMO when return to spontaneous circulation is not achieved by 20 minutes of resuscitation or longer.[45] ECPR is increasingly used for in-hospital pediatric cardiac arrest (IHCA) and has been associated with improved survival compared with conventional CPR for IHCA.[46,47] Most children who undergo ECPR are those with congenital or acquired heart disease.[45] Survival to hospital discharge in children who undergo ECPR is 31% to 64%.[48] Patient selection is important, but no randomized controlled trial has been conducted to compare conventional CPR with ECPR. There is no consensus on how long conventional CPR should be performed before initiation of ECPR, but most institutions have developed protocols for the most senior clinician on the team to initiate ECPR within 5 to 10 minutes of conventional CPR. Improved outcomes are achieved with cannulation in less than 40 minutes. However, survival has been reported with high-quality CPR provided for ≥60 minutes.[48]

CONTRAINDICATIONS

There are few absolute contraindications to ECMO (**Table 2**). ECMO should not be offered in situations wherein the patient has an overall poor prognosis or is unlikely to survive without unacceptable disability.[43,44] Other considerations are technical and are related to occluded or abnormal vessels from previous ECMO runs, or the use of VA ECMO in a patient who is unlikely to have cardiac recovery and is not a candidate for ventricular assist device or heart transplant. Finally, careful consideration must be given for disease processes associated with increased mortality on ECMO.[44] Relative contraindications to ECPR include unwitnessed cardiopulmonary arrest and out-of-hospital pediatric cardiopulmonary arrest.[48]

MANAGEMENT DURING EXTRACORPOREAL MEMBRANE OXYGENATION
Hemostatic Alterations During Extracorporeal Membrane Oxygenation/Anticoagulation

The introduction of the ECMO circuit induces disruption of the hemostatic balance. As the flowing blood interacts with the artificial surface of the cannula, an acute inflammatory response occurs. This response triggers activation of coagulation and a

Table 2
Contraindications to extracorporeal membrane oxygenation

Absolute Contraindications	Relative Contraindications
• Lethal chromosomal abnormalities • Severe neurologic deficit (including intracranial hemorrhage with mass effect) • Incurable malignancy • Severe coagulopathy • Extreme prematurity • Irreversible primary disease	• Prolonged duration of mechanical ventilation • Recent neurosurgical procedure or intracranial hemorrhage (<7 d) • Preexisting chronic illness with poor prognosis

prothrombotic state.[49] The use of continuous anticoagulation is then necessary to prevent thrombosis in the circuit and in the patient. This increases the risk for major bleeding events. In infants and young children, it is important to note that most of the procoagulant and anticoagulant factors are significantly lower than those in older children and adults.[50] These differences can lead to difficulties in management of the critically ill infant or young child.

To date, unfractionated heparin (UFH) remains the most widely used anticoagulant in ECMO.[51] UFH has been used for more than 5 decades, is low-cost, and has a short half-life, and its effects are reversible.[52] The use of direct thrombin inhibitors for ECMO is increasing with bivalirudin being the most common. Bivalirudin inhibits free or fibrin-bound thrombin and has only a minor component of renal clearance and a half-life of about 25 minutes. Ranucci and colleagues[53] reported that in pediatric VA ECMO, patients given bivalirudin for anticoagulation in ECMO had lower mortality (31%) than the group given UFH (62.5%). However, studies overall have found no difference in survival.[54] Clinical trials comparing UFH and bivalirudin in pediatric ECMO are limited. Current anticoagulation monitoring and therapeutic targets vary between institutions. In general, centers use a combination of whole blood tests (activating clotting time or thromboelastography/thromboelastometry) and plasma-based tests (antifactor Xa activity [anti-Xa] or activated partial thromboplastin time). The Pediatric ECMO Anticoagulation Collaborative is a multidisciplinary team of experts developing evidence-informed consensus statements for management of anticoagulation for infants and children on ECMO. Although these guidelines do not replace clinical trials, they will provide much-needed guidance for all clinicians providing care for children on ECMO.

Gas Exchange and Mechanical Ventilation During Extracorporeal Membrane Oxygenation

During ECMO, oxygenation is determined by circuit flow, total cardiac output, and hemoglobin level. Hyperoxia is associated with increased mortality in pediatric VA and VV ECMO patients and should be avoided.[55] In VV ECMO, the mixing of blood results in systemic saturations as low as 75% to 85%, and systemic saturation targets are dependent on end-organ perfusion. As the patient's native lung function recovers, the systemic arterial oxygen saturation will increase.[43] During VV and VA ECMO, hypercarbia should be corrected slowly and is determined by the sweep gas flow from the mechanical lung. In contrast to VV ECMO, VA ECMO provides hemodynamic support, and higher oxygen saturations can be achieved. The amount of blood flow depends on the cannula size, native cardiac output, and systemic vascular resistance. The mechanical ventilator settings are often decreased to "rest settings" that varies according to disease process and center preference. The goal for mechanical ventilation is to reduce barotrauma and volutrauma and minimize oxygen toxicity.[43] Low normal peak inspiratory pressure, lower fraction of inspired oxygen less than 0.5, low respiratory rate, and positive end-expiratory pressure between 5 and 15 cm H_2O titrated for lung recruitment are recommended.[43]

Weaning

Weaning from ECMO should be considered when the underlying disease process that led to ECMO has improved. In both VA and VV ECMO, intravascular volume status, ventilation, and oxygenation should be optimal before weaning trials. In VV ECMO, the ECMO sweep and Fio_2 are reduced, before reduction of ECMO flow and "capping" the oxygenator. In VA ECMO, more rapid weaning can be started once myocardial recovery is evident. ECMO flow can be reduced sequentially to a level that maintains circuit flow without thrombosis. Physiologic monitoring is needed to determine the adequacy of end-organ perfusion during the weaning trial. An echocardiogram may be obtained at a prespecified time to determine if a patient is ready for decannulation.[56]

Complications

Hematologic complications during ECMO include bleeding, thrombosis, and hemolysis. The Bleeding and Thrombosis during Pediatric ECMO study was a prospective observational study that included more than 500 children supported with ECMO.[57] Bleeding occurred in 70% of patients, and intracranial hemorrhage occurred in 16%. Predictors of bleeding included the need for CPR or ECPR, direct transition from cardiopulmonary bypass to ECMO, older age, and higher organ failure index. Thrombotic events occurred in 37.5% of patients. Of these, 31.1% involved circuit thrombosis, and 12.8% were patient related. Thrombus formation may occur during periods of low ECMO flow, at sites of stasis or turbulent flow, and during periods of inadequate anticoagulation.[58] More than 33% of all patients were reported as having some degree of hemolysis, but this was limited by low number of sites routinely screened for hemolysis. Other complications, including acute renal failure, have been associated with increased mortality.

OUTCOMES
Short-Term Outcome/Survival

Survival to hospital discharge is listed by age and indication for ECMO in **Table 1**. Variables affecting short-term survival include diagnosis, disease severity, type of support, comorbidities, and complications. Two pediatric risk estimate scores to predict mortality have been published using ELSO registry data, the ped-RESCUERS and the P-PREP scores.[57,59] These scoring systems cannot help clinicians to decide when, or if, a patient should be placed on ECMO, but they help to measure center performance, aid in research, and help inform discussions regarding mortality risk with families.

Morbidity/Neurologic Outcome

In children supported with ECMO, the Functional Status Score at discharge was good, mildly abnormal, or moderately abnormal in greater than 50% of patients. As expected, characteristics reflecting increased chronicity and severity of illness were associated with worse functional status.[60] A population-based retrospective cohort study found that hospital readmission occurred in 36% of ECMO survivors within 1 year of discharge, and 3% of these children died.[61] This study supports previous work suggesting that readmission is common, yet intermediate and late mortality are low in this population.

In survivors, morbidity is common, and many studies focus on neurologic outcomes. Overall, standardized cognitive testing performance falls within 1 to 2 standard deviations of the mean.[62] Fourteen percent to 89% of patients who had cardiac arrest had favorable neurologic outcome. There was a wide range of disabilities that included deficits in overall cognition, behavior, motor skills, and school performance.[63]

Long-Term Outcome

Robust longitudinal outcome data with detailed neuropsychologic testing are lacking in the pediatric respiratory ECMO and neonatal and pediatric cardiac ECMO populations. In studies using age-appropriate neuropsychiatric testing in cardiac ECMO patients 2 to 6 years after discharge, a wide range of disability was reported with 28% to 50% of patients having motor or sensory impairment and 25% to 50% of patients having cognitive impairment or IQ < 2 standard deviations from the mean.[62–66] Recommendations for follow-up testing and care are available from the ELSO registry, but additional long-term outcome studies are needed.

ADVANCES IN EXTRACORPOREAL MEMBRANE OXYGENATION
Awake Extracorporeal Membrane Oxygenation

Reports of successful management of adult patients on ECMO while extubated, without adverse events, led to attempts to replicate this in children. The ELSO registry provides guidance on indications and considerations for extubation in VV ECMO for respiratory failure. A case series in neonates and case reports of children with respiratory and cardiac insufficiency requiring ECMO suggest that extubation is feasible and not associated with complications.[67–70] The benefits of this approach are avoidance of complications from mechanical ventilation, decreased need for sedation, and early mobilization and rehabilitation. In a recent international survey of ECMO programs, 27% of pediatric centers report extubating patients on ECMO.[70] More studies are needed to guide patient selection and determine safety.

Early Mobilization and Rehabilitation

The benefits of early mobilization and lower sedative use in critically ill pediatric patients have been the focus of recent work. The PICU Up! Initiative (a bundled mobilization intervention) is currently being studied by Pediatric Acute Lung Injury and Sepsis Investigators using a stepped-wedge cluster randomized trial design.[71] Ambulatory ECMO has been reported in children with respiratory failure awaiting lung transplantation and in a patient with cardiomyopathy on VA ECMO while awaiting heart transplantation.[72,73] Although ambulatory ECMO may not be feasible in many children, earlier physical rehabilitation should be the goal, and care bundles specifically designed for patients on ECMO warrant investigation.

Mobile Extracorporeal Membrane Oxygenation

Interfacility ECMO transport teams have been developed to retrieve patients who were cannulated for ECMO by a referring facility or to send a team to cannulate a patient for ECMO. The major priority for transport is patient safety, and team composition varies by center. Centers with neonatal and pediatric ECMO transport teams report few adverse events and outcomes consistent with the ELSO registry.[74]

Severe Acute Respiratory Syndrome Coronavirus 2 Pandemic/COVID-19

Over the course of the COVID-19 pandemic, the use of ECMO has increased. Early experience indicated high mortality. An adult ELSO Registry report included 4812 patients from international centers and showed that patients who received ECMO earlier in the pandemic had improved survival rates and decreased duration of ECMO support. The more recent cohort (after May 1, 2020) had a higher likelihood of treatment-refractory disease despite conventional risk factors, and centers with lower volume of patients with COVID-19 who required ECMO had higher mortality. These data suggest that the changing mortality profile in this population needs continued study. Outcome may be related to patient selection, disease phenotype, and center factors.[75]

ECMO for children with COVID-19 has been used infrequently. In a large multicenter report of children with multisystem inflammatory syndrome in children, ECMO was used in 4% of cases.[76] The ELSO registry maintains an active dashboard with neonatal/pediatric ECMO cases. To date, 174 confirmed COVID-19–associated cases have been reported internationally with 32% in-hospital mortality. Of these ECMO patients, 43% had no comorbidity reported. Acute respiratory distress syndrome was the most common acute illness followed by acute heart failure/myocarditis. Sixty-nine percent of patients were supported with respiratory ECMO, and 26% were supported with cardiac ECMO. Fifteen percent of patients suffered pre-ECMO cardiac arrest. Thus, although the numbers are small, ECMO for children with COVID-19 has been associated with excellent short-term outcome.[77]

FUTURE DIRECTIONS
Precision Medicine and Targeted Therapeutics

Precision medicine focused on identifying similar groups of patients into biologic subgroups that may differ in response to therapeutics is an important area under investigation. In children supported with ECMO, this may involve more detailed understanding of individual patient risk of bleeding and thrombosis during ECMO by identification of biologic subgroups. Therapeutics that target different pathways that contribute to bleeding and thrombosis could then be individualized. For example, novel therapeutics, including selective inhibition of the contact pathway by factor XI and factor XII, are currently under investigation and may be beneficial for all patients requiring ECMO, or precisely applied to a subgroup of patients.[78] Larsson and colleagues[79] have developed recombinant anti-human XIIa antibodies, which have been shown to be an effective and safe alternative to UFH in animal models. The major advantage of these antibodies is their specificity to FXIIa. By inhibiting FXIIa, they affect only direct downstream targets, providing a more complete inhibition of thrombin formation and thrombin-mediated activation of platelets and inflammation on the circuit without increasing the risk of bleeding.

Other areas of investigation include novel monitoring with point-of-care microfluidic devices that generate essential information regarding homeostatic parameters of platelet activation and clot formation under flow conditions. In addition, assessment of prothrombotic platelet-derived microparticle production on the extracorporeal circuit may help ascertain the risk of thromboembolic complications.[80]

Inert Circuits

To minimize bleeding and thrombotic complications, there are ongoing studies to modify the ECMO circuit to make it as nonthrombogenic as the vascular endothelium. Endothelial cells produce many surface anticoagulation biological substances, including prostacyclin and nitric oxide (NO), which inhibit thrombin-mediated platelet recruitment and activation. The addition of exogenous prostacyclin or NO to extracorporeal circuits along with UFH has been shown to reduce platelet activation and consumption. Recently, an ECMO circuit made of NO-releasing polymers has been shown to decrease thrombin formation in an animal model of VV ECLS.[81]

SUMMARY

In conclusion, ECMO is a valuable modality in the care of critically ill children. Indications for its use have increased, but mortality is unchanged, likely because of use in sicker patients. Optimal anticoagulation remains challenging, and additional studies are needed. There are many reports on short-term outcomes, but neurologic morbidity and long-term outcomes warrant additional investigation. Advances in awake ECMO and a paradigm shift to early mobilization have been reported in recent years without adverse effects. Most recently, excellent outcomes have been reported with the use of ECMO in a small number of children during the COVID-19 pandemic. Finally, precision medicine with targeted therapeutics and novel monitoring techniques are under investigation and show promise.

CLINICS CARE POINTS

- Though the number of extracorporeal membrane oxygenation centers continues to grow, mortality rates have remained static, likely because of increased complexity of children supported with extracorporeal membrane oxygenation.
- The Extracorporeal Life Support Organization Registry provides readily available guidelines for clinicians.
- Neonatal and pediatric extracorporeal membrane oxygenation survivors have significant morbidity but low late mortality.
- Awake and extubated extracorporeal membrane oxygenation has been used in children without adverse events.
- A small number of children with COVID-19 have been supported with extracorporeal membrane oxygenation with excellent outcome.
- Precision medicine may be an area of promise in applying anticoagulation therapeutics to neonatal and pediatric extracorporeal membrane oxygenation patients.

DISCLOSURE

The authors have nothing to disclose.

REFERENCES

1. Gibbon JH Jr. Application of a mechanical heart and lung apparatus to cardiac surgery. Minn Med 1954;37:171–85.
2. Rashkind WJ, Freeman A, Klein D, et al. Evaluation of a disposable plastic, low volume, pumpless oxygenator as a lung substitute. J Pediatr 1965;66:94–102.
3. Dorson W Jr, Baker E, Cohen ML, et al. A perfusion system for infants. Trans Am Soc Artif Intern Organs 1969;15:155–60.
4. Fortenberry JD, Lorusso R. "The history and development of extracorporeal life support" in Extracorporeal Life Support: the ELSO Red Book 5th edition, edited by Brogan RV, Lequier L, Lorusso R, et al, Ann Arbor, MI 2017; 1-15.
5. Aird WC. Discovery of the cardiovascular system: from Galen to William Harvey. J Thromb Haemost 2011;9(Suppl 1):118–29.
6. Davies A, Jones D, Bailey M, et al. Australia and New Zealand Extracorporeal Membrane Oxygenation (ANZ ECMO) influenza investigators. JAMA 2009; 302(17):1888–95.

7. Bartlett RH. Esperanza: the first neonatal ECMO patient. ASAIO J 2017;63(6): 832–43.
8. Bartlett RH. Extracorporeal life support: history and new directions. ASAIO J 2005;51(5):487–9.
9. Boettcher W, Merkle F. History of extracorporeal circulation: the conceptional and developmental period. J Extra-Corpor Technol 2003;35(3):172–0183.
10. Cavarocchi NC. Introduction to extracorporeal membrane oxygenation. Crit Care Clin 2017;33(4):763–6.
11. Combes A, Hajage D, Capellier G, Demoule A, Lavoué S, Guervilly C, Da Silva D, Zafrani L, Tirot P, Veber B, Maury E, Levy B, Cohen Y, Richard C, Kalfon P, Bouadma L, Mehdaoui H, Beduneau G, Lebreton G, Brochard L, Ferguson ND, Fan E, Slutsky AS, Brodie D, Mercat A, EOLIA Trial Group, REVA, ECMONet. Extracorporeal membrane oxygenation for severe acute respiratory distress syndrome. N Engl J Med 2018;378(21):1965–75.
12. Extracorporeal Life Support Organization. ELSO homepage. 2021. Available at: https://www.elso.org/TrainingCourses.aspx. Last Accessed (January/3/2021).
13. Hessel EA 2nd. A brief history of cardiopulmonary bypass. Semin Cardiothorac Vasc Anesth 2014;18(2):87–100.
14. Longmore DB, Wyatt R. Towards safer cardiac surgery: chapter 29 long term extracorporeal membrane oxygenation. MTP Press; 1981. p. 475.
15. Passaroni AC, Silva MA, Yoshida WB. Cardiopulmonary bypass: development of John Gibbon's heart-lung machine. Rev Bras Cir Cardiovasc 2015;30(2):235–45.
16. Peek GJ, Mugford M, Tiruvoipati R, et al. CESAR trial collaboration. Efficacy and economic assessment of conventional ventilatory support versus extracorporeal membrane oxygenation for severe adult respiratory failure (CESAR): a multicentre randomised controlled trial. Lancet 2009;374(9698):1351–63.
17. Stoney WS. Evolution of cardiopulmonary bypass. Circulation 2009;119(21): 2844–53.
18. Wolfson PJ. The development and use of extracorporeal membrane oxygenation in neonates. Ann Thorac Surg 2003;76(6):S2224–9.
19. Yeager T, Roy S. Evolution of gas permeable membranes for extracorporeal membrane oxygenation. Artif Organs 2017;41(8):700–9.
20. International Summary Extracorporeal Life Support Organization 2021. Available at: https://www.elso.org/Registry/Statistics/InternationalSummary.aspx. Accessed November 7, 2021.
21. Lequier L, Horton SB, McMullan MD, et al. Extracorporeal membrane oxygenation circuity. Pediatr Crit Care Med 2013;14:S7–12.
22. O'Halloran CP, Thiagarajan RR, Yarlagadda VV, et al. Outcomes of infants supported with extracorporeal membrane oxygenation using centrifugal versus roller pumps: an analysis from the ELSO registry. Pediatr Crit Care Med 2019;12: 1177–84.
23. Green TP, Kriesmer P, Steinhorn RH, et al. Comparison of pressure-volume-flow relationships in centrifugal and roller pump extracorporeal membrane oxygenation systems for neonates. ASAIO Trans 1991;37:572–6.
24. O'Brien C, Monteagudo J, Shad C, et al. Centrifugal pumps and hemolysis in pediatric extracorporeal membrane oxygenation (ECMO) patients: an analysis of Extracorporeal Life Support Organization (ELSO) Registry Data. J Pediatr Surg 2017;52:975–8.
25. Toomasian JM, Vercaemst L, Bottrell S, et al. "The circuit" in extracorporeal life support: the ELSO red book 5th edition, edited by Brogan RV, Lequier L, Lorusso R, et al, Ann Arbor, MI 2017; 49-80.

26. Barbaro RP, Paden ML, Guner YS, et al. Pediatric Extracorporeal Life Support Organization registry international report 2016. ASAIO J 2017;63:456–63.

27. Barbaro RP, Paden ML, Guner YS, et al. Pediatric Extracorporeal Life Support Organization Registry International Report. ASAIO J 2017;63:456–63.

28. Mangoush O, Purkayastha S, Haj-Yathia S, et al. Heparin-bonded circuits versus nonheparin-bonded circuits: an evaluation of their effect on clinical outcomes. Eur J Cardiothorac Surg 2007;31:1058–69.

29. Fan E, Gattinoni L, Combes A, et al. Venovenous extracorporeal membrane oxygenation for acute respiratory failure: a clinical review from an international group of experts. Intensive Care Med 2016;42:712–24.

30. Brown KL, Ridout DA, Shaw M, et al. Healthcare-associated infection in pediatric patients on extracorporeal life support: the role of multidisciplinary surveillance. Pediatr Crit Care Med 2006;7:546–50.

31. Skinner SC, Iocono JA, Ballard HO, et al. Improved survival in venovenous versus venoarterial extracorporeal membrane oxygenation for pediatric noncardiac sepsis patients: a study of the Extracorporeal Life Support Organization registry. J Pediatr Surg 2012;47:63–7.

32. Jaber B, Bembea MM, Loftis LL, et al. Venovenous versus venoarterial extracorporeal membrane oxygenation in inotrope dependent pediatric patients with respiratory failure. ASAIO J 2021;67:457–62.

33. Ruth A, Vogel AM, Adachi I, et al. Central venoarterial extracorporeal life support in pediatric refractory septic shock: a single center experience. Perfusion 2021. https://doi.org/10.1177/02676591211001782.

34. McClaren G, Butt W, Best D, et al. Extracorporeal membrane oxygenation for refractory septic shock in children: one institution's experience. Pediatr Crit Care Med 2007;8:447–51.

35. Raffa GM, Kowalewski M, Brodie D, et al. Meta-analysis of peripheral or central extracorporeal membrane oxygenation in postcardiotomy and non-postcardiotomy shock. Ann Thorac Surg 2019;107:311–21.

36. Hacking DF, Best D, d'Udekem Y, et al. Elective decompression of the left ventricle in pediatric patients may reduce the duration of venoarterial extracorporeal membrane oxygenation. Artif Organs 2015;39:319–26.

37. Jarboe MD, Gadepalli SK, Church JT, et al. Avalon catheters in pediatric patients requiring ECMO: placement and migration problems. J Pediatr Surg 2018;53:159–62.

38. Kouch M, Green A, Damuth E, et al. Rapid development and deployment of an intensivist-led venovenous extracorporeal membrane oxygenation cannulation program. Crit Care Med 2022;50(2):e154–61.

39. Burns J, Cooper E, Salt G, et al. Retrospective observational review of percutaneous cannulation for extracorporeal membrane oxygenation. ASAIO J 2016;62:325–8.

40. Conrad SA, Grier LR, Scott SL, et al. Percutaneous cannulation for extracorporeal membrane oxygenation by intensivists: a retrospective single-institution case series. Crit Care Med 2015;43:1010–5.

41. Drucker NA, Wang SK, Markel TA, et al. Practice patterns in imaging guidance for ECMO cannulation: a survey of the American Pediatric Surgical Association. J Pediatr Surg 2020;55:1457–62.

42. Fletcher K, Chapman R, Keene S. An overview of medical ECMO for neonates. Semin Perinatol 2018;42:68–79.

43. Maratta C, Petera RM, Leeuwen GV, et al. Extracorporeal Life Support Organization (ELSO): 2020 pediatric respiratory ELSO guideline. ASAIO J 2020;66:975–9.

44. MacLaren G, Conrad S, Peek G. Indications for pediatric respiratory extracorporeal life support. Extracorporeal Life Support Organization Guidelines. Available at: https://www.elso.org/portals/0/Files/ELSO%20guidelines%20paeds%20resp_May2015.pdf Accessed November10, 2021.

45. Esangbedo ID, Brunnetti MA, Campbell FM, et al. Pediatric extracorporeal cardiopulmonary resuscitation: a systematic review. Pediatr Crit Care Med 2020; 21:e934–43.

46. Meaney PA, Nadkarni VM, Cook EF, et al. American Heart Association National Registry of Cardiopulmonary Resuscitation Investigators: higher survival rates among younger patients after pediatric intensive care unit cardiac arrests. Pediatrics 2006;118:2424–33.

47. Lasa JJ, Rogers RS, Localio R, et al. Extracorporeal cardiopulmonary resuscitation (E-CPR) during pediatric in-hospital cardiopulmonary arrest is associated with improved survival to discharge: a report from the American Heart Association's Get With The Guidelines Resuscitation (GWTG-R) Registry. Circulation 2016;133:165–76.

48. Guerguerian AM, Sano M, Mark T, et al. Pediatric extracorporeal cardiopulmonary resuscitation ELSO guidelines 2021;67:229–37.

49. Oliver WC. Anticoagulation and coagulation management for ECMO. Semin Cardiothorac Vasc Anesth 2009;13(3):154–75.

50. Andrew M, Vegh M, Johnston M, et al. Maturation of the hemostatic system during childhood 1992;80:1998–2005.

51. Martin AA, Bhat R, Chitlur M. Hemostasis in pediatric extracorporeal life support: overview and challenges. Pediatr Clin N Am 2022;69(3). in press.

52. Hirsh J, Anand SS, Halperin JL, et al. Mechanism of action and pharmacology of unfractionated heparin. Arterioscler Thromb Vasc Biol 2001;1:1094–6.

53. Ranucci M, Ballotta A, Kandil H, et al, Surgical and Clinical Outcome Research Group. Bivalirudin-based versus conventional heparin anticoagulation for postcardiotomy extracorporeal membrane oxygenation. Crit Care 2011;15(6):R275.

54. Schill MR, Douds MT, Burns EL, et al. Is anticoagulation with bivalirudin comparable to heparin for pediatric extracorporeal life support? Results from a high-volume center. Artif Organs 2021;45:15–21.

55. Cashen K, Reeder R, Dalton HJ, et al. Hyperoxia and hypocapnia during pediatric extracorporeal membrane oxygenation: associations with complications, mortality, and functional status among survivors. Pediatr Crit Care Med 2018;19: 245–53.

56. Larson C, Chiletti R, d'Udekem Y. "Weaning pediatric cardiac ECMO" "in extracorporeal life support: the ELSO red book 5th edition, edited by Brogan RV, Lequier L, Lorusso R, et al, Ann Arbor, MI 2017; 387-393

57. Barbaro RM, Boonstra PS, Paden ML, et al. Development and validation of the pediatric risk estimate score for children using extracorporeal respiratory support (Ped-RESCUERS). Intensive Care Med 2016;42:879–88.

58. Dalton HJ, Reeder R, Garcia-Filion P, et al. Factors associated with bleeding and thrombosis in children receiving extracorporeal membrane oxygenation. Am J Respir Crit Care Med 2017;196:762–71.

59. Bailly DK, Reeder RW, Zabrocki LA, et al. Development and validation of a score to predict mortality in children undergoing ECMO for respiratory failure: pediatric pulmonary rescue with extracorporeal membrane oxygenation (P-PREP) score. Crit Care Med 2017;45:e58–66.

60. Cashen K, Reeder R, Dalton HJ, et al. Functional status of neonatal and pediatric patients after extracorporeal membrane oxygenation. Pediatr Crit Care Med 2017;18:561–70.
61. Lawrence AE, Sebastio YV, Deans KJ, et al. Beyond survival: readmissions and late mortality in pediatric ECMO survivors. J Pediatr Surg 2021;56:187–91.
62. Boyle K, Felling R, You A, et al. Neurologic outcomes after extracorporeal membrane oxygenation-a systematic review. Pediatr Crit Care Med 2018;19:76–766.
63. Hamrick SE, Gremmels DB, Keet CA, et al. Neurodevelopmental outcome of infants supported with extracorporeal membrane oxygenation after cardiac surgery. Pediatrics 2003;111:e671–5.
64. Wagner K, Risnes I, Bernsten T, et al. Clinical and psychosocial follow-up study of children treated with extracorporeal membrane oxygenation. Ann Thorac Surg 2007;84:1349–55.
65. Lequier L, Joffe AR, Robertson CM, et al. Two-year survival mental, and motor outcomes after cardiac extracorporeal life support at less than five years of age. J Thorac Cardiovasc Surg 2008;136:976–83.
66. Ryerson LM, Guerra GG, Joffe AR, et al. Survival and neurocognitive outcomes after cardiac extracorporeal life support in children less than 5 years of age: a ten-year cohort. Circ Heart Fail 2015;8:312–21.
67. Schmidt F, Jack T, Sasse M, et al. Awake veno-arterial extracorporeal membrane oxygenation" in pediatric cardiogenic shock: a single-center experience. Pediatr Cardiol 2015;36:1647–56.
68. Costa J, Dirnberger DR, Froehlich CD, et al. Awake neonatal extracorporeal membrane oxygenation. ASAIO J 2020;66:e70–3.
69. Schmidt F, Sasse M, Boehne M, et al. Concept of "awake venovenous extracorporeal membrane oxygenation" in pediatric patients awaiting lung transplantation. Pediatr Transplant 2013;17:224–30.
70. Jenks CL, Tweed J, Gigli KH, et al. An international survey on ventilator practices among extracorporeal membrane oxygenation centers. ASAIO J 2017;63:787–92.
71. Wieczorek B, Acscenzi J, Kims Y, et al. PICU Up!: impact of quality improvement intervention to promote early mobilization in critically ill children. Pediatr Crit Care Med 2016;17:e559–66.
72. Turner DA, Rehder KJ, Bonadonna D, et al. Ambulatory ECMO as a bridge to lung transplant in a previously well pediatric patient with ARDS. Pediatrics 2014;134:e583–5.
73. Shudo Y, Wang H, Ha RV, et al. Heart transplant after profoundly extended ambulatory central venoarterial extracorporeal membrane oxygenation. J Thorac Cardiovasc Surg 2018;156:e7–9.
74. Direnberger D, Fiser R, Harvey C, et al. Guidelines for ECMO Transport Extracorporeal Life Support Organization (ELSO), Ann Arbor, MI. Available online at: https://www.elso.org/Portals/0/Files/ELSO%20GUIDELINES%20FOR%20ECMO%20TRANSPORT_May2015.pdf. Accessed November 11, 2021.
75. Barbaro RP, MacLaren G, Boonstra PS, et al. Extracorporeal membrane oxygenation for COVID-19: evolving outcomes from the International Extracorporeal Life Support Organization Registry. Lancet 2021;398:1230–8.
76. Feldstein LR, Rose EB, Horwitz SM, et al. Overcoming COVID-19 Investigators; CDC COVID-19 Response Team. Multisystem inflammatory syndrome in U.S. children and adolescents. N Engl J Med 2020;383:334–46.
77. COVID-19 registry dashboard. Available at: https://www.elso.org/Registry/FullCOVID19RegistryDashboard.aspx?goHash=1&sO=1&all=true&NA=false&

Eur=false&Asia=false&La=false&Africa=false&AA=false&Neo=true&Ped= true&Adlt=false#TheFilter. Accessed November 11, 2021.

78. DeLoughery EP, Olson SR, McCarty OJ, et al. The safety and efficacy of novel agents targeting factors XI and XII in early phase human trials. Semin Thromb Hemost 2019;45:502–8.

79. Larsson M, Rayzman V, Nolte MW, et al. A factor XIIa inhibitory antibody provides thromboprotection in extracorporeal circulation without increasing bleeding risk. Sci Transl Med 2014;222(6):222ra17.

80. Meyer AD, Gelfond JA, Wiles AA, et al. Platelet-derived microparticles generated by neonatal extracorporeal membrane oxygenation systems. ASAIO J 2015; 61(1):37–42.

81. Annich GM, Meinhardt JP, Mowery KA, et al. Reduced platelet activation and thrombosis in extracorporeal circuits coated with nitric oxide release polymers. Crit Care Med 2000;28:915–20.

Hemostasis in Pediatric Extracorporeal Life Support
Overview and Challenges

Amarilis A. Martin, MD[a],*, Rukhmi Bhat, MD, MS[b],
Meera Chitlur, MD[c]

KEYWORDS

- Mechanical circulatory support • Mechanical circulatory devices
- Extracorporeal membrane oxygenation • ECMO • Ventricular assist device • VAD
- Pediatrics • Anticoagulation

KEY POINTS

- Hemostatic complications from mechanical circulatory support (MCS) are an important cause of morbidity and mortality in critically ill children.
- There is a poor correlation between monitoring assays and anticoagulation safety and efficacy in pediatric MCS.
- Although alternative anticoagulants such as bivalirudin are being increasingly used in children on MCS, experience is limited to a few case reports or case series.
- Differences in coatings, anticoagulants, monitoring assays, and therapeutic target ranges across centers have made the systematic study of hemostatic outcomes of pediatric MCS difficult.
- Development of standardized anticoagulation protocols, monitoring assays, and definitions may improve the outcomes in pediatric MCS.

INTRODUCTION

Extracorporeal membrane oxygenation (ECMO) is indicated as a bridge to recovery or transplantation in patients with refractory cardiac and/or respiratory failure. During ECMO, deoxygenated blood from the patient passes through an oxygenator and

[a] Division of Pediatric Critical Care Medicine, Central Michigan University College of Medicine, Children's Hospital of Michigan, Carl's Building Suite 4114, 3901 Beaubien Street, Detroit, MI 48201, USA; [b] Division of Hematology, Oncology and Stem Cell Transplantation, Northwestern University Feinberg School of Medicine, Ann & Robert H. Lurie Children's Hospital of Chicago, 225 E. Chicago, Box #30, Chicago, IL 60611, USA; [c] Wayne State University, Central Michigan University, Hemophilia Treatment Center and Hemostasis Program, Special Coagulation Laboratory, Division of Hematology/Oncology, Children's Hospital of Michigan, 3901 Beaubien Street, Detroit, MI 48201, USA
* Corresponding author.
E-mail address: aamartin@dmc.org

Pediatr Clin N Am 69 (2022) 441–464
https://doi.org/10.1016/j.pcl.2022.01.009
0031-3955/22/© 2022 Elsevier Inc. All rights reserved.
pediatric.theclinics.com

oxygenated blood is returned to the patient. There are two types of ECMO pumps: the roller pump whereby the blood in the cannula is squeezed between two rollers and pumped back to the patient, and the centrifugal pump whereby the pump generates an outward centrifugal force resulting in a forward movement of the blood back into the patient. As their names imply, venous-arterial (VA) ECMO receives deoxygenated blood from a vein and delivers oxygenated blood into an artery, and veno-venous (VV) ECMO takes deoxygenated blood from and delivers blood back into a vein. VA ECMO is used in patients with cardiovascular compromise with or without pulmonary disease and VV ECMO is used in patients with pulmonary failure but with otherwise appropriate cardiovascular function. Extracorporeal cardiopulmonary resuscitation (ECPR) uses ECMO in patients with refractory cardiac and/or respiratory failure during cardiopulmonary resuscitation or immediately after the return of spontaneous circulation.

Ventricular assist devices (VADs) are indicated as a bridge to cardiac transplantation, bridge to recovery, or destination therapy in children with end-stage heart failure. A VAD receives blood directly from the ventricle of the heart and delivers it into the pulmonary or systemic circulation. A VAD can assist the right ventricle (RVAD), the left ventricle (LVAD), both ventricles (BiVAD), or the systemic ventricle (SVAD) in patients with single ventricle physiology to maintain adequate cardiac output. VADs can be either paracorporeal (the pump is outside the patient's body) or intracorporeal (the pump is inside the thoracic cavity), and they can be either pulsatile (blood is pumped into the circulation) or continuous (blood is spun into the circulation via axial or centrifugal force). **Table 1** summarizes the different types of VADs currently used in children.

Incidence and Risk Factors of Extracorporeal Membrane Oxygenation and Ventricular Assist Device-associated Thromboembolic and Hemorrhagic Events

Thromboembolic and hemorrhagic complications from both ECMO and VADs are unfortunately common and important contributors to morbidity and mortality. The rate of thrombosis and hemorrhage is relatively constant for each ECMO day.[13] Based on the Extracorporeal Life Support Organization (ELSO) Registry Report, mechanical clots occur in 47% and 29% of neonatal and pediatric ECMO runs, respectively; ischemic stroke accounts for 5.9% of neonatal and 5.4% of pediatric ECMO runs; and limb ischemia occurs in less than 1% of neonatal and pediatric ECMO runs.[14] The incidence of ischemic stroke in pediatric VAD is slightly higher at 8%.[15]

Hemorrhage is more common at 35% and 55% in neonatal and pediatric ECMO runs, respectively, and include cannula or surgical site bleeding, hemorrhagic stroke, gastrointestinal (GI) hemorrhage, hemopericardium-induced tamponade, and pulmonary hemorrhage. Hemorrhagic stroke is seen in 8% of neonatal and 6% of pediatric ECMO runs, accounting for 24% and 11% of the neonatal and pediatric ECMO hemorrhagic complications, respectively.[14] The incidence of hemorrhagic complications in children on VAD is 29%, with 4% being hemorrhagic stroke and 7% GI hemorrhage.[15]

The risks for thrombosis and bleeding in patients on mechanical circulatory support (MCS) depend on multiple factors, which can be divided into patient-specific, circuit-specific, and institution-specific. These are summarized in **Table 2**.

Patient-specific risk factors

Patient-specific factors include the patient's age, size, underlying medical condition, and overall health. Younger patients have an immature inflammatory and coagulation system. Smaller children (1) have lower patient-to-circuit blood volume ratios, which increases their risk for hemodilution and the need for blood priming of the circuit, (2) have lower patient-to-circuit surface area, which increases the amount of blood that interacts with the nonepithelialized circuit surface, (3) have smaller ventricular and

Table 1
VADs currently available for the pediatric population[1-12]

VAD	Support Type	Support Duration	Patient Population
Short-Term			
RotaFlow® (Maquet Cardiovascular, Wayne, NJ)	Paracorporeal Centrifugal Uni- and biventricular	≤ 6 hours	Patent's size: all Priming volume: 32 mL Flow delivery: ≤ 10 L/min
PediMag® (Thoratec, Pleasanton, CA)	Paracorporeal Centrifugal Uni- and biventricular	≤ 6 hours	Patient's size: < 20 kg; < 0.5 m² Priming volume: 14mL Flow delivery: ≤ 1.5 L/min
CentriMag® (Thoratec, Pleasanton, CA)	Paracorporeal Centrifugal Uni- and biventricular	≤ 6 hours - 30 days	Patient's size: > 10 kg Priming volume: 31 mL Flow delivery: ≤ 10 L/min
TandemHeart® (CardiacAssist, Pittsburgh, PA)	Paracorporeal Centrifugal Univentricular Percutaneous insertion	≤ 6 hours	Patient's size: > 1.3 m² Priming volume: 10 mL Flow delivery: ≤ 5 L/min
TandemHeart® (CardiacAssist, Pittsburgh, PA)	Intracorporeal Axial Univentricular Percutaneous insertion	≤ 4-14 days	Patient's size: >0.7-1.5 m² Pump size: 12-21 French Flow delivery: 2.5-5 L/min
Long-Term			
Berlin Heart EXCOR® (Berlin Heart, Berlin, Germany)	Paracorporeal Pulsatile Uni- and biventricular	Years	Patient's size: 3-60kg; 0.2-1.3m² Pump volume: 10-60 mL Flow delivery: 0.5-6 L/min
Thoratec VAD (Thoratec, Pleasanton, CA)	Para- or intracorporeal Pulsatile Uni- and biventricular	Years	Patient's size: ≥ 1.3 m² Pump volume: 65 mL Flow delivery: 1.2-7.2 L/min

(continued on next page)

Table 1
(continued)

VAD	Support Type	Support Duration	Patient Population
SynCardia Total Artificial Heart (TAH) (SynCardia Systems, Tucson, AZ)	Intracorporea Pulsatile Biventricular	Years	Patient's size: > 1.2-1.7 m^2 Pump volume: 50-70 mL Flow delivery: $\leq$ 9.5 L/min
HeartMate III™ (Thoratec, Pleasanton, CA)	Intracorporeal Centrifugal Univentricular	Years	Patient's size: > 1.0 m^2 Priming volume: 21 mL Flow delivery: 3-10 L/min
HeartWare, HVAD® (HeartWare Systems, Framingham, MA)	Intracorporeal Centrifugal Uni- and biventricular	Years	Patient's size: > 1.0-1.2 m^2 Priming volume: 15 mL Flow delivery: $\leq$ 10 L/min
Jarvik 2000®; Jarvik 2015® (Jarvik Heart, New York, NY	Intracorporeal Axial Uni- and biventricular	Years	Patient's size: > 8 kg Priming volume: 10 mL Flow delivery: 2-8.5 L/min
HeartMate II® (Thoratec, Pleasanton, CA)	Intracorporeal Axial Univentricular	Years	Patient's size: > 1.4 m^2 Priming volume: 7 mL Flow delivery: 2.5-10 L/min

Table 2		
Risk factors for thromboembolic and hemorrhagic events in pediatric ECMO and VAD		
Patient-Specific	**Circuit-Specific**	**Institution-Specific**
Age • Maturity of the hemostatic system in neonates infants vs. older children	Brand • Rough vs. smooth surfaces • Type of surface coating	Institution's Expertise Availability of Multidisciplinary Team
Size • Patient-to-circuit surface area • Ventricular size	Size • Patient-to-circuit surface area • Cannula size	Type of Anticoagulant Used

Medical Condition and State of Health
• Critical illness, systemic illness, shock-like states
• Specific organ pathology
• Cardiovascular physiology
  ○ single vs. two ventricle
  ○ mechanical vs. tissue valves
  ○ types and sizes of patches, conduits, shunts
  ○ congenital vs. acquired
  ○ chronic vs. acute
  ○ syndromic vs. nonsyndromic
• Arrhythmias, cardiac pulsatility
• Genetic predispositions
• Environmental influences
• Type and doses of medications
• Other medical therapies
  ○ RRT
  ○ blood product transfusions
  ○ recent CPB
  ○ recent ECMO
	Type of Support
	• VA vs. VV ECMO
	• Central vs. peripheral ECMO
	• Centrifugal vs. roller ECM° pump
	• Continuous vs. pulsatile VAD
	• Paracorporeal vs. intracorporeal VAD
	• Single vs. dual chamber VAD
		Anticoagulation Management Strategy

Abbreviations: CPB, cardiopulmonary bypass; RRT, renal replacement therapy.

vascular diameters, requiring smaller cannulas and pumps which may increase turbulent flow and shear stress, (4) have decreased ability to tolerate even low amounts of blood loss, and (5) have clinically significant hemorrahgic and thromboembolic events with relatively smaller clots. Small left ventricular size has been associated with increased shear stress and thrombosis incidence in patients with an LVAD.[16]

The patient's current and overall medical condition also plays a factor in the risk for bleeding and thrombosis. Critical illness itself presents a coagulopathic milieu, and ongoing medical conditions, genetic predispositions, environmental influences, type and dose of medications, recent or ongoing medical therapies, and duration of MCS can further influence prothrombotic and anticoagulant states. Studies report increased bleeding and thrombosis risk with a need for greater platelet transfusion volume and longer ECMO runs.[17,18] The anatomy and physiology of the cardiovascular circulation, the cause of the patient's heart failure, and ongoing arrhythmias may further alter the risk for bleeding or clotting. Cardiac lesions producing high-shear stress can lead to an acquired von Willebrand disease (vWD) and bleeding.[19] Patients with a right-to-left shunt (eg, atrial and ventricular septal defects, pulmonary arteriovenous malformation) and a clot in the reinfusing cannula of the VV ECMO circuit are at high risk for thromboembolic stroke. Furthermore, patients with poor atrial or ventricular contraction have higher risk for cardiac thrombosis and thromboembolic events regardless of the MCS used.

Circuit-specific risk factors
ECMO and VAD-specific risk factors for coagulopathy include the type, brand, and size of the VAD and ECMO circuits. Unfortunately, many pediatric studies have reported inconclusive circuit-specific risks for bleeding and thrombosis.[18,20] Nevertheless, it is important to remember that patients with a clot within the arterial cannula during VA ECMO and anywhere on a VAD are at high risk for ischemic stroke.

Institution-specific risk factors
Institution-specific factors include anticoagulant and antiplatelet choice, the overall management of anticoagulation, and the institution's expertise in pediatric MCS. The heterogeneous patient population on mechanical circulatory devices, types and brands of circuits used, and institutional practices have made quantification of thrombosis and hemorrhage risks in pediatric ECMO and VAD difficult.[21,22]

Mechanisms for Coagulopathy in Pediatric Extracorporeal Membrane Oxygenation and Ventricular Assist Device

Hemostasis is achieved by a complex interplay between platelets, endothelium and coagulation factors. While factor VIII (FVIII), von Willebrand factor (vWF), prostacyclin, thrombomodulin, and plasminogen activator inhibitor type 1 (PAI-1) are produced by the endothelium, most of the procoagulant and anticoagulant factors are produced in the liver.[23]

During normal resting conditions, (1) the inflammatory system is dormant and (2) a balance between procoagulant and anticoagulant factors is such that some anticoagulation is achieved to prevent spontaneous thrombosis while minimizing the risk of bleeding at rest (**Fig. 1**). Platelets, which mediate inflammation and aid in the coagulation cascade while stabilizing a clot, are also dormant.

NORMAL CONDITIONS AT REST

Procoagulant/Antifibrinolytic Factors	Anticoagulant/Profibrinolytic Factors
Inflammatory system	Protein C, Protein S
Platelets	Thrombomodulin
TF, Factors I-XII	Antithrombin, Heparin
PAI-1, TAFI	tPA, uPA, Urokinase

Fig. 1. Prevention of spontaneous thrombosis and hemorrhage at rest. PA1-1 = plasminogen activator inhibitor type 1; TAR = thrombin activatable fibrinolysis inhibitor; TF = tissue factor; tPA = tissue plasminogen activator; uPA = uroplasminogen activator.

Regardless of the underlying inflammatory and coagulopathic milieu of the patient, the ECMO and VAD circuits themselves promote a proinflammatory and coagulopathic state through three main mechanisms: (1) activation of the contact system by the nonendothelialized circuit, (2) shear stress during the passage of blood through the circuit, and (3) activation of the complement system by the nonself-circuit (**Fig. 2**).

The contact system (ie, factor XI, factor XII, high molecular weight kininogen, and prekallikrein) is immediately activated when the patient's blood comes in contact with the nonendothelialized circuit.[24] In addition to producing the proinflammatory and procoagulant molecules bradykinin and kallikrein, this pathway triggers the intrinsic coagulation cascade with eventual production of factor Xa (FXa), thrombin, and fibrin. Fibrin is insoluble, adheres to the circuit or vasculature, and activates platelets. A clot forms when fibrin strands cross-link (ie, fibrin clot) trapping platelets and erythrocytes within this network (ie, platelet clot).

Platelets are the key mediators of inflammation and coagulation in MCS. Proinflammatory cytokines, fibrin, exposure to the large foreign circuit surface, shear stress, and adenosine diphosphate (ADP) each independently activate platelets. Shear stress from the rough and uneven circuit results in hemolysis and release of ADP. Turbulence from abnormal blood flow by the failing heart and in areas whereby fibrin and platelet

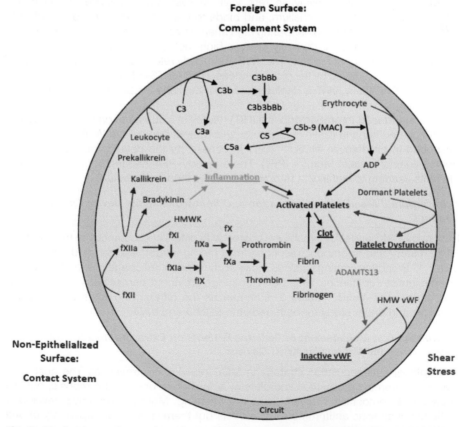

Fig. 2. Mechanisms of coagulopathy in ECMO and VAD. *ADP = adenosine diphosphate; HMW = high molecular weight; HMWK = high molecular weight kininogen; MAC = membrane attack complex; vWF = von Willebrand factor.*

thrombi form promotes further platelet activation.[25,26] Platelet activation is followed by degranulation and release of its proinflammatory and procoagulant contents, which promote inflammation and coagulation.

Leukocytes are activated by shear stress and by binding to activated platelets and procoagulant factors. Organ damage from arterial and venous thrombotic and embolic events also enhances the inflammatory response. The complement system (ie, C3, C5-C9), which is part of the innate immune response, is immediately activated by the nonself-circuit, and its products (eg, C3a, C5a) activate the endothelium and augment inflammation.[24] The inflammatory state that results may exacerbate the underlying critical state of the patient.

Despite an increasing number of platelets that are activated over longer circuit runs, platelets are often dysfunctional in ECMO and VAD.[27,28] Excessive shear stress can shear off the surface receptors of platelets (eg, GPIbα, GPVI), making them inactive or dysfunctional.[29] Increased risk for bleeding results when platelets, fibrin, and coagulation factors are dysfunctional or depleted from the circulation.

An acquired vWD is commonly seen in pediatric patients on MCS.[30–33] Chronic platelet activation may lead to a constant low-level release of vWF and A Disintegrin and Metalloprotease With Thrombospondin Type 1 Repeats-13 (ADAMTS-13) into the circulation.[31] In contrast to platelets which secrete vWF only when activated, endothelial cells constitutively secrete vWF at rest. vWF circulates through the body, binds to injured endothelium, and binds to platelet surface receptor GPIb-IX-V to facilitate platelet adhesion. During high shear stress, vWF also stimulates platelet aggregation. ADAMTS-13 normally cleaves high-molecular-weight vWF into smaller subunits to render them inactive. The vWF chronically released by platelets in patients on MCS is either cleaved by the platelet-released ADAMTS-13 or by the circuit's shear stress.[19,31] Eventually, vWF is depleted, which may place the patient at increased risk for bleeding.

Heparin-induced thrombocytopenia (HIT) occurs in a subset of patients exposed to unfractionated heparin (UFH) or low-molecular-weight heparin (LMWH) and has been described in children on MCS.[34,35] HIT is caused by the development of autoantibodies against platelet factor 4 (PF4). The antibody–PF4–heparin complex activates platelets, leading to significant thrombosis and thrombocytopenia.

Extracorporeal Membrane Oxygenation and Ventricular Assist Device Circuit Coatings

Pediatric ECMO and VAD circuits are coated with different substances to minimize the inflammatory and thrombotic response from the nonendothelialized and nonself-circuit.[36–38] Bioactive coatings include those composed of anticoagulant, profibrinolytic, or antiplatelet substances. Biopassive coatings provide a barrier between the blood and the nonself-circuit. **Tables 3** summarizes the different coatings commercially available and under study for both pediatric ECMO and VAD.

Anticoagulation Management of Pediatric Patients on Extracorporeal Membrane Oxygenation and Ventricular Assist Devices

The optimal anticoagulation strategy in MCS remains controversial. The goal is to decrease thrombin production and platelet activation to prevent thrombosis, but still allow some hemostasis to avert excessive bleeding. Most centers have developed institutional-specific antithrombotic protocols but there is no clear superiority of one approach over the other.

Among the antithrombotic agents, UFH is the most widely used agent in extracorporeal circuits. In cases of HIT, or true heparin resistance, other agents such as direct

Table 3 ECMO and VAD surface coatings			
		Commercially available	Under study

ECMO	Bioactive	• Heparin (anticoagulant)	• Heparin-based[a]
			• NO-based (antiplatelet, bacteriostatic)
			  ○ NO-releasing
			  ○ NO + other bioactives
			• Complement inhibitors
			  ○ C1-esterase inhibitors

	Biopassive	• Albumin (passivation) • PC (endothelialization) • PEG (hydrophilicity) • PEO/sulfate/sulfonate (endothelialization) • PMEA (low platelet adhesion) • Silicone (Passivation) • Smart-X (low protein & cellular adhesion) • Softline (low surface tension))	• Non-ionic polymers (passivation) • Organosilanes (superhydrophobic) • TLP (superhydrophobic) • Zwitterionic polymers (endothelialization)
	Bioactive + Biopassive	• Heparin + albumin • PEO/sulfate/sulfonate/heparin	
VAD	Bioactive	• Heparin	
	Biopassive		• TLP • Zwitterionic polymers

Abbreviations: NO, nitric oxide; PC, phosphorylcholine; PEG, polyethylene glycol; PEO, polethylene oxide; PMEA, poly-2-methoxyethyl acrylate; Smart-X (brand), polycaprolactone-polysiloxane block copolymers; Softline (brand), glycerol-PEG-ricinoleate; TLP, tethered liquid perfluorocarbon
[a] Heparin bound to the circuit by different mechanisms

thrombin inhibitors (DTIs) have been used. Following initial postoperative anticoagulation with short-acting anticoagulants (eg, UFH, DTIs), patients requiring long-term VAD have been transitioned to longer-acting agents (ie, warfarin in children older than 12 months, LMWH in children younger than 12 months). **Table 4** lists specific anticoagulant and antiplatelet drugs used in pediatric ECMO and VADs.

Unfractionated heparin
Heparin is a member of the glycosaminoglycan family of carbohydrates and consists of variably sulfated repeating disaccharide units. About a third of the heparin binds to antithrombin (AT), and this fraction is responsible for most of its anticoagulant effect.[39,40] The remaining two-thirds have minimal anticoagulant activity at therapeutic concentrations, but at high concentrations (greater than those usually obtained clinically), it catalyzes the AT effect of a second plasma protein cofactor, heparin cofactor II.[41] UFH action is mediated by interacting with AT and tissue factor pathway inhibitor (TFPI). It binds to AT via a specific pentasaccharide sulfation sequence contained

Table 4
Systemic anticoagulant and antiplatelet drug used in pediatric ECMO and VAD

Drug	MOA	Time to peak/half life	Clearance	Test	Reversal agent(s)	Suggested dosing	Target Ranges	Indication
UFH	Indirect via AT inhibition of IIa and Xa	1 hr/1–2 hrs	Renal	APTT Anti-Xa ACT	Protamine	LD: 50–100 u/kg prior to insertion of arterial cannula CI: 10–30 units/kg/hr titrated to effect	APTT 60–80 sec Anti-Xa 0.5–1 U/ml	ECMO Short-term VAD Long-term VAD
LMWH	Indirect via AT inhibition of Xa	3–4 hrs/7 hrs (after multiple doses)	Renal	Anti-Xa	Partially with protamine	1 mg/kg	Anti-Xa 0.5–1 U/ml	Long-term VAD
VKA	Inhibition Vit K factors II, VII, IX, X	24–72 hrs/variable, mean 40 hrs	Hepatic	INR	Vitamin K FFP		INR 2–3	ECMO Short-term VAD Long-term VAD
Bivalirudin	Direct thrombin inhibitor	Immediate/25 mins	Proteolysis Renal	APTT DTT	None	LD: 0.15–0.5 mg/kg CI: 0.15–0.25 mg/kg/hr	APTT 1.5–2 × nl ACT> 200 sec	Short-term VAD Long-term VAD
Aspirin	Liver			TEG AA Inhibition	Platelet transfusion	1–5 mg /kg/d	TEG MA <70 mm TEG AA inhibition 70%	Short-term VAD Long-term VAD
Dipyridamole	Liver			TEG	Platelet transfusion	1.5 mg /kg/d	TEG MA <70 mm	Short-term VAD Long-term VAD
Clopidogrel	Liver			TEG	Platelet transfusion	0.2 mg /kg/d	TEG MA <70 mm TG ADP net G 4–8	Short-term VAD Long-term VAD

Abbreviations: AA, arachidonic acid; APTT, activated partial thromboplastin time; AT, antithrombin; CI, continuous infusion; DTT, dilute thrombin time; FFP, fresh frozen plasma; INR, international normalised ratio; LD, loading dose; LMWH, low molecular weight heparin; TEG, thromboelastography; UFH, unfractionated heparin; VKA, vitamin K antagonist;

within the heparin polymer. By binding to AT, UFH increases its inhibitory action on thrombin (FIIa) and FXa by a thousand-fold. In addition, binding to TFPI catalyzes its inhibitory action on FXa and potentiates its inhibitory action two- to four-fold as compared with TFPI alone. Differences in the concentration of these proteins account for the need for dose variations among neonates and infants compared with children. *In vitro* analysis of the UFH effect shows that the ratio of UFH inhibition of FIIa and FXa varies with age, with infants and younger children having greater anti-FIIa activity for any given dose of UFH.[42]

Anticoagulant activity of UFH is monitored using the activated partial thromboplastin time (APTT) or the anti-FXa (anti-Xa) activity. Challenges to the use of UFH include increased clearance and physiologically lower levels of AT in sick infants.[43,44] UFH also binds to plasma proteins accounting for its variable bioavailability. This is problematic in infants and young children as they have a high volume of distribution compared with body surface area, which may explain their need for a higher dose compared with older children.[45] The marked variation in the reported incidence of bleeding associated with UFH in ECMO and VAD is another challenge, which is partly due to differing definitions for major and minor bleeding. Furthermore, while rare in children, HIT has nonetheless been reported with UFH use.[13,22,46]

The major advantages of UFH are its short half-life, reversibility with protamine, and extensive experience with its use. Frequent need for monitoring, poor correlation between dose and APTT or anti-Xa level, and variable time to the therapeutic range is some of its main disadvantages.

Bivalirudin

Bivalirudin is a 20 amino acid derivative of leech-derived hirudin that has target specificity for thrombin. It is a divalent DTI that binds both the substrate and catalytic site of thrombin and acts by preventing thrombin-mediated platelet activation. As a potent anticoagulant, it inhibits both circulating and clot bound thrombin, is reversible and, has a short half-life of 30 minutes.[47] It is cleared primarily by plasma peptidases with only 20% cleared by the kidneys, and can therefore be used in patients with mild to moderate renal dysfunction, albeit with dose modification. It has a relatively predictable anticoagulant effect as it does not bind to plasma proteins, interact with platelets, or require AT for its effect. It is an attractive option for patients with HIT, true heparin resistance, or liver dysfunction. However, unlike UFH, it does not inhibit the intrinsic pathway coagulation proteins.

There is limited experience of bivalirudin use in pediatrics. The possibility of drug degradation with stasis of blood flow, especially in stagnant areas in the ECMO circuit is a concern.[48] In addition, laboratory monitoring of bivalirudin is difficult. Despite these limitations, some centers have shifted to primarily bivalirudin-based anticoagulation protocols for antithrombotic management in VAD because of its predictable anticoagulant effect.[21] A few case series reports of bivalirudin use in ECMO have been reported to date.[49–52]

Low-molecular-weight heparin

LMWH is a polysaccharide prepared by the chemical or enzymatic digestion of UFH by depolymerization. The resultant molecular weight is between 4 and 8 kDa and has predominantly anti-Xa activity and minimal anti-FIIa activity. The different preparations of LMWH are formulated based on the ratio of FXa to FIIa activity and interaction with platelet factor 4 and heparin cofactor II, but very few studies have evaluated their use in the pediatric population.[53,54] Among the different LMWH, enoxaparin is the more commonly used LMWH. It has relatively stable pharmacokinetics and thus a more predictable response than UFH.

Similar to UFH, LMWH exerts its anticoagulant effect by binding to AT via a penta-saccharide sequence. It potentiates the action of AT on thrombin and FXa. Unlike UFH, its anti-Xa inhibition is greater than thrombin inhibition. Both UFH and LMWH release TFPI from vascular sites, which explains some of the antithrombotic effects of subcutaneously administered LMWH.[55]

Warfarin
Warfarin is a vitamin K antagonist that inhibits the vitamin K-dependent coagulation factors (FII, FVII, FIX, and FX). It is available only in oral form, limiting its use to those patients that can take oral medications. Additionally, physiologically low levels of vitamin K-dependent coagulation factors in infants and underlying medical conditions limiting gut absorption make its use challenging in this population.

Alternative anticoagulants
Other anticoagulant agents such as argatroban (a DTI) and FU-175 (a serine protease inhibitor) have been reported in pediatric MCD but data are limited to a small number of children.[56–58]

Antiplatelet agents
Antiplatelet therapy in combination with antithrombotics has been used in VADs to provide platelet inhibition. Its utility has been extended from its successful use with other artificial devices such as stents and mechanical heart valves.

Aspirin is an irreversible inhibitor of platelets that affects cyclooxygenase-1 that blocks thromboxane production.[59] It is used alone or in combination with other anti-platelet agents in patients on VAD. Its use in ECMO has been reported in smaller studies.[60]

Other antiplatelet agents used include dipyridamole and clopidogrel. Dipyridamole is a phosphodiesterase inhibitor that prevents the breakdown of cAMP, preventing signal transduction in platelet activation.[61] Clopidogrel undergoes in vivo biotransfor-mation to an active thiol metabolite which irreversibly blocks the P2Y12 component of the ADP receptors on the platelet surface. This prevents the activation of the GPIIa/IIIb complex and reduces platelet aggregation for the remainder of the lifespan of the platelet (7–10 days). It has been used in combination with antiplatelet therapy as well as with antithrombotic therapy to prevent pump thrombosis in children on VAD.[62]

There are three published anticoagulation therapy protocols for VADs. The Berlin Heart EXCOR protocol list two antiplatelet regimens (aspirin and dipyridamole), while the Stanford protocol lists triple antiplatelet therapy (aspirin, dipyridamole, clopidog-rel). Both protocols use UFH for anticoagulation.[63,64] The recent Advanced Cardiac Therapies Improving Outcomes Network (ACTION) protocol does not specify the an-tiplatelet regimen but uses bivalirudin as its main antithrombotic therapy.[65] Despite these published guidelines, most institutions have developed their own individualized approach, making it difficult to compare outcomes.[21] Adherence to protocol-driven anticoagulation therapy has been associated with a lower incidence of hemorrhagic and thrombotic complications.[66,67]

Antithrombin
AT is a serine protease synthesized in the liver. This naturally occurring AT inhibits thrombin, FXa, FIXa, and to a lesser extent FXIa, FXIIa, and FVIIa. When heparin binds to AT a conformational change occurs in the reactive sites of AT, neutralizing the ac-tivities of these coagulation factors by more than a thousand-fold. In addition to its

effect on coagulation, AT modulates the inflammatory response of the endothelium via heparan sulfate proteoglycans embedded along its surface.[68] Newborns, infants, and patients with liver disease, consumptive process (eg, disseminated intravascular coagulation), or sepsis have physiologically lower levels of AT.[69]

Practices regarding the use of antithrombin-III (ATIII) in ECMO are varied, and data regarding its use are inconsistent. Stansfield and colleagues[70] reported outcomes following routine ATIII replacement during neonatal ECMO before and after the initiation of a supplemental AT protocol. Patients in the AT group required less blood products and had lower rates of clots in the oxygenator and in other locations. However, total circuit lifespan was not different between groups, and there were no significant differences in rates of hemorrhagic complications of cerebral infarcts. Additionally, there was a lack of matching between groups as there were more patients on VV ECMO in the AT group. Furthermore, the study did not address the changes in circuit technology. Gordon and colleagues[71] reported a case series of 28 neonates and pediatric patients on ECMO receiving AT for functional AT activity less than 60% and/or signs of heparin resistance defined at the discretion of the clinician. Patients receiving AT experienced a small but significant increase in anti-Xa levels; however, they had a higher incidence of intracranial hemorrhage. In a multicenter pediatric cohort study by Wong and colleagues,[72] AT administration was associated with a 55% increase in thrombosis risk ($P < .001$), 27% increase in hemorrhage risk ($P < .001$), 37% increase in the risk of either thrombosis or hemorrhage ($P < .001$), and longer hospitalization stay without an increase in mortality.

Currently, the paucity of evidence for the efficacy of AT supplementation on clinical outcomes, paired with its potential risks and high costs, AT supplementation in neonatal and pediatric patients on ECMO should be approached with caution.

Anticoagulation Monitoring Assays in Extracorporeal Membrane Oxygenation and Ventricular Assist Device

Systemic anticoagulation is a tightrope between preventing bleeding related to excessive anticoagulation and thrombosis from the insufficient inhibition of coagulation. A good understanding of the assays used to monitor anticoagulation, including the variables influencing the tests and pitfalls, is beneficial to ensure successful anticoagulation without increased risk of bleeding or thrombosis. While the activated clotting time (ACT) and APTT are time-tested assays, especially for monitoring anticoagulation on ECMO, data suggest that they may not correlate with the clinical outcomes of bleeding and thrombosis.[73–75] Despite an increasing number of tests to monitor systemic anticoagulation, not one test has been found to be predictive of bleeding and thrombosis, leading to recommendations to consider multiple tests to determine effective anticoagulation without increased risk of bleeding.[18] In patients on VAD, the use of systemic anticoagulation with antiplatelet agents makes monitoring of anticoagulation even more difficult and reinforces the need for more than one test to predict the risk of bleeding or thrombosis. **Table 5** provides an overview of the common tests used, what the test measures, and factors influencing the results. While choosing the best anticoagulation monitoring assay, it is important to know that there is a poor correlation between ACT, APTT, and anti-Xa assays.[76] Therefore, these assays should not be used interchangeably.

Coagulation Assays

Activated clotting time

This is the most commonly used bedside assay for monitoring anticoagulation with UFH on ECMO. It is a global assay that measures the effects of platelet count,

Table 5
Anticoagulation and antiplatelet assays in pediatric ECMO and VAD

Test	Method	What It Measures	Variables Other than Anticoagulation, Affecting the Results
Activated Clotting Time (ACT)	Whole blood activated by an intrinsic activator kaolin/celite/glass	Time from FXII activation to clot formation	• Type of activator: kaolin vs. celite vs. glass • Platelet count and function • Lupus anticoagulant • Coagulation factor deficiency • Elevated levels/activity of coagulation proteins • Hypothermia
Activated Partial Thromboplastin Time (APTT)	Recalcified platelet-poor plasma activated with an intrinsic activator such as kaolin, silica, or ellagic acid and phospholipid	Time from FXII activation to clot formation	• Coagulation factor deficiency or dysfunction • Elevated levels/activity of coagulation proteins • Hyperlipidemia • Hyperbilirubinemia • Antiphospholipid antibody • Elevated CRP • Hemodilution
Anti-Xa Assay (aka, Heparin level)	Chromogenic or APTT based assay that measures residual activated Factor X (FXa) in patient plasma. The residual FX activity is inversely proportional to the heparin concentration	Heparin concentration in patient plasma	• Elevated plasma free hemoglobin • Hyperlipidemia (chromogenic assay only) • Hyperbilirubinemia (chromogenic assay only)
Dilute Thrombin Time (DTT)	Patient plasma diluted with pooled normal plasma, followed by the addition of thrombin to initiate clotting	Time to conversion of fibrinogen to fibrin Clotting time may be compared with a drug-specific reference curve to calculate the concentration of the direct thrombin inhibitor	• Elevated plasma free hemoglobin • Hyperlipidemia (chromogenic assay only) • Hyperbilirubinemia (chromogenic assay only)

Viscoelastic Testing TEG®/ROTEM®	Whole Blood Assays measuring from clot initiation, formation to lysis using specific intrinsic and/or extrinsic activators	Time to clot formation, strength of clot, and degree of fibrinolysis	Brand of thrombin reagent used factors that affect the thrombin time such as hypoalbuminemia, elevated levels of FDPs and fibrinogen, and acquired deficiencies of fibrinogen
Platelet Mapping on TEG®	Comparison of clot strength with thrombin activation vs ADP or AA activation	Measurement of percent inhibition of ADP or AA receptors on platelets	• Coagulation factor deficiency/dysfunction • Platelet dysfunction/thrombocytopenia
Platelet Aggregation studies	Platelet aggregation in whole blood or Platelet rich plasma in response to agonists such as ADP, AA, collagen, and epinephrine	Measure of platelet inhibition compared with a normal control	• Unclear dose–response relationship • Significant intraindividual variation

Abbreviations: AA, arachidonic acid; ADP, adenosine diphosphate; CRP, c-reactive protein; FDP, fibrin degradation products; ROTEM, rotational thromboelastometry; TEG, thromboelastography.

fibrinogen activity and function, and coagulation protein deficiencies or dysfunction. ELSO guidelines recommend titrating ACTs between 180 and 220 seconds in patients on UFH to minimize risks of bleeding or thrombosis. The major advantage is that it is a point-of-care test that is inexpensive and easy to perform. However, there are different ACT instruments that yield different results, making comparisons between centers and systems difficult.[77] Studies comparing the ACT to the UFH or bivalirudin dose show poor correlation, suggesting that the ACT may not be an accurate measure of anticoagulation in patients on UFH or bivalirudin.[78,79]

Activated partial thromboplastin time

APTT is a time-tested assay to monitor anticoagulation with UFH and, recently, bivalirudin. The correlation between UFH and APTT is dependent on a baseline APTT in the normal range, from which the relationship between the APTT and UFH is linear. However, patients on MCS are critically ill with associated hypo- or hypercoagulability, coagulation factor inhibitors, and elevated FVIII levels resulting in abnormal APTT at baseline. Hence, several studies have shown a poor correlation between the APTT and the UFH or bivalirudin dose.[78,80] Some centers now using the anti-Xa assay to monitor anticoagulation with UFH instead of the APTT. In ECMO, the target ranges recommended are 1.5 to 2.5 times the baseline, assuming that the baseline APTT is in the normal range. Because this is not always the case in critically ill patients, alternative monitoring methods have to be considered for bivalirudin.

Specific Assays to Measure Heparin Activity

Anti-Xa assay

This assay measures the degree of inhibition of FXa by UFH via ATIII. Even though this assay does not measure the inhibition of thrombin by the UFH-AT complex, it is used as a surrogate measure of the overall anticoagulant activity of UFH.[77] There are two types of anti-Xa assays available: one depends on the patient's endogenous AT levels, the other has added AT. Assays without the added AT are recommended, as this provides a more accurate assessment of the anticoagulant effect of the UFH.[81] The target anti-Xa activity recommended is 0.3 to 0.7 units per milliliter.[82] Although single-center studies have shown a better correlation between the UFH dose and anti-Xa levels than APTT in children on ECLS, others have not.[77,83]

Prothrombin Time and International Normalized Ratio

Prothrombin time (PT) and international normalized ratio (INR) are prolonged by warfarin, argatroban, and bivalirudin. PT measures the activity of the extrinsic and common pathways of coagulation and, therefore, is dependent on the functional activity of FVII, FX, FV, FII (prothrombin), and fibrinogen. The PT varies with the type of thromboplastin (eg, rabbit, human, bovine, etc.) used in the assay. The INR is the PT ratio of a test sample compared with a normal PT corrected for the sensitivity of the thromboplastin used in the test. The target INR levels are between 2.7 and 3.5 in the Berlin Heart EXCOR protocols and between 2 and 3.5 for other devices.[22] The PT and INR are primarily used for monitoring warfarin in patients on oral anticoagulation in older children on VADs in outpatient settings. While bivalirudin causes the prolongation of the PT and INR, this test is not used to monitor its anticoagulant effect. This can result in challenges when trying to bridge from bivalirudin to warfarin.[84]

Specific Assays to Measure Direct Thrombin Inhibitors

Dilute thrombin time and ecarin clotting time

These assays are limited to specialized laboratories and recommendations for target levels are still under investigation. Both assays have been shown to have a dose-dependent response to increasing concentrations of DTIs. While PTT is also pro-longed with increasing concentrations of DTI, the PTT reaches a maximum prolonga-tion above a certain level; therefore, overdoses cannot be reliably predicted or measured using standard assays.[85] Studies are still ongoing to determine the appro-priate assay for monitoring DTIs in the setting of MCS.

Anti-IIa assay

This assay is similar in principle to the anti-Xa assay, whereby the amount of thrombin neutralized is proportional to the amount of DTI in the sample. A chromogenic sub-strate is added to bind to the residual thrombin which can then be measured by a chro-mogenic assay. The amount of residual thrombin activity is, therefore, inversely proportional to the amount of bivalirudin in the sample. This assay is not currently FDA approved for the measurement of bivalirudin concentration.

Viscoelastic testing thromboelastography and rotational thromboelastometry

Both are whole blood assays being investigated for their ability to monitor anticoagu-lation in MCS. They measure the viscoelastic properties of blood and can measure the dynamics of clot formation from initiation to lysis. The major difference is their ability to measure clot strength in a more physiologic milieu in the presence of both cellular and enzymatic factors of coagulation. However, the lack of flow and shear force and the lack of an endothelial surface still renders the assay nonphysiologic. The limited avail-ability of these assays is a major drawback to studying their utility in MCS and estab-lishing guidelines. While some centers use these assays during MCS and have documented a better correlation between these tests and the APTT, no studies have compared outcomes.[86] Furthermore, there are no established guidelines for target ranges for any of the parameters on viscoelastic testing thromboelastography or rotational thromboelastometry.

Specific Assays to Measure Platelet Activity

Thromboelastography platelet mapping

The addition of antiplatelet agents to the anticoagulation regimens for VADs makes the monitoring of anticoagulation even more challenging. The Edmonton protocol for the Berlin Heart established guidelines for platelet inhibition with both aspirin and dipyri-damole.[63] However, this has not been validated for use with other forms of VADs. Recent reviews have indicated that many centers use modified versions of the proto-col and abandoned the use of the platelet mapping assay.[63] The interindividual vari-ability is another major drawback of this assay.

Platelet aggregation studies

This assay measures platelet function and/or inhibition related to antiplatelet agents. The time required to perform this assay and the technical expertise required for inter-pretation is a major limiting factor to its utilization. Few studies have looked at its uti-lization in the management of antiplatelet agents in patients on MCS.[87] While these tests may be predictive of platelet dysfunction, the time required in obtaining the re-sults and the volume of blood needed make the assay less useful.

Practical Considerations for Clinicians

Physical examination and imaging must be monitored closely to identify early signs of thrombosis or hemorrhage and need to adjust anticoagulation to prevent significant adverse events, morbidity, and mortality.

Stroke assessment in infants with an open fontanelle is usually performed using daily head ultrasounds. Fullness of fontanelle is highly suspicious for increased intracranial pressure. For patients of all ages, a thorough neurologic examination must be obtained at regular and frequent intervals. If the patient requires neuromuscular blockade (NMB), pupillary reflex and vital sign changes should be monitored closely. Discontinuation of the NMB when feasible will allow the assessment of the neurologic status of the patient. If there are new neurologic deficits or significant bleeding or thrombosis elsewhere, computed tomography or magnetic resonance imaging of the brain should be obtained as early as possible to assess for dural sinus thrombosis and to better delineate intracranial ischemic or hemorrhagic changes.

Decreased filling of the VAD with hemodynamic changes or new-onset reduction in pulse pressure on VA ECMO may be signs of cardiac stun or hemopericardium with tamponade. Emergent echocardiogram may help confirm the diagnosis.

Bright red blood output from any orifice including at the cannula and central access sites, as well as through chest tubes, nasogastric tubes, and other drains should be monitored carefully. With excessive bleeding, anticoagulation should be reduced, and further imaging obtained to assess the extent of bleeding (eg, imaging to assess for hemothorax or adequate cannula placement) must be considered.

Skin and digit discoloration may be due to arterial thrombosis and should be monitored closely by a vascular surgeon and hand or foot specialist. Limb swelling or discoloration should also prompt evaluation for deep venous thrombosis with Doppler ultrasound.

Management of Thrombosis and Hemorrhage

Most institutions have a multidisciplinary approach to managing anticoagulation and hemostatic complications in patients on MCS. Monitoring of anticoagulation by the hematology specialist is necessary to manage the reversal or modification of anticoagulation in the presence of bleeding or thrombotic events. Management depends on the site of ischemia and hemorrhage and may involve consultation with specialists such as vascular surgeons for limb ischemia, neurologists and neurosurgeons for ischemic or hemorrhagic stroke, and GI and general surgery for GI hemorrhage. Additionally, hemorrhage can be treated with judicious blood product administration, and appropriate cannula position should be evaluated with significant cannula site bleeding.

With excessive thrombosis in the circuit, it is imperative to exchange the circuit in a timely manner in the operating room (ECMO, VAD) or at the bedside (ECMO). Appropriate measures must be taken to decrease the risk for bleeding and hypoxemia or cardiac arrest during the exchange. Ready availability of blood products and other resuscitative measures during the circuit change is critical. It is imperative to consider the risks and benefits of continuing and discontinuing MCS.

Challenges and Future Studies

A significant gap remains in understanding and managing bleeding and thrombosis in pediatric MCS. The heterogeneity of patients on MCS and the ongoing introduction of new ECMO and VAD circuits with differing sizes and antithrombotic coatings make the management of coagulopathy unpredictable and challenging. This is confounded by the fact that no center uses the same equipment or anticoagulation regimen. Centers also vary greatly in pediatric MCS expertise.[21,22] Furthermore, anticoagulant or antiplatelet monitoring is difficult with the difference in availability and the number and variety of assays, and the conventional coagulation profile has not been found to be a predictor of cerebrovascular events in pediatric ECMO.[75]

Multi-institutional collaborations have attempted to address these issues and improve knowledge gaps. The international ELSO registry has been tracking pediatric and neonatal ECMO runs for several decades and has provided much insight needed to improve ECMO outcomes in this. Pediatric VAD registries have been developed for similar reasons and include the Advanced Cardiac Therapies Improving Outcomes Network (ACTION), the European Registry for Patients with Mechanical Circulatory Support (EUROMACS), and the Pediatric Registry for Mechanical Circulatory Support (PediMACS).[88] Importantly, the ACTION network has defined guidelines for pediatric VAD anticoagulation with promising results.[65,66] Perhaps, similar guidelines and long-term studies are needed for pediatric ECMO. In addition, standardization of ECMO and VAD circuits, standard definitions for bleeding and thrombotic complications, and monitoring assays for antithrombotic and antiplatelet therapy may further improve the delivery of MCS and patient outcomes.

SUMMARY

Management of pediatric patients on MCS is complex. It requires a clear understanding of hemostatic principles, the safety and efficacy of different anticoagulant and antiplatelet agents, and the pitfalls of different monitoring assays. Standardizing ECMO and VAD circuits can help improve the study and delivery of these modalities. A multidisciplinary approach with intensivists, surgeons, and hematologists is beneficial during the management of bleeding and thrombotic complications, as well as in the development of management protocols. Finally, uniformity in reporting patient outcomes, including the definition of bleeding and thrombotic complications, will allow for comparisons across centers.

CLINICS CARE POINTS

- Hemorrhage and thrombosis are important complications of pediatric MCS.
- Hemostatis in pediatric MCS is complex and requires a multidisciplinary team approach.
- More research is needed to better evaluate and manage hemostatis in pediatric patients on MCS.
- Efforts to standardize definitions, MCS devices, anticoagulation protocols, and hemostatic assays may improve pediatric MCS outcomes.

DISCLOSURE

A.A. Martin has no disclosures to report. R. Bhat has no disclosures to report. M. Chitlur has no relevant disclosures to report.

REFERENCES

1. Abbott. CentriMag™ and PediMag™ blood pumps. 2019. Available at: https://www.cardiovascular.abbott/content/dam/bss/divisionalsites/cv/hcp/products/heart-failure/centrimag/documents/hf-centrimag-pedimag-pumps-spec-sheet.pdf. Accessed November 8, 2021.
2. Abiomed®. Impella: Ventricular support systems for use during cardiogenic shock and high-risk PCI: Instructions for use and clinical reference manual (Unites States only). 2017. Available at: https://www.accessdata.fda.gov/cdrh_docs/pdf14/p140003s018d.pdf. Accessed November 8, 2021.
3. Berlin Heart EXCOR® Pediatric. The ventricular assist device for children product catalog. 2018. Available at: https://www.berlinheart.com/fileadmin/user_upload/

Berlin_Heart/Bilder/US_Website/Berlin_Heart_Inc_Product_Catalog_MPC21_6_
zusammengefuehrte_Seiten.pdf. Accessed November 8, 2021.

4. Slaughter MS, Tsui SS, El-Banayosy A, et al. Results of a multicenter clinical trial with the Thoratec Implantable Ventricular Assist Device. J Thorac Cardiovasc Surg 2007;133(6):1573–80.

5. OPTUM®. Mechanical circulatory support devices clinical guideline. 2021. Available at: https://www.uhcprovider.com/content/dam/provider/docs/public/policies/clinical-guidelines/mechanical-circulatory-support-device.pdf. Accessed November 8, 2021.

6. Abbott. HeartMate 3™ Left Ventricular Assist System instructions for use. 2020. Available at: https://www.google.com/url?sa=t&rct=j&q=&esrc=s&source=web&cd=&cad=rja&uact=8&ved=2ahUKEwjsr87b4vnzAhVeB50JHUvpAL8QFnoECAgQAQ&url=https%3A%2F%2Fmanuals.sjm.com%2F~%2Fmedia%2Fmanuals%2Fproduct-manual-pdfs%2F8%2Fd%2F8de80de7-8a05-4acb-928d-840d01ef9aad.pdf&usg=AOvVaw0kCQP8HhSh-dxJmNB92VMb. Accessed November 8, 2021.

7. HeartWare®. HeartWare® Ventricular Assist System instructions for use. 2014. Available at: http://www.cvicu.co.nz/assets/cvicu/IFU00308-rev01-OUS-IFU-EN.pdf. Accessed November 8, 2021.

8. Medtronic. 2020 Cardiac rhythm and heart failure hospital and physician reimbursement guide for mechanical circulatory support devices. 2020. Available in. https://asiapac.medtronic.com/content/dam/medtronic-com/us-en/hcp/reimbursement/documents/crhf-reimbursement-guide-mcs-devices.pdf. Accessed November 8, 2021.

9. Kilic A, Nolan TD, Li T, et al. Early in vivo experience with the pediatric Jarvik 2000 heart. ASAIO J 2007;53(3):374–8.

10. Baldwin JT, Adachi I, Teal J, et al. Closing in on the PumpKIN Trial of the Jarvik 2015 Ventricular Assist Device. Semin Thorac Cardiovasc Surg Pediatr Card Surg Annu 2017;20:9–15.

11. Abbott. HeartMate II® Left Ventricular Assist System (LVAS) instructions for use. 2020. Available at: https://www.google.com/url?sa=t&rct=j&q=&esrc=s&source=web&cd=&ved=2ahUKEwi5maL37_nzAhVmAZ0JHQ5OAKIQFnoECAMQAQ&url=https%3A%2F%2Fmanuals.sjm.com%2F~%2Fmedia%2Fmanuals%2Fproduct-manual-pdfs%2F5%2F2%2F5254ce76-8073-4b54-a7d8-6c057a3678aa.pdf&usg=AOvVaw1JPMsBS4dnlhXkzPxRY204. Accessed November 8, 2021.

12. Mascio CE. Mechanical circulatory support in congenital heart disease. In: American college of cardiology. 2018. Available at: https://www.acc.org/latest-in-cardiology/articles/2018/03/28/12/51/mechanical-circulatory-support-in-congenital-heart-disease. Accessed November 8, 2021.

13. Dalton HJ, Reeder R, Garcia-Filion P, et al. Factors associated with bleeding and thrombosis in children receiving extracorporeal membrane oxygenation. Am J Respir Crit Care Med 2017;196(6):762–71.

14. ECLS registry report, International Summary. Ann Arbor: Extracorporeal Life Support Organization; 2017. p. 1–34. Available at: https://www.elso.org/Portals/0/Files/Reports/2017/International%20Summary%20January%202017.pdf.

15. Morales DLS, Adachi I, Peng DM, et al. Fourth annual pediatric interagency registry for mechanical circulatory support (pedimacs) report. Ann Thorac Surg 2020;110(6):1819–31.

16. Chivukula VK, Beckman JA, Prisco AR, et al. Small left ventricular size is an independent risk factor for ventricular assist device thrombosis. ASAIO J 2019;65(2):152–9.

17. Cashen K, Dalton H, Reeder RW, et al. Platelet transfusion practice and related outcomes in pediatric extracorporeal membrane oxygenation. Pediatr Crit Care Med 2020;21(2):178–85.

18. Drop JGF, Wildschut ED, Gunput STG, et al. Challenges in maintaining the hemostatic balance in children undergoing extracorporeal membrane oxygenation: a systematic literature review. Front Pediatr 2020;8:612467.

19. Horiuchi H, Doman T, Kokame K, et al. Acquired von willebrand syndrome associated with cardiovascular diseases. J Atheroscler Thromb 2019;26(4):303–14.

20. George AN, Hsia TY, Schievano S, et al. Complications in children with ventricular assist devices: systematic review and meta-analyses. Heart Fail Rev 2021. https://doi.org/10.1007/s10741-021-10093-x.

21. May LJ, Lorts A, VanderPluym C, et al. Marked Practice variation in antithrombotic care with the berlin heart EXCOR pediatric ventricular assist device. ASAIO J 2019;65(7):731–7.

22. Huang JY, Monagle P, Massicotte MP, et al. Antithrombotic therapies in children on durable ventricular assist devices: a literature review. Thromb Res 2018; 172:194–203.

23.. Trung C, Nguyen JAC. Endothelial interactions and coagulation. In: Steven E, Lucking F, Tamburro RF, et al, editors. Pediatric critical care: text and study guide. 2nd edition. Switzerland: Springer; 2021. p. 55–76.

24. Millar JE, Fanning JP, McDonald CI, et al. The inflammatory response to extracorporeal membrane oxygenation (ECMO): a review of the pathophysiology. Crit Care 2016;20(1):387.

25. Linneweber J, Dohmen PM, Kertzscher U, et al. The effect of surface roughness on activation of the coagulation system and platelet adhesion in rotary blood pumps. Artif Organs 2007;31(5):345–51.

26. Ghbeis MB, Vander Pluym CJ, Thiagarajan RR. Hemostatic challenges in pediatric critical care medicine-hemostatic balance in VAD. Front Pediatr 2021;9: 625632.

27. Cheung PY, Sawicki G, Salas E, et al. The mechanisms of platelet dysfunction during extracorporeal membrane oxygenation in critically ill neonates. Crit Care Med 2000;28(7):2584–90.

28. Baghai M, Heilmann C, Beyersdorf F, et al. Platelet dysfunction and acquired von Willebrand syndrome in patients with left ventricular assist devices. Eur J Cardiothorac Surg 2015;48(3):421–7.

29. Sun W, Wang S, Chen Z, et al. Impact of high mechanical shear stress and oxygenator membrane surface on blood damage relevant to thrombosis and bleeding in a pediatric ECMO circuit. Artif Organs 2020;44(7):717–26.

30. Gossai N, Brown NM, Ameduri R, et al. Pediatric acquired von willebrand disease with berlin heart excor ventricular assist device support. World J Pediatr Congenit Heart Surg 2016;7(5):614–8.

31. Dassanayaka S, Slaughter MS, Bartoli CR. Mechanistic pathway(s) of acquired von willebrand syndrome with a continuous-flow ventricular assist device: in vitro findings. ASAIO J 2013;59(2):123–9.

32. Ruth A, Meador M, Hui R, et al. Acquired von willebrand syndrome in pediatric extracorporeal membrane oxygenation patients: a single institution's experience. Pediatr Crit Care Med 2019;20(10):980–5.

33. Kubicki R, Stiller B, Kroll J, et al. Acquired von Willebrand syndrome in paediatric patients during mechanical circulatory support. Eur J Cardiothorac Surg 2019; 55(6):1194–201.

34. Scott LK, Grier LR, Conrad SA. Heparin-induced thrombocytopenia in a pediatric patient receiving extracorporeal membrane oxygenation managed with argatroban. Pediatr Crit Care Med 2006;7(5):473–5.
35. Eghtesady P, Nelson D, Schwartz SM, et al. Heparin-induced thrombocytopenia complicating support by the Berlin Heart. ASAIO J 2005;51(6):820–5.
36. Ontaneda A, Annich GM. Novel surfaces in extracorporeal membrane oxygenation circuits. Front Med (Lausanne) 2018;5:321.
37. Zhang M, Pauls JP, Bartnikowski N, et al. Anti-thrombogenic surface coatings for extracorporeal membrane oxygenation: a narrative review. ACS Biomater Sci Eng 2021;7(9):4402–19.
38. Leslie DC, Waterhouse A, Ingber DE. New anticoagulant coatings and hemostasis assessment tools to avoid complications with pediatric left ventricular assist devices. J Thorac Cardiovasc Surg 2017;154(4):1364–6.
39. Lam LH, Silbert JE, Rosenberg RD. The separation of active and inactive forms of heparin. Biochem Biophys Res Commun 1976;69(2):570–7.
40. Andersson LO, Barrowcliffe TW, Holmer E, et al. Anticoagulant properties of heparin fractionated by affinity chromatography on matrix-bound antithrombin iii and by gel filtration. Thromb Res 1976;9(6):575–83.
41. Hirsh J. Heparin. N Engl J Med 1991;324(22):1565–74.
42. Newall F, Ignjatovic V, Summerhayes R, et al. In vivo age dependency of unfractionated heparin in infants and children. Thromb Res 2009;123(5):710–4.
43. Andrew M, Paes B, Johnston M. Development of the hemostatic system in the neonate and young infant. Am J Pediatr Hematol Oncol 1990;12(1):95–104.
44. Andrew M, Paes B, Milner R, et al. Development of the human coagulation system in the full-term infant. Blood 1987;70(1):165–72.
45. McDonald MM, Jacobson LJ, Hay WW, et al. Heparin clearance in the newborn. Pediatr Res 1981;15(7):1015–8.
46. Vakil NH, Kanaan AO, Donovan JL. Heparin-induced thrombocytopenia in the pediatric population: a review of current literature. J Pediatr Pharmacol Ther 2012;17(1):12–30.
47. Sylvia LM, Ordway L, Pham DT, et al. Bivalirudin for treatment of LVAD thrombosis: a case series. ASAIO J 2014;60(6):744–7.
48. Ranucci M. Bivalirudin and post-cardiotomy ECMO: a word of caution. Crit Care 2012;16(3):427.
49. Jyoti A, Maheshwari A, Daniel E, et al. Bivalirudin in venovenous extracorporeal membrane oxygenation. J Extra Corpor Technol 2014;46(1):94–7.
50. Nagle EL, Dager WE, Duby JJ, et al. Bivalirudin in pediatric patients maintained on extracorporeal life support. Pediatr Crit Care Med 2013;14(4):e182–8.
51. Ranucci M, Ballotta A, Kandil H, et al. Bivalirudin-based versus conventional heparin anticoagulation for postcardiotomy extracorporeal membrane oxygenation. Crit Care 2011;15(6):R275.
52. Pieri M, Agracheva N, Bonaveglio E, et al. Bivalirudin versus heparin as an anticoagulant during extracorporeal membrane oxygenation: a case-control study. J Cardiothorac Vasc Anesth 2013;27(1):30–4.
53. Eriksson BI, Söderberg K, Widlund L, et al. A comparative study of three low-molecular weight heparins (LMWH) and unfractionated heparin (UH) in healthy volunteers. Thromb Haemost 1995;73(3):398–401.
54. Samama MM, Gerotziafas GT. Comparative pharmacokinetics of LMWHs. Semin Thromb Hemost 2000;26(Suppl 1):31–8.

55. Hoppensteadt DA, Jeske W, Fareed J, et al. The role of tissue factor pathway inhibitor in the mediation of the antithrombotic actions of heparin and low-molecular-weight heparin. Blood Coagul Fibrinolysis 1995;6(Suppl 1):S57–64.

56. VanderPluym CJ, Cantor RS, Machado D, et al. Utilization and outcomes of children treated with direct thrombin inhibitors on paracorporeal ventricular assist device support. ASAIO J 2020;66(8):939–45.

57. Potter KE, Raj A, Sullivan JE. Argatroban for anticoagulation in pediatric patients with heparin-induced thrombocytopenia requiring extracorporeal life support. J Pediatr Hematol Oncol 2007;29(4):265–8.

58. Nagaya M, Futamura M, Kato J, et al. Application of a new anticoagulant (Nafamostat Mesilate) to control hemorrhagic complications during extracorporeal membrane oxygenation–a preliminary report. J Pediatr Surg 1997;32(4):531–5.

59. Blanco FJ, Guitian R, Moreno J, et al. Effect of antiinflammatory drugs on COX-1 and COX-2 activity in human articular chondrocytes. J Rheumatol 1999;26(6):1366–73.

60. Bein T, Zimmermann M, Philipp A, et al. Addition of acetylsalicylic acid to heparin for anticoagulation management during pumpless extracorporeal lung assist. ASAIO J 2011;57(3):164–8.

61. Michelson AD. Antiplatelet therapies for the treatment of cardiovascular disease. Nat Rev Drug Discov 2010;9(2):154–69.

62. Rutledge JM, Chakravarti S, Massicotte MP, et al. Antithrombotic strategies in children receiving long-term Berlin Heart EXCOR ventricular assist device therapy. J Heart Lung Transplant 2013;32(5):569–73.

63. Steiner ME, Bomgaars LR, Massicotte MP. Berlin Heart EXCOR Pediatric VAD IDE study investigators. Antithrombotic therapy in a prospective trial of a pediatric ventricular assist device. ASAIO J 2016;62(6):719–27.

64. Rosenthal DN, Lancaster CA, McElhinney DB, et al. Impact of a modified antithrombotic guideline on stroke in children supported with a pediatric ventricular assist device. J Heart Lung Transplant 2017;36(11):1250–7.

65. Villa CR, VanderPluym CJ. Investigators* A. ABCs of stroke prevention: improving stroke outcomes in children supported with a ventricular assist device in a quality improvement network. Circ Cardiovasc Qual Outcomes 2020;13(12):e006663.

66. Auerbach SR, Simpson KE, Investigators ALN. HVAD usage and outcomes in the current pediatric ventricular assist device field: an advanced cardiac therapies improving outcomes network (ACTION) analysis. ASAIO J 2021;67(6):675–80.

67. Northrop MS, Sidonio RF, Phillips SE, et al. The use of an extracorporeal membrane oxygenation anticoagulation laboratory protocol is associated with decreased blood product use, decreased hemorrhagic complications, and increased circuit life. Pediatr Crit Care Med 2015;16(1):66–74.

68. Wiedermann CJ. Clinical review: molecular mechanisms underlying the role of antithrombin in sepsis. Crit Care 2006;10(1):209.

69. Monagle P, Barnes C, Ignjatovic V, et al. Developmental haemostasis. Impact for clinical haemostasis laboratories. Thromb Haemost 2006;95(2):362–72.

70. Stansfield BK, Wise L, Ham PB, et al. Outcomes following routine antithrombin III replacement during neonatal extracorporeal membrane oxygenation. J Pediatr Surg 2017;52(4):609–13.

71. Gordon SE, Heath TS, McMichael ABV, et al. Evaluation of heparin anti-factor Xa levels following antithrombin supplementation in pediatric patients supported with extracorporeal membrane oxygenation. J Pediatr Pharmacol Ther 2020;25(8):717–22.

72. Wong TE, Nguyen T, Shah SS, et al. Antithrombin concentrate use in pediatric extracorporeal membrane oxygenation: a multicenter cohort study. Pediatr Crit Care Med 2016;17(12):1170–8.
73. Reed RC, Rutledge JC. Laboratory and clinical predictors of thrombosis and hemorrhage in 29 pediatric extracorporeal membrane oxygenation nonsurvivors. Pediatr Dev Pathol 2010;13(5):385–92.
74. McMichael ABV, Hornik CP, Hupp SR, et al. Correlation among antifactor Xa, activated partial thromboplastin time, and heparin dose and association with pediatric extracorporeal membrane oxygenation complications. ASAIO J 2020;66(3): 307–13.
75. Anton-Martin P, Journeycake J, Modem V, et al. Coagulation profile is not a predictor of acute cerebrovascular events in pediatric extracorporeal membrane oxygenation patients. ASAIO J 2017;63(6):793–801.
76. Bembea MM, Schwartz JM, Shah N, et al. Anticoagulation monitoring during pediatric extracorporeal membrane oxygenation. ASAIO J 2013;59(1):63–8.
77. Ryerson LM, Lequier LL. Anticoagulation management and monitoring during pediatric extracorporeal life support: a review of current issues. Front Pediatr 2016; 4:67.
78. Liveris A, Bello RA, Friedmann P, et al. Anti-factor Xa assay is a superior correlate of heparin dose than activated partial thromboplastin time or activated clotting time in pediatric extracorporeal membrane oxygenation*. Pediatr Crit Care Med 2014;15(2):e72–9.
79. Moynihan K, Johnson K, Straney L, et al. Coagulation monitoring correlation with heparin dose in pediatric extracorporeal life support. Perfusion 2017;32(8): 675–85.
80. Arachchillage DRJ, Kamani F, Deplano S, et al. Should we abandon the APTT for monitoring unfractionated heparin? Thromb Res 2017;157:157–61.
81. Funk DM. Coagulation assays and anticoagulant monitoring. Hematol Am Soc Hematol Educ Program 2012;2012:460–5.
82. Basu D, Gallus A, Hirsh J, et al. A prospective study of the value of monitoring heparin treatment with the activated partial thromboplastin time. N Engl J Med 1972;287(7):324–7.
83. Ranucci M, Cotza M, Isgrò G, et al, Surgical clinical outcome REsearch (SCORE) Group. Anti-factor Xa-based anticoagulation during extracorporeal membrane oxygenation: potential problems and possible solutions. Semin Thromb Hemost 2020;46(4):419–27.
84. Hohlfelder B, Sylvester KW, Rimsans J, et al. Prospective evaluation of a bivalirudin to warfarin transition nomogram. J Thromb Thrombolysis 2017;43(4): 498–504.
85. Curvers J, van de Kerkhof D, Stroobants AK, et al. Measuring direct thrombin inhibitors with routine and dedicated coagulation assays: which assay is helpful? Am J Clin Pathol 2012;138(4):551–8.
86. Teruya J, Hensch L, Bruzdoski K, et al. Monitoring bivalirudin therapy in children on extracorporeal circulatory support devices: thromboelastometry versus routine coagulation testing. Thromb Res 2020;186:54–7.
87. Görlinger K, Bergmann L, Dirkmann D. Coagulation management in patients undergoing mechanical circulatory support. Best Pract Res Clin Anaesthesiol 2012; 26(2):179–98.
88. Lichtenstein KM, Tunuguntla HP, Peng DM, et al. Pediatric ventricular assist device registries: update and perspectives in the era of miniaturized continuous-flow pumps. Ann Cardiothorac Surg 2021;10(3):329–38.

Acute Liver Failure in Children

Divya G. Sabapathy, MD[a], Moreshwar S. Desai, MBBS[a],*

KEYWORDS

- Critical care hepatology • Extracorporeal liver support • Liver transplantation

KEY POINTS

- Pediatric acute liver failure is rare but catastrophic, with variable clinical presentations often resulting in rapid decline with multiorgan failure.
- Age and etiology-based approach is key to prompt identification of acute liver failure (ALF).
- The commonest cause of ALF in pediatrics is indeterminate, where there is no identifiable cause and comprises of 50% of all presentations.
- Etiology-specific treatment with general supportive care may reverse liver injury and prevent the need for liver transplantation.
- Extrahepatic complications are life threatening and need anticipation, surveillance, and quick judicious deployment of available therapies to optimize outcomes.

INTRODUCTION

The liver is the largest solid organ in a human body comprising ~2% of the bodyweight, and uniquely receiving blood supply from two sources: the portal vein (~75%) and hepatic artery (25%). Composed of hepatocytes, stellate cells, Kupffer cells, and sinusoidal endothelial cells, this organ is critical in maintaining whole body energy metabolism and homeostasis. Hepatocytes form the bulk (~70%) of the liver mass, and have several essential functions: (1) synthesis of plasma proteins (albumin and clotting factors); (2) production and excretion of bile; (3) detoxification of ammonia to urea; (4) production of glucose; (5) conjugation and excretion of bilirubin; (6) metabolism of fats, proteins, and carbohydrates; and (7) storage of glycogen.[1,2] Liver injury impairs organ function and negatively affects whole body and tissue metabolism and can induce organ failure in the brain, heart, lungs, and kidneys, which lead to the life-threatening complications seen in ALF.[3] The major comorbidities that affect short-term and long-term survival in patients with ALF include: hepatic

[a] Department of Pediatrics, Division of Pediatric Critical Care Medicine and Liver ICU, Baylor College of Medicine, 1, Baylor Plaza, Houston, TX 77030, USA
* Corresponding author.
E-mail address: mdesai@bcm.edu

Pediatr Clin N Am 69 (2022) 465–495
https://doi.org/10.1016/j.pcl.2022.02.003
0031-3955/22/© 2022 Elsevier Inc. All rights reserved.
pediatric.theclinics.com

encephalopathy (HE), hepatic cardiopathy, hepatorenal syndrome, coagulopathy, metabolic derangements, electrolyte and acid–base disturbance, and infections (**Fig. 1**). Supporting a child with acute liver failure (ALF) through liver transplantation (LT) or natural recovery of native liver is indeed challenging for clinicians, with transplant free survival in pediatric acute liver failure (PALF) of only 50% to 60%.[4,5] Deeper insights into the triggers and progression of liver failure, the pathophysiologic mechanisms driving extrahepatic organ failure, as well as knowledge of available support systems and their limitations are essential to optimize health care delivery and improve outcomes beyond the current status quo - such is the *premise* of this review.

DEFINITION AND EPIDEMIOLOGY OF PEDIATRIC LIVER FAILURE

The PALF study group[6] has defined PALF as, *"coagulopathy with INR $\geq$ 1.5 with encephalopathy or INR $\geq$2 without encephalopathy due to a liver cause, not correctable by intravenous Vitamin K, with biochemical evidence of acute liver injury and no evidence of chronic liver disease."* Based on the duration between onset of jaundice and development of coagulopathy and/or encephalopathy, ALF (interchangeably also termed fulminant ALF) has been further subdivided into: hyperacute (within 1 week), acute (8–28 days), and subacute (4–12 weeks). The estimated frequency of ALF in all age groups in the United States is approximately 17 cases per 100,000 population per year ($\sim$ 500–600 admissions/y),[7] but the frequency in children is unknown. PALF accounts for approximately 10% of pediatric liver transplants (LTs) performed in the United States annually.[8]

Etiology and Causes of Pediatric Acute Liver Failure

Causes of PALF can be broadly categorized by the insult that induces hepatocyte injury, or, by age of the child at presentation with the liver injury. **Table 1** lists PALF etiologies classified by the inciting trigger (toxins, infection, ischemia, autoimmune, genetic, inflammatory), whereas **Table 2** lists etiologies based on age of presentation

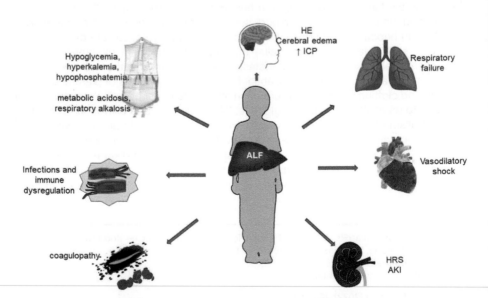

Fig. 1. *Extrahepatic complications of PALF:* Figure depicts effects of liver injury on brain, heart, lungs, kidneys, coagulation, immunity, and metabolism in a child.

Table 1 Etiologies of PALF by category[3,6]	
Etiologies of PALF	
Drugs	*Dose dependent*: APAP; halothane. *Idiosyncratic/synergistic*: Ketoconazole, Allopurinol, propylthiouracil, Amiodarone, Troglitazone, Diclofenac/Sulindac/Mefenamic acid, Tolcapone, Valproic acid, Amiodarone); Simvastatin, Isoniazid, Dantrolene, Fialuridine/Stavudine, amoxycillin/clavulinic acid, herbal medicines
Toxins	*Amanita phalloides* (mushroom poisoning), yellow phosphorus, industrial solvents
Infectious (viral)	HSV, hepatitis (A, B, B + D, and E), adenovirus, EBV, CMV, Echovirus, Varicella, Measles, Flavivirus (yellow fever), Ebola, Lassa, Dengue virus, Toga virus, Marburg virus
Infectious (nonviral)	Salmonellosis, tuberculosis, malaria, *Bartonella*, leptospirosis, gram-negative bacteria causing intraabdominal infections
Ischemia	Budd-Chiari syndrome, Acute circulatory failure/cardiac failure, myocarditis, tissue hypoxia due to respiratory failure or shock, low cardiac output states (myocarditis, Fontan circulation, dysrhythmias, cardio-pulmonary bypass)
Genetic/ metabolic	Galactosemia, tyrosinemia, hereditary fructose intolerance, Niemann-Pick disease type C, Wilson disease, mitochondrial cytopathies, fatty oxidation defects, α1-antitrypsin deficiency, inborn defects in bile acid synthesis, inborn urea cycle defects
Infiltrative	HLH, leukemia, lymphoma
Idiopathic	Unclear cause, thought to be cytotoxic T cell mediated

(neonatal, infancy, early childhood, adolescent). Classification of the causes of ALF in these 2 broad categories allows clinicians to rapidly review the differential diagnosis for ALF and respond with the appropriate management in a timely manner.

The most common causes of ALF that present in the pediatric intensive care unit (ICU) are briefly described with their respective treatments listed in **Table 3**.

Table 2 Etiologies of PALF by age of presentation[3,6]	
Etiologies of PALF	
Infants (0–1 y)	GALD (neonatal hemochromatosis), Galactosemia, tyrosinemia, fructose intolerance, fatty acid defects, Niemann-Pick type C, urea cycle defects, congenital HLH, mitochondrial defects, hypoplastic left heart syndrome, myocarditis, low cardiac output, shock states, sepsis, herpes virus (maternally acquired), adenovirus, TORCH infections, maternally transmitted HBV, therapeutic misadventure from medications (APAP).
Child (1–12 y)	Urea cycle defects, fatty oxidation defects, Wilson disease, sepsis, shock states, HSV, CMV, adenovirus, viral-mediated pathologic immune activation, macrophage activation syndrome (secondary HLH), AIH, leukemia, Budd-Chiari syndrome, idiopathic PALF, antiepileptics, ingestion (drugs, APAP)
Adolescents (12–18 y)	Wilson disease, HSV, adenovirus, CMV, EBV, AIH, secondary HLH, fatty liver disease (FLD) of pregnancy, leukemia, cardiomyopathy, failed Fontan circulation, sepsis, heat stroke, intentional APAP overdose, mushroom poisoning, psychedelic drug ingestion, herbal medicines

Acetaminophen (N-acetyl-p-aminophenol [APAP]; paracetamol): APAP, a universally prescribed medicine for childhood fever and pain, can induce hepatotoxicity and lead to ALF, either with acute intentional (suicidal) ingestion of large quantity (greater than 100 mg/kg) or by chronic ingestion of excessive amounts of APAP (greater than 100 mg/kg/d or greater than 15 mg/kg every 4 hours) for more than 1 day.[9,10] Children present with marked elevation of aspartate aminotransferase (AST), alanine aminotransferase (ALT), and prothrombin time/international normalized ratio (PT/INR), accompanied by a modest increase in total bilirubin levels. APAP overdose results in accumulation of the noxious NAPQI metabolite within the hepatocyte, which leads to depleted glutathione content, mitochondrial oxidative stress, mitochondrial dysfunction, depleted ATP stores, and cell death. APAP toxicity is potentiated by coexisting chronic liver disease, coingestion of alcohol, or herbs and medications that impair hepatic glucuronidation, and malnutrition which also reduces glutathione stores. N-acetylcysteine (NAC) replenishes and maintains hepatic glutathione stores by providing cysteine, the substrate which detoxifies reactive metabolites of APAP[11] and reverses liver injury. NAC should be administered immediately in patients with established or suspected APAP hepatotoxicity (see **Table 3**).

Non-APAP Drug-induced Liver Injury: Idiosyncratic (non-dose dependent) hepatoxicity has been reported with exposure to certain anesthetics, antiepileptics, antibiotics, isoniazid, propylthiouracil, chemotherapy agents, recreational drugs, and alternative herbal medicines.[12–15] Accidental ingestion of certain wild mushrooms (*Amanita phalloides*) can cause ALF because of hepatotoxins within the mushroom.[16]

Autoimmune Hepatitis (AIH): AIH has a wide clinical spectrum, ranging from indolent subclinical disease to fulminant hepatic failure. The diagnostic criteria are based on elevations of immunoglobulins, demonstration of positive autoimmune markers (antinuclear antibody, antismooth muscle antibody, and/or liver-kidney microsomal antibody), histologic features of liver inflammation, absence of viral disease, and therapeutic response to steroids and anti-inflammatory agents.[17] True frequency of AIH is unknown, but more than 25% of cases in the PALF database/registry had AIH as a diagnosis.[18] AIH is more frequent in adolescents and adults with a female predominance, although it should be considered among all age groups, including in infants 9 weeks to 12 months of age. Early diagnosis allows for early treatment and LT can be avoided.[18]

Hemophagocytic Lymphohistiocytosis (HLH): HLH is a rare systemic condition that leads to pathologic, immune-mediated damage to the liver caused by infiltration and overactivation of cytotoxic T lymphocytes and macrophages which exhibit hemophagocytic activity and overproducet proinflammatory cytokines (interferon-gamma). HLH can be congenital (autosomal recessive), affecting perforin-mediated cytolytic pathway, or acquired from inappropriate hyperinflammatory response triggered by acute viral infection, specifically Epstein-Barr virus (EBV).[19,20] HLH-induced ALF most commonly presents in the first 5 years of life, often accompanied with fever, hepatosplenomegaly, marked elevation in serum aminotransferase levels, hepato-biliary dysfunction, cholestasis, cytopenia, hypertriglyceridemia, hyperferritinemia (often more than 5000 ng/mL), hypofibrinogenemia, and elevated levels of soluble IL-2 receptor alpha.[19,20]

Gestational Alloimmune Liver Disease (GALD): GALD, earlier termed neonatal hemochromatosis, is characterized by alloimmune-mediated hepatocyte injury and ALF accompanied by iron accumulation (hemosiderosis) in liver and extrahepatic organs. GALD presents during the neonatal period and is thought to be mediated by maternal IgG antibodies directed against fetal hepatocytes, activating fetal complement cascade. Such activity leads to hepatocyte death, refractory hypoglycemia, severe coagulopathy,

Table 3
Etiology-specific therapies for PALF[7]

Etiology	Specific Treatment	Critical Care Considerations
APAP toxicity	NAC loading dose of 150 mg/ kg IV in D5W over 1 h, followed by 50 mg/kg IV in D5W over 4 h, then 100 mg/ kg IV over 16 h	Treatment should be continued, preferably intravenously, until INR and transaminases normalize. Watch for coexisting chronic liver disease and coingestions if liver injury worsens despite appropriately dosed and timed NAC administration. Follow Kings College Criteria for APAP prognosis
Mushroom (amatoxin from species *Amanita*)	Silibinin; penicillin 1,000,000 U/ kg/d; or thioctic acid 300 mg/ kg/d	The complications depend on dose of ingested toxin. NAC can be considered as an adjunct
HSV	Acyclovir 10 mg/kg IV every 8 h for at least 7 d	Start acyclovir pending HSV results in neonatal PALF, evidence of clinical findings, and sexually high-risk adolescents. Rule out HSV before starting steroids or anti-HLH therapy
Adenovirus CMV	Cidofovir 5 mg/kg weekly, or renally adjusted dose based on creatinine clearance	Renal toxicity is a major concern, thus prehydration and use of probenecid is recommended. Monitor blood/stool/respiratory secretions titers. Immunosuppressive agents worsen adenoviral load. It is ideal to clear and control systemic adenoviral load before LT
HBV	Antivirals such as Entecavir, Tenofovir, Adefovir Interferon α-2b Immunoglobulins for exposure	Vaccination has decreased the frequency of HBV in children in developed countries. Vertically acquired HBV can be seen in neonatal period
AIH	Corticosteroids (Methylprednisolone 2 mg/kg/ d, to a max of 60 mg/d)	Rule out HSV, adenovirus, and cancer, before starting steroids. Often, resolution of PALF with steroids may confirm the diagnosis. Despite preexisting liver disease, acute decompensation of AIH gets highest priority (Status 1A) for organ allocation

(*continued on next page*)

Table 3
(*continued*)

Etiology	Specific Treatment	Critical Care Considerations
Wilson disease	Chelating agents (Penicillamine, Trientine) Low Cu diet Total plasma exchange (TPE) Albumin-assisted dialysis LT for decompensated Wilson disease	Chelating therapy works if Wilson disease is diagnosed early. In fulminant phase of ALF, it is advisable to avoid chelating agents because of sudden, systemic Cu overload. Despite the disease being an inherited, preexisting liver condition, acute decompensation gets highest priority (Status 1A) for organ allocation
Urea cycle defects	Low protein, high fat, and carbohydrate diet with amino acid supplements, and ammonia scavengers (sodium benzoate, sodium phenylacetate, sodium phenylbutyrate) Prevent catabolic states in acute crisis (glucose-insulin drip) Dialysis for refractory, symptomatic hyperammonemia LT for multiple metabolic crisis despite medical therapy	Ammonia is the only mediator of encephalopathy in these disorders (as hepatocytes can clear other protein-bound toxins). Thus, ammonia has a dose-dependent effect on encephalopathy and can be treated by lowering ammonia alone with scavenger therapy and/or dialysis (because ammonia is water soluble). In contrast, dialysis alone is not beneficial in PALF and albumin-assisted dialysis and/or TPE is needed to manage encephalopathy Dialysis is initiated at much higher ammonia levels in urea cycle defects (greater than 300 μmol/L) than in PALF (greater than 150 μmol/L)
iPALF	Antithymocyte Globulin Corticosteroids	This is under clinical trial www.clinicalTrials.gov Identifier NCT04862221. Opportunistic infections should be ruled out before starting therapy
Tyrosinemia type-1	Elimination of tyrosine and phenylalanine in diet Oral NCTB, carnitine, and Vitamin D	LT is the definitive therapy Yearly surveillance for development of hepatocellular carcinoma is needed
Galactosemia	Remove dietary lactose	Aggressive surveillance and treatment of gram-negative bacteremia and sepsis is important
Hemophagocytic lymphohistiocytosis (HLH)	IVIG (pending diagnosis) Decadron: 10 mg/m^2/ d followed by taper	Rule out herpes, adenovirus, CMV, and lymphoma before embarking on

(*continued on next page*)

	Table 3	
(continued)		
Etiology	**Specific Treatment**	**Critical Care Considerations**
	Etoposide: 150 mg/m²/wk, followed by taper Anakinra (IL-1 receptor antibody): 6–10 mg/kg/d Emapalumab (monoclonal antibody against interferon gamma): 3 mg/kg/dose twice weekly LT if liver injury is irreversible Bone marrow transplant for congenital HLH	immunosuppressives. Such infections require nuanced use/dosing of therapies The immunomodulation should be titrated to effect considering risk for opportunistic infection, with concurrent prophylaxis against fungus and *Pneumocystis jirovecii* Monoclonal antibody therapies will be removed by TPE thus should be dosed after but can be given during CRRT and albumin-assisted dialysis
GALD	Double volume exchange transfusion and IVIG (1 g/kg)	As opposed to other neonatal ALF, GALD patients have modest elevations in AST and ALT compared with degree of coagulopathy and cholestasis
FLD of pregnancy	Deliver fetus	Must co-manage with obstetric services. Watch for HELLP (hemolysis, elevated liver enzymes, and low platelets) which can mimic FLD of pregnancy

hypoalbuminemia, elevated serum ferritin, ascites, and a pathognomonic hemosiderin deposition in liver and extrahepatic organs such as salivary glands, brain, heart, pancreas, and spleen. Normal/modest elevations of ALT differentiates GALD from other forms of neonatal hepatitis. Immediate neutralization (binding) with immune-globulins (IVIG) and steroids, and/or removal of the alloantibodies via exchange transfusion is successful in reversing ongoing liver damage[21,22] and avoiding LT.

Inherited/Congenital Metabolic Conditions: Overall, metabolic diseases account for at least 10% of PALF cases in the United States, Canada, and the United Kingdom. Most patients with metabolic ALF present in infancy and early childhood, except for Wilson disease, which presents after 5 years of age.[23,24]

Galactosemia presents as ALF associated with gram-negative sepsis in a neonate consuming breast milk or other lactose-containing formulas. Despite early detection by newborn screening, it should be suspected in any critically ill neonate with a negative screen, yet presents with multisystem organ failure, ALF, and reducing substances in the urine. Hereditary tyrosinemia type-1 also can present with gram-negative sepsis, profound coagulopathy, and modest transaminitis with a positive newborn state screen. Niemann-Pick type C is a lysosomal storage disease which presents with ALF, splenomegaly, and progressive neurologic deterioration.[23,24]

Urea cycle disorders, which include ornithine transcarbamylase deficiency, citrullinemia type-1, and carbamoyl phosphate synthetase deficiency, are inborn errors of ammonia detoxification/arginine synthesis due to inherited deficiencies in core enzymes of the Krebs-Henseleit cycle. Urea cycle disorders present in the neonatal period and early infancy with hyperammonemia, refusal to eat, excessive vomiting and hyperammonemia-associated brain damage, cerebral edema, seizures, or regression of milestones. Gluconeogenesis, coagulation, and bilirubin profiles are characteristically normal and differentiate hyperammonemia and encephalopathy in hepatocyte destruction-induced ALF from metabolic liver failure.[24,25]

Mitochondrial hepatopathies present with progressive neurologic deficiencies, cardiomyopathy, myopathy, severe lactic acidosis, and an elevated molar ratio of lactate to pyruvate (greater than 25) due to deficiencies in respiratory complexes I, III, or IV or mitochondrial DNA depletion. These often carry a poor prognosis, as children may not be considered good candidates for LT especially if brain injury is irreversible.[26–28]

Wilson disease, an autosomal recessive disorder of copper (Cu) metabolism caused by mutation of the ATP7B gene, is the most common, inherited metabolic condition associated with PALF in children more than 5 years of age. Presence of Coombs-negative hemolytic anemia, coagulopathy, renal dysfunction, modest transaminitis, and significant cholestasis with low alkaline phosphatase is suggestive of this diagnosis. Wilson disease is also associated with low serum ceruloplasmin (less than 20 mg/dL), elevated urine Cu, and increased Cu content in the liver and circulation. Demonstration of Kayser-Fleischer rings on slit lamp examination is diagnostic of the disease but may be present only 50% of the time.[29,30] Most patients require LT, although a subset may respond to chelating therapy, high volume plasma exchange, and albumin dialysis.[29–31]

Infectious (viral) causes: Hepatitis A (HAV), hepatitis B (HBV), herpes simplex (HSV), parvovirus, adenovirus, and enterovirus are directly linked to the development of ALF. With childhood immunizations for HAV and HBV, the frequency of these viruses has decreased in developed countries but remain major causes of liver failure in developing countries.[3] Hepatitis C virus, cytomegalovirus (CMV), EBV, human herpes virus 6 (HHV6), and HIV, are also associated with ALF, but it is uncertain whether they are the cause or effect (reactivation) of ALF. There is substantial evidence that pathologic immune activation/HLH/MAS may be triggered by EBV, HHV6, and CMV that can cause hepatobiliary dysfunction and ALF (see **Table 1**).[32]

The global pandemic caused by COVID-19 has not been linked to fulminant ALF. Children with COVID-19 pneumonia have shown mild elevations in ALT and AST, possibly from cardiopulmonary complications, tissue hypoxia, or medication (remdesivir)-induced transaminitis.[33]

Infectious (nonviral) causes: Nonviral infectious causes such as gram-positive and gram-negative bacteria, or any events that lead to sepsis and septic shock can lead to ALF. *Neisseria meningitides*, enteric bacteria that cause intraabdominal abscesses and bacterial peritonitis, also increases ALF susceptibility (see **Table 1**). Spirochetal infection (syphilis) and leptospirosis are some of the rare but reported causes of ALF. Children with Brucellosis, Q-fever (*Coxiella burnetii*), malaria (*Plasmodium falciparum*), and *Entamoeba histolytica* infections have presented with ALF in developing countries, sub-Saharan Africa and nations where these diseases are endemic.[8]

Hypoperfusion and shock states: Because the liver derives ~75% of its blood flow from the portal vein, it is prone to ischemic insult in low flow states where cardiac output is compromised. Septic shock or cardiogenic shock (cardiomyopathy, cardiopulmonary bypass, hypoplastic left heart syndrome), conditions that impeded the hepatic drainage into the heart (Fontan circulation, or veno-occlusive diseases such as Budd-Chiari syndrome) also induce ischemic liver damage.[34,35] Ischemic hepatitis (previously termed "shock liver"), uniquely presents with transaminitis where AST is higher than ALT, and usually resolves with resolution of shock, though is exacerbated if there is preexisting liver disease.

Indeterminate (iPALF): This subgroup, where there is no identifiable cause, is the most common cause (50%) of PALF.[36] Attempts to identify hepatotrophic viruses, potential autoimmune mediated damage, APAP exposure (APAP-cysteine biomarkers), evidence of hyperinflammation, macrophage activation, or HLH have proved futile. Histopathologic studies on previously collected liver biopsies from children with iPALF show an abundance of cytotoxic T lymphocytes (CD8) cells suggesting that immune dysregulation could be the basis of iPALF.[37–39] Clinical trials with corticosteroids[40] and antithymocyte globulin directed against cytotoxic T lymphocytes have now begun in the United States.

CLINICAL PRESENTATION IN THE INTENSIVE CARE UNIT

Presentation: Children with ALF usually present with progressive jaundice, lack of appetite, malaise, viral prodrome, vomiting, and abdominal pain. Altered mental status, irritability, poor feeding, change in sleep/wake cycle is often a sign of HE. Except for acute ingestions of hepatotoxins, most children are previously healthy, making it difficult to ascertain the time of initial insult.[5] Thereafter, ALF can progress rapidly. In the PALF registry, patients with encephalopathy (53%), seizures (7%), and ascites (22%)[6,8,41] needed ICU care.

Clinical examination: Findings of acute onset jaundice, ascites, and hepatomegaly (acute liver edema) often suggest ALF. In the ICU, a complete neurologic examination is key in determining the New Haven stage (grade) of HE (**Table 4**), the presence of which guides management decisions and urgency to list for transplantation is based on presence/absence of HE. Presence of vasodilatory shock suggests an advanced stage of ALF and exacerbates encephalopathy and coagulopathy. Although uncommon in ALF, bruising or clinical bleeding indicates associated trauma (surgical procedure), sepsis, and thrombocytopenia. Certain etiology-specific clinical findings include presence of Kayser-Fleischer rings seen with a slit lamp in the Descemet membrane of the cornea indicates Cu deposition in Wilson disease (seen 50% of times), vesicles (HSV), nonspecific rash, conjunctivitis (viral), and lymphadenopathy (malignancy/HLH). Dysmorphic features and growth retardation may suggest genetic/metabolic disease. Foul breath (fetor hepaticus) indicates advanced stage ALF with hepatocyte destruction.[5,41]

Organ-specific signs and symptoms and pathophysiology: The liver controls host metabolism and homeostasis. ALF disrupts tissue metabolism and impairs function of the extrahepatic organs (see **Fig. 1**). Multisystem organ failure increases mortality and morbidity in PALF; hence, a detailed understanding of the pathophysiologic processes that drive extrahepatic organ dysfunction is essential for the selection of appropriate treatment options and successful management of the critically ill child.

HE: HE is a constellation of neuropsychiatric disturbances associated with ALF in a patient without preexisting brain disease. HE is evident on admission ~50% of times per PALF registry data.[6,8] Initial recognition of HE is difficult as it may initially present as nonspecific irritability, poor feeding, change in sleep/wake cycles, or disturbances of consciousness or motor functioning (see **Table 4**). Irreversible brain injury secondary to cerebral edema and raised intracranial pressure (ICP), often seen in late HE, is the most dreaded and life-threatening complication of ALF.[42,43]

Pathophysiology of HE: Ammonia plays a central role in the pathophysiologic processes that lead to HE (**Fig. 2**). Ammonia is a by-product of nitrogen metabolism,

Table 4
New haven criteria for HE

Grade	Clinical Symptoms	Pertinent Examination	Critical Care Considerations
I	*Infants/children:* Inconsolable, irritable, "not acting self" *Adolescents/Adults:* Trivial lack of awareness, euphoria/anxiety, decreased attention span, impaired addition, and handwriting	Often have normal neurologic examination, normal/hyperreflexia GCS 14–15	Seldom have cerebral edema; EEG often unremarkable
II	*Infants/children:* drowsy, inconsolable, "more sleepy than usual" *Adolescents/adults:* Lethargy or apathy, disorientation, subtle personality change, inappropriate behaviors, lack of inhibition	Hyperreflexia, tremors, impaired handwriting GCS 12–14	<25% of patients have cerebral edema; EEG may be normal or show diffuse slowing; will need frequent neuro-monitoring preferably in the ICU
III	*Infants/children:* Stuporous, somnolent, sleepy but arousable, combative, obeys commands *Adolescents/adults:* Somnolence or semistupor, confusion, disorientation, cannot do a simple tasks	Hyperreflexia, ataxia, abnormal gait, abnormal hand–eye coordination, positive Babinski GCS 8–12	Cerebral edema in 25%–35% of patients; EEG with triphasic waves and slowing; end tidal CO_2 monitoring needed Consider enhanced blood purification, and pharmacologic ammonia control
IV-A IV-B	*Infants/children:* Comatose but responds to painful stimulus *Adolescents/adults:* Comatose but responds to painful stimulus *Infants/children:* Comatose with no response to painful stimulus *Adolescents/adults:* Comatose with no response to painful stimulus	Areflexia, decerebrate/decorticate posturing, signs of raised ICP, pupillary changes, GCS = 3–7	More than 75% of patients will have cerebral edema and raised ICP; EEG slow; intubation necessary for airway protection Catastrophic brain injury likely in this stage; liver transplant often urgent Advise enhanced blood purification, ammonia control, hyperosmolar therapy, prevention of secondary brain injury

generated within the small intestine and transported to the liver via portal circulation. In intact hepatocytes, ammonia is incorporated into the urea cycle and detoxified by conversion to urea—a water-soluble compound excreted by the kidneys. In ALF, when hepatocytes are destroyed, ammonia content in the blood increases and is taken up by astrocytes of the brain. Astrocytes, whose primary role is to protect brain neurons against excitotoxicity, converts ammonia into glutamine via the enzyme glutamine synthetase. With prolonged and persistent exposure to pathologically high quantities of ammonia, intracellular glutamine concentrations increase, thereby increasing intracellular osmolarity. Osmotic stress in turn leads to an influx of extracellular water into the astrocytes, causing cerebral edema, raised ICP, coma, brain herniation, and

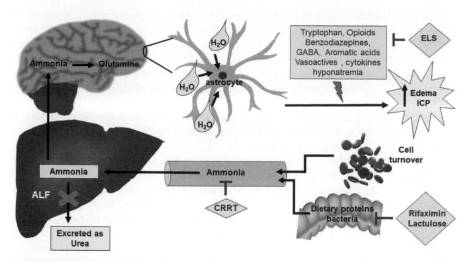

Fig. 2. *Pathophysiology of HE:* An injured liver fails to convert ammonia generated from the gut (dietary and activity of coliform bacteria) and cell turnover into nontoxic urea. Excess ammonia is metabolized to glutamine within the astrocytes of the brain, which increases intracellular osmolarity and draws water (H_2O) into the cell leading to cerebral edema and increased ICP. Brain injury is further potentiated by other unmeasured protein bound toxins, inflammation, and hemodynamic instability. Lactulose and Rifaximin are used to lower the ammonia generated in the gut. CRRT assists in removal of water-soluble ammonia, whereas albumin-assisted dialysis (ELS: extracorporeal liver support) is needed to remove protein-bound toxins.

eventual death (see **Fig. 2**). The critical contribution of ammonia in the pathogenesis and progression of HE is highlighted by clinical observations that more than half of the patients with ammonia levels more than 200 μmol/L develop HE and intracranial hypertension, whereas levels more than 150 μmol/L result in cerebral herniation. Moreover, persistent elevations of ammonia during 3 days of hospital stay are associated with death.[4,44–47]

Although ammonia plays a central role, it is not the only mediator of HE in ALF, thus levels do not always correlate with the degree of HE. In addition to ammonia, a failed liver also fails to detoxify countless other known and unknown circulating albumin and water-bound toxins, such as glutamine, gamma-aminobutyric acid, benzodiazepine-like substances, tryptophan/serotonin, aromatic amino acids, opioid substances, bile acids, and manganese all of which potentiate brain injury.[4,44–47] Here, extracorporeal albumin-assisted dialysis and/or plasma exchange are needed to attempt control of HE. In contrast, isolated hyperammonemia seen in inborn urea cycle defects, where encephalopathy and cerebral edema are seen only at much higher concentrations of ammonia (greater than 300–400 μmol/L), is reversible with decreasing ammonia levels (a water-bound substance) via dialysis and nitrogen scavengers. Additionally, ongoing inflammation, circulating chemokines and cytokines, vasodilators, hemodynamic compromise, hyponatremia, and acid–base disturbances further disrupt cerebral microvascular endothelial cells and alter the permeability of the blood–brain barrier to induce vasogenic edema, ultimately exacerbating HE (see **Fig. 2**). These pathophysiologic processes inform our approach in managing HE.[4,44–47]

Hepatic cardiopathy: Although cardiac dysfunction, injury, and failure are features of cirrhosis (cirrhotic cardiomyopathy),[48–50] subtle evidence of damage to cardiomyocytes (elevations in cardiac troponin I) and echocardiographic evidence of left ventricular stress have been documented in ~75% of adults with ALF.[51] Myocardial involvement is associated with higher odds of developing advanced HE and death.[51] Acute myocardial injury has not been reported in children with ALF; however, myocardial failure and cardiovascular collapse are observed with fulminant liver necrosis and multisystem organ failure. The systemic release of toxic mediators and cytokines by the rapidly dying and necrotic hepatocytes, compounded by the inability of the liver to clear them, leads to vasoplegia and vasodilatory shock refractory to fluids.[52,53] In addition, direct myocardial damage may also be seen in viral (adenovirus, CMV, HSV, EBV) mediated liver failure.

Hepato-renal syndrome (HRS): HRS is defined as Stage 2 or 3 acute kidney injury (AKI) in liver failure that is a reversible, functional deterioration of renal function without structural or histologic abnormality in the absence of shock, hypotension, hemorrhage, sepsis, or nephrotoxic medication.[54] HRS can progress either rapidly during the course of 2 weeks (Type 1) or indolently during a longer period (Type II). HRS remains difficult to define in children, with a speculated incidence between 6% and 11% or higher.[4,55,56]

The most widely accepted primary mechanism of HRS is development of splanchnic vasodilatation from mediators such as nitric oxide, carbon monoxide, and other vasodilator peptides released into the blood stream from a failing liver and portal hypertension (a complication of cirrhosis). Splanchnic vasodilatation steals blood flow away from the kidneys resulting in dramatic reduction in effective blood volume delivered to the kidneys. In presence of hepatic cardiopathy, the renovascular system compensates by stimulating the renin–angiotensin–aldosterone axis, sympathetic nervous system, and nonosmotic release of arginine vasopressin, which lead to water retention, hyponatremia, and severe vasoconstriction of the renal vasculature. These cascades of events further exacerbate renal hypoperfusion, ultimately precipitating AKI[4,57] (**Fig. 3**). Although associated with higher mortality, resolution of liver injury (spontaneous or after LT) has been shown to reverse HRS.[55,58]

Hepatic coagulopathy: One of the primary roles of the liver is synthesis of plasma proteins, including procoagulants (Factors II, V, IX, XI, and fibrinogen) and anticoagulants (Protein C, S, and antithrombin III). Hence, despite prolongation of INR/PT (one of the key defining parameters of ALF) overall bleeding risk is low (~5%) unless there is procedural or surgical trauma. This is due to "rebalanced hemostasis" from simultaneous reductions in both procoagulant and anticoagulant factors. Thromboelastography (TEG), which qualitatively assesses the clotting ability of the whole blood suggests that the homeostatic milieu of ALF in children may be slightly hypercoagulable because there is also a concomitant increase in circulating von Willebrand factor from low-grade endothelial cell activation and an increase in Factor VIII levels (because it is produced by endothelial cells).[59–63] Understanding this unique pathophysiologic context of liver-induced coagulopathy is essential in contemplating the pros and cons of plasma transfusions.

Metabolic derangements and acid–base abnormalities: Hypoglycemia, resulting from impaired hepatic gluconeogenesis and depleted glycogen stores, is one of the presenting symptoms of PALF often necessitating ICU admission for frequent monitoring and therapy with high glucose infusion rates (GIR). Hyperkalemia and hyperphosphatemia are seen if there is ongoing hepatocyte destruction and are worsened by concomitant AKI. Hypophosphatemia may also be seen as phosphorus is consumed during the regeneration of hepatocytes. Whole body acid–base balance can be impaired by ongoing active hepatic necrosis, shock, and increased anaerobic metabolism, which leads to lactic acidosis, or as the result of inborn errors of

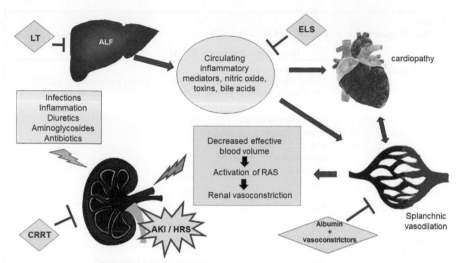

Fig. 3. *Pathophysiology of HRS and AKI:* Inflammatory mediators and vasodilatory toxins induce hepatic cardiopathy and vasoplegia. Splanchnic vasodilation steals cardiac output, lowering effective blood volume. Renin–angiotensin axis gets activated, which leads to constriction of renal vessels, kidney hypoperfusion, and HRS/AKI. Infections, inflammation, use of diuretics, and aminoglycoside further potentiate AKI. Splanchnic vasodilation is treated with albumin infusions and use of vasoconstrictors. Albumin-assisted dialysis (ELS) has a potential benefit in removing circulation vasodilators and toxins. CRRT is indicated in managing advanced HRS and AKI. LT reverses HRS.

metabolism resulting in accumulation of certain amino acids. Respiratory alkalosis is seen with hyperventilation associated with early hyperammonemia and raised ICP, whereas respiratory acidosis is seen with hypoventilation and respiratory failure in advanced stages of HE.

MANAGEMENT IN THE INTENSIVE CARE UNIT

Indications for ICU transfer: ALF can evolve rapidly into multisystem organ failure and death without close monitoring and transfer to higher level of care centers that can quickly and judiciously deploy cardiorespiratory and liver support systems. Indications for transferring to an ICU in a hospital capable of listing and providing LT for children include (1) respiratory insufficiency and impending respiratory failure, (2) shock needing vasoactive support, (3) worsening mental status with or without hyperammonemia, (4) coagulopathy needing multiple blood and plasma products, and (5) AKI needing dialysis or continuous renal replacement therapy (CRRT).

Fundamentals of ICU management: Despite scientific advancements, there are yet no proven therapies to reverse hepatocyte injury or hasten hepatocyte regeneration. The guiding principles for managing a critically ill child with ALF are rapid and accurate diagnosis; early recognition and surveillance of extrahepatic organ injury; nuanced use of available therapies to support the liver and other failing organs; optimizing homeostasis and hemodynamics to prevent catastrophic, irreversible insults to remote organs while awaiting spontaneous recovery of native liver function or LT.

Laboratory investigations: Early diagnosis and prompt intervention is essential in a child presenting with ALF to ensure optimal outcomes. **Table 5** lists the laboratory tests needed to (1) diagnose the presence and degree of liver dysfunction, (2) identify

Table 5
Diagnostic studies for a child with PALF in the ICU

	Diagnostic Approach to PALF
Routine laboratory tests	Chemistry panel Comprehensive electrolytes (calcium, phosphorus, magnesium) Glucose (particularly in infants)[a] Complete blood count Reticulocyte count Blood type and crossmatch Direct Coombs Cholesterol/triglyceride Amylase Uric acid Arterial blood gas Lactate Blood cultures Urinalysis and urine culture
Tests designed to diagnose ALF	ALT,[a] AST,[a] GGT[a] Total,[a] conjugated,[a] and unconjugated bilirubin[a] PT/INR Factors II, VII,[a] IX, X (Vitamin K dependent) Factor V[a] Factor VIII (if Factor VIII is low too then consider DIC) Fibrinogen[a] Fibrin split products Albumin[a] Ammonia[a]
Etiology-specific tests	Acetaminophen levels (APAP poisoning) Serum amino acids (inborn errors of metabolism) Alpha-1-Antitrypsin phenotype Plasma acyl carnitines (fatty oxidation defects) Lactate/pyruvate ratio (mitochondrial disease) Galactose-1-phosphate uridyl transferase (Galactosemia) Urine reducing substances (Galactosemia) Serum quantitative IgG, alpha-smooth muscle actin antibody (AIH) ANA, Liver–kidney microsomal antibody (AIH) Results of newborn screening, serum amino, and organic acids (inborn errors) Ferritin, total iron-binding capacity (GALD) Ferritin, triglycerides, fibrinogen, soluble IL-2 receptor (HLH) NK cell activity, perforin expression (HLH) Viral titers: Hepatitis (A, B, C, D, E), CMV, adenovirus, HSV Urine and serum drug screen Serum Cu and ceruloplasmin (Wilson disease) 24-h urinary Cu (Wilson disease)
To assess PALF complications	*CNS:* Ammonia, EEG, transcranial Doppler, head imaging (CT) *Cardiac:* ECG, BNP, troponin, echocardiography *Renal:* Renal ultrasound, creatinine, urine output, urinalysis, urine sodium *Pancreatic:* amylase, lipase *Hematologic:* DIC panel, INR, TEG *Endocrine:* Cortisol levels *Infectious:* Blood, urine, and sputum cultures

(continued on next page)

Table 5 (continued)	
Diagnostic Approach to PALF	
Imaging	Abdominal ultrasound with Doppler
	CT angiography (liver vasculature)
	Brain CT (cerebral edema/bleed)
	Brain MRI (metabolic disease)
	Body MRI (extrahepatic iron deposition in GALD)
Biopsy	Bone marrow aspiration/biopsy (HLH, hematologic malignancy)
	Liver biopsy (rarely performed except to diagnose AIH)
	Salivary gland biopsy (iron deposition in GALD)
	Muscle or skin biopsy (mitochondrial disease)
Additional studies determine readiness for LT	ECG
	Echocardiography
	Albumin and prealbumin
	Blood type and cross
	Anti-A and B antibodies (for potential need for ABO incompatible liver)
	COVID testing for operating room

[a] Identifies tests that can assess severity of PALF. See **Table 6** for prognostic markers.

the potential causes of liver injury, (3) assess the presence and severity of extrahepatic complications, and (4) test for candidacy for LT.

General supportive care: Intravenous access including central venous catheters should be promptly established for fluid management with the goal of euvolemia, euglycemia (targeting blood sugar between 110 and 130 mg/dL), and normal acid–base status. Comprehensive vital signs and fluid balance should be monitored and documented.

Established disease-specific management: Few diseases and triggers that induce ALF, if identified early, can be successfully treated before hepato-cellular destruction becomes irreversible. Etiology-specific management of ALF is listed in **Table 3**.

Organ-specific management of complications: The challenge for every intensivist lies in anticipating complications, supporting multiorgan dysfunction, preventing secondary injury and using technology designed to support the liver and sustain life until recovery of native liver function or LT. Most of therapeutic interventions used in the ICU are based on sound pathophysiologic basis, biologic plausibility, experience and expertise of bedside clinicians. Pediatric care also relies on knowledge extrapolated from adult, American Association for the Study of Liver Diseases guidelines,[44,64,65] as there are no robust clinical trials for PALF. **Table 6** outlines the recommended interventions to manage complications of ALF.

ICU management of HE: Basic neurocritical care measures should be instituted to prevent secondary injury such as elevation of the head of bed, midline positioning of neck, and prevention of hypoxemia, hypercarbia, hypotension, hyperglycemia, or hypoglycemia. Aggressive fever and infection control, targeting normal acid–base and electrolyte balance, and appropriate use of sedation and analgesia are important in preventing the worsening of encephalopathy. In this effort, avoidance of hepatically cleared agents like benzodiazepines is crucial. For cerebral edema and increased ICP, intubation is indicated to protect the airway and maintain normocarbia. Sedation, neuromuscular blockade, pentobarbital induced coma and hypothermia may be indicated in cases of severe cerebral edema and raised ICP. Hyperosmolar therapy with hypertonic saline and maintenance of relative hypernatremia (145–150 mEq/L) can

Table 6
System based interventions for complications of ALF in the ICU.[4,5,7,44,64,65]

System	Approach	Critical Care Considerations
CNS	Lactulose (0.5 cc/kg/dose), titrate to produce 2–4 soft stools daily Rifaximin Elevate head of bed to 30° Intubate for airway protection for Grade 3–4 HE Minimal stimulation Hypothermia for severe HE Hypertonic saline to goal Na 145–155. Barbiturates to decrease ICP If ICP monitor is placed, then keep ICP <20 mm Hg and CPP that is age appropriate Transfer to centers with the resources to concuct LT ± albumin-assisted dialysis	Lactulose can cause abdominal bloating. Diarrhea can cause dehydration and electrolyte imbalance Conduct rapid sequence intubation For sedation/paralysis avoid benzodiazepines, and preferentially use cisatracurium Consider empirical antibiotics (ceftriaxone) Treat sepsis, shock, and electrolyte imbalance that potentiate HE ICP monitor should be weighed against risks; if present correct coagulopathy aggressively Pharmacologic therapies used in urea cycle defects have not been found effective Steroids are strongly contraindicated.
RESPIRATORY	Intubate for airway protection (see above) Aim for Paco$_2$ between 40 and 45	Aggressive hyperventilation should be reserved for acute management of intracranial hypertension
CARDIOVASCULAR	Target age-appropriate MAP Fluid resuscitation: Crystalloid, 5% albumin Vasoactive agents: first line norepinephrine, second line vasopressin Test for adrenal insufficiency and use stress steroids for refractory shock	There is no benefit to starch/gelatin-based products Use established sepsis guidelines for management of septic shock
METABOLIC	Avoid hypoglycemia, hyperglycemia, hyponatremia, hyperkalemia Maintain normal serum phosphorus Glucose infusion rate: 10–12 mg/kg/min Maintain 1–2 mg/kg/d of protein intake 1–2 mg/kg/d Avoid catabolic states Use isotonic fluids	Avoid lactated ringers and acetate containing fluids Avoid hypotonic fluids, in effort to prevent hyponatremia Central venous access is often needed for high GIR and medication administration

RENAL	Avoid nephrotoxic medications	Maintaining acid–base balance is imperative
	Avoid excessive diuresis	If dialysis is indicated, then CRRT is advised over intermittent HD
	Terlipressin (not approved yet in North America), vasopressin, norepinephrine, midodrine or octreotide along with albumin expanders should be used in HRS	High clearance on CRRT may be needed to control hyperammonemia
	CRRT for advanced AKI and HRS	CRRT may be indicated to allow administration of blood products and nutrition without fluid overload
		Watch for citrate accumulation and hypocalcemia on CRRT
		Intraoperative CRRT may be indicated in anuric renal failure and if excessive blood loss is perceived during LT
HEMATOLOGIC	Vitamin K should be started at least for 3 d unless proven ineffective	TEG/ROTEM-based correction is preferred over relying on INR alone
	FFP, cryoprecipitate for clinical bleeding or elective procedures	Consider prothrombin complex to prevent fluid overload
	Aminocaproic acid/antifibrinolytics for mucosal oozing	Use fibrinogen concentrate to increase fibrinogen, as cryoprecipitate has factor VIII and could be thrombogenic
	Factor VII is reserved for invasive bolt placemen or life-threatening bleeding	
	Octreotide for GI bleed (rare in ALF)	

help prevent worsening brain edema and herniation.[66] Vasoactive infusions are used to maintain cerebral perfusion pressure, although age-specific targets are unknown in HE.[45,47] Use of ICP monitoring is controversial as it has not offered any survival benefits in adults and children, thus should be considered only in centers with expertise in device placement after considering risks of intracranial bleeding and infection.[67] Noninvasive options to monitor ICP, such as transcranial dopplers, continuous electroencephalography and ultrasonographic evaluations of optic nerve sheath diameters are under investigation.

As ammonia is a critical mediator of HE, pharmacologic agents known to lower ammonia are started early to prevent rapid increases in blood concentrations that may lead to the need for dialysis. Rifaximin, an oral, nonabsorbable antibiotic, decreases intestinal ammonia production from gut bacteria, and lactulose decreases enterohepatic circulation of ammonia by decreasing intraluminal pH in the intestines thereby limiting ammonia uptake by the portal system. Additionally, high diffusive clearance or high-volume hemofiltration might be necessary to maintain ammonia less than 100 μmol/L, especially if the rate of regeneration or degree of hepatocyte failure is high.[44,64,65] Blood purification via albumin-assisted dialysis may be needed to successfully reduce water soluble and protein bound toxins to manage HE.[68,69]

ICU management of hepatic cardiopathy and shock: Hemodynamic imbalance, circulatory shock and inflammation potentiate the toxic effects of hyperammonemia on the astrocytes, and directly contribute to worsening HE and cerebral edema.[70] Hypovolemia, often present in children with ALF on arrival to the ICU, can be treated with judicious fluid resuscitation using isotonic solutions, while vasodilatory shock can be managed with vasoconstrictors, preferably alpha-adrenergic agents like norepinephrine and vasopressin.[53,71] As adrenal insufficiency can occur in ALF, hydrocortisone should be considered for the treatment of shock.[72,73] Current pediatric sepsis guidelines[74] suggest the use of extracorporeal membrane oxygenation (ECMO) for fluid, vasopressor, and steroid nonresponsive shock. However, the outcomes for use of ECMO in PALF are dismal.[75–77] In children with ALF who required hemodynamic support, we and others[55,68] have reported modest success with early institution of total plasmapheresis, high flux CRRT and albumin dialysis with charcoal adsorption—a combination therapy we term hybrid extracorporeal therapy[68]

ICU management of AKI: HRS type I is treated by withholding diuretics, improving renal blood flow to the kidneys with albumin loading and reversing splanchnic pooling of blood with vasoconstrictors such as terlipressin (not available in the United States), vasopressin, norepinephrine and octreotide. Use of nephrotoxic agents (NSAIDS, contrast medium, aminoglycosides), and aggressive use of diuretics should be avoided. If oliguria persists despite adequate intravascular volume and use of vasopressors, high dose (clearance) CRRT should be initiated before the child progresses to overt renal failure.[78–80] CRRT is preferred over intermittent hemodialysis, as it maintains a steady acid–base and electrolyte balance, particularly sodium and ammonia clearance. The circuit prevents rapid fluid shifts, and end-organ consequences of fluid overload, cerebral and pulmonary edema with administration of blood/plasma products and nutritional support.[55]

ICU management of coagulopathy: Clinical bleeding is rare due to "balanced deficiencies" of the proteins that regulate the coagulation cascade. However, functional coagulation monitoring such as thromboelastography is recommended rather than relying on plasma-based INR or fibrinogen thresholds for blood product replacement.[59–63] If coagulopathy is suspected, Vitamin K is given initially (1 mg for infants or 5 mg for adolescents) to empirically correct potential vitamin K deficiency and should be discontinued if there is no response. Fresh frozen plasma (FFP) is ideal to correct coagulopathy; however, to avoid fluid overload, prothrombin complex, fibrinogen concentrates, cryoprecipitate or antifibrinolytics (aminocaproic acid/tranexamic acid) may be considered in patients with active bleeding or mucosal oozing or planned surgical procedures including vascular access. Recombinant factor VII is rarely used unless there is evidence of life-threatening bleeding. For uncontrolled coagulopathy, therapeutic plasma exchange (TPE) is beneficial to rapidly correct abnormalities in coagulation factors and maintain homeostasis while minimizing exogenous protein and fluid overload. TPE however should be performed in tandem with CRRT with awareness that FFP used in TPE could lead to acute citrate overload and citrate toxicity in ALF. There is a universal consensus that in the absence of DIC, sepsis, surgical procedures, and infections that lead to thrombocytopenia, over enthusiastic use of prophylactic blood products is discouraged as it may artificially lower the INR, thus interfering in the assessment of the ALF severity. This in turn confounds treatment plans and transplant listing decisions.[59–63]

ICU management of fluids, electrolytes, and nutrition: After appropriate correction of shock, fluids are used judiciously in ALF given significant risk for fluid overload. Total fluid goal should be ~ 80% to 90% maintenance, considering potential need for blood products. Hypoglycemia is corrected with a continuous infusion of high GIR, whereas hyponatremia is avoided by use of isotonic fluids containing sodium concentration of 150 mEq/L. Hypertonic saline boluses and continuous infusion may be needed to maintain higher sodium levels in advanced HE.[66] Nutrition support with appropriate carbohydrate and fat calories should be initiated as resting energy expenditure is high in ALF. Enteral feeds are advised if mental status and airway status allow safe administration. Gastric pH is maintained above 4 with intravenous proton pump inhibitor agents or an H_2 receptor antagonist to prevent gastrointestinal bleeding. If enteral feeds are not feasible, total parenteral nutrition is indicated.[81]

In hyperacute ALF and Grade 3 to 4 HE, where ammonia generation is high and difficult to manage, protein content in TPN can be restricted to ~ 1 g/kg/d. The avoidance of protein is no longer recommended as catabolic states are more deleterious to the patient. Intravenous administration of branched-chain amino acids has been reported to paradoxically increase ammonia production and is not recommended at this time. Trace elements such as Cu, manganese, molybdenum, chromium, and selenium should be eliminated as they may accumulate in patients with ALF.[81]

ICU management of infections: Patients with ALF have impaired immune response and are particularly prone to bacterial and fungal infections. Thus, close surveillance and prompt initiation of antifungal and/or antibacterial agents is paramount.

Extracorporeal Liver Support

Unmetabolized circulating toxins and vasodilators (water soluble and protein bound) are responsible for the catastrophic complications seen in ALF (HE, vasodilatory shock, and HRS), which often coexist. Blood purification (removal of toxins from the blood) is therefore key to survival of a child with ALF until recovery of basic functions or LT. Current extracorporeal liver support (ELS) systems have been designed to compensate for a failing liver by attempting to prevent encephalopathy by clearing and controlling spikes in ammonia levels; removing unmeasured protein bound toxins, maintaining hemodynamic stability by reducing circulating vasodilators and bile acids, maintaining fluid and homeostatic balance between procoagulant and anticoagulant factors, and facilitating delivery of optimal nutrition and blood products. Based on technology used to remove protein bound toxins, there are multiple noncellular and cellular (biologic) extracorporeal modalities (**Table 7**). Of note, no single system is superior to another, and there are no head-to-head comparisons of these modalities in

Table 7
Noncellular and cellular extracorporeal liver support systems[4,31,68,69,82,83]

ELS System	Biologic Principles	Key Features	Critical Care Considerations
Noncellular/nonbiologic			
CRRT only	AKI is common in PALF Hyperammonemia is key in the development of HE Fluid overload, metabolic acidosis and electrolyte imbalance must be avoided Blood products and nutrition needs must be met without causing fluid overload	Reduces ammonia levels without rapid fluid shifts, with ability to increase clearance to control ammonia levels Maintains acid–base and electrolyte balance Allows administration of blood products and nutrition without causing fluid overload Very efficacious in urea cycle defects	Does not remove albumin-bound toxins, bile acids, or bilirubin Continuous anticoagulation (heparin, citrate or prostacyclin) is required for preventing circuit clotting Blood priming is needed for infants CRRT may be needed intraoperatively if excessive blood loss or metabolic disturbances are expected during LT Dialysis catheter is required, thereby increasing risk of bleeding, clotting, infections, and need for sedation (to keep child immobile to effectively run the circuit)
TPE only (High volume plasma exchange)	PALF leads to coagulopathy which is often refractory to blood and plasma products Albumin-bound toxins contribute to HE and hemodynamic impairment in ALF	Patient plasma is separated and eliminated from whole blood, and replaced by FFP Assists with coagulopathy and SIRS Maintains fluid and protein neutrality	Because TPE is intermittent, the effect is short-lived There is exposure to plasma products since exogenous FFP is given Should be ideally done in tandem to CRRT, as FFP contains citrate, which accumulates in the circulation and can cause hypocalcemia Monoclonal antibodies, immunoglobulins, and beneficial growth factors may be removed
TPE + CRRT	Albumin-bound and water-soluble toxins need to be removed with control of coagulopathy	CRRT and TPE done in tandem	Although there is continuous removal of ammonia and water soluble toxins, removal of protein-bound toxins is intermittent Risk for citrate accumulation is high (although not as high as if TPE were done alone)

Molecular adsorbent recirculating system (MARS; Gambro, Sweden)	Albumin-bound and water-soluble toxins need to be removed Native albumin needs to be rejuvenated/restored to improve its function and its ability to bind to toxins Minimize exogenous protein (albumin/plasma) load	Blood is circulated across an albumin permeable (5–60 kDa) membrane against a 20% human albumin dialysate Toxins bind to albumin in the dialysate, which is then subject to hemodialysis to remove water-soluble toxins. The albumin passes through a charcoal column where protein-bound toxins are adsorbed and cleansed in an anion exchange resin column before being recirculated	Protein neutral since exogenous albumin is not used Has neither positive nor negative effect on coagulopathy Watch for thrombocytopenia and drop in fibrinogen levels Ability of exogenous albumin to adsorb toxins wanes with time Maintains fluid balance. Beneficial in HE. Resource intensive Has been studied and found to be efficacious in PALF
TPE + CRRT + MARS (hybrid extracorporeal liver support)	Management of coagulopathy, HE, AKI, inflammation and hemodynamic instability are crucial for better outcomes	TPE is done in tandem with CRRT, after which child is placed on MARS circuit	Facilitates control of coagulopathy, HE, hyperammonemia, AKI and fluid overload Resource intensive Frequent circuit changes are required when switching from TPE + CRRT to MARS
Single pass albumin dialysis (SPAD)	Basic principles are similar to MARS	Combination of hemodialysis and albumin dialysis After passing through the filter, the albumin is discarded	Relatively simple to perform Watch for thrombocytopenia Pediatric studies found SPAD to be well tolerated, and effective in detoxification, with improved hemodynamics and HE Cost and efficacy depend on patient weight and severity of ALF. Namely, very expensive in adolescents and adults because of high volume of albumin needed
Fractionated plasma separation adsorption	Fundamental principles are similar to MARS	Plasma (albumin) separated from whole blood using 250–300 kDa membrane filter	Improves bilirubin, creatinine and ammonia. However, there has been no

(continued on next page)

Table 7
(continued)

ELS System	Biologic Principles	Key Features	Critical Care Considerations
(Prometheus; Fresenius Medical Care, St. Wendel, Germany)		Plasma then enters secondary circuit where albumin-bound toxins are adsorbed Finally, plasma goes through a hemodialyzer where water-soluble toxins are removed	survival benefit in adults Not tested in children
Albumin exchange and replenishment system (Dialive; Yaqrit University College, London, UK)	ALF damages native albumin, which cannot be rejuvenated (recharged) completely despite MARS. Damaged albumin can induce inflammatory response, which could be detrimental. Damage-associated and pathogen-associated molecular proteins (DAMPS and PAMPS) contribute to immune paralysis and death	Two-membrane filter system: One membrane (60 kDa) removes damaged albumin which is then replaced by infusion of fresh human albumin 60 kDa membrane also removes circulating pro-inflammatory and anti-inflammatory cytokines, as well as chemokines, thus resetting the immune balance Second heparin-coated membrane removes DAMPs and PAMPs, thus preventing immune paralysis	Preclinical studies in swine model of APAP induced ALF demonstrated improved survival, heart and lung function and endotoxemia reduction Data analysis in multicenter adult trial is ongoing. Not studied in pediatrics.
Cellular/Biologic			
Extracorporeal-assisted device (ELAD; Vital Therapies; San Diego, CA)	Hepatocytes obtained from a cancer cell line are integrated into a device to provide functional activity to a patient with ALF	Comprised of hollow fiber dialysis cartridges that are lined with the cells. Blood comes in contact with the cells while flowing through the cartridges	Can generate albumin and metabolize drugs Not efficient for ammonia detoxification No added benefit in survival compared with standard therapy, thus production of these devices has been halted
Spheroid reservoir bioartificial liver (SRBAL; Mayo Clinic, Jacksonville, FL)	Primary healthy swine hepatocytes in a bioreactor are capable of providing functional activity	Hollow fiber dialyzer to detoxifies blood, whereas primary swine hepatocytes spheroids enhance detoxification and protein synthesis	Can generate albumin, metabolize drugs and reduce ICP in swine models of D-galactosamine-induced ALF Human trials pending

children, although data from adult patients suggest advantages in resolving enceph-alopathy, albeit without any survival benefit. Hence, use of these devices in children is not recommended outside the setting of clinical trials.[4,31,68,69,82,83]

LIVER TRANSPLANTATION

Current statistics suggest ~55% to 60% chance of spontaneous recovery of native liver function, suggesting that ~40% to 45% of children will die without LT. Even those with potentially recoverable ALF (ie, APAP toxicity) may still need LT if hepatocyte destruction exceeds the point of recovery. Indeed, reports from Europe and the United States have shown that about 45% to 50% of patients with ALF undergo liver trans-plantation, whereas it was contraindicated in 13% to 27% of cases at the time of admission. About 6% to 18% of cases were removed from the LT waiting list because of development of a contraindication or improvement in the clinical and prognostic status or death before availability of a donor liver.[84,85]

Criteria to determine listing for LT in PALF: Criteria to determine prognosis and or-gan allocation have always been a challenge. Scores have been developed based on the prediction of need for LT for survival. In the United States, United Network for Or-gan Sharing uses pediatric end-stage liver disease (PELD; less than 12 years) or model for end-stage liver disease (MELD; more than 12 years) scores for organ allocation, based on degree of severity of liver failure (**Table 8**). PELD and MELD however do not reflect the urgency of LT for children with PALF, as scores do not account for extra-hepatic organ failure. Certain children with ALF are given a priority over their PELD/MELD score and are listed at the highest LT priority of Status 1A.[84,85] The specific uni-versally accepted criteria to determine Status 1A are listed in **Table 8**. Other scoring systems used to determine criteria are the Kings College criteria for APAP toxicity, non-APAP toxicity, Clichy criteria, and the liver injury units[86–90] (see **Table 8**). Venti-lator requirement, hemodynamic status, and presence of active infection also deter-mine timing of the LT because LT is a major high-risk surgical procedure involving massive fluid shifts. LT is contraindicated if there is irreversible neurologic damage, where chances of meaningful survival despite a new liver are poor.

Types of grafts—Advent of LT and immunosuppressive therapy post-LT has dramatically improved survival in PALF. Considering ongoing organ shortage and a mismatch of donor to recipient ratio, surgical techniques have advanced to increase the number of donor organs in multiple ways. A child can receive an organ from (1) a deceased donor (either whole organ or a split organ with left lobe for the child and right lobe for an adult recipient), termed orthotopic LT[91,92], or, (2) living related or un-related donor (usually the left lobe).[93–95] Today, advanced knowledge and medica-tions available for post-LT immunosuppression allow successful transplantation of ABO-incompatible organs in children.[96]

Auxiliary liver transplant: In this technique, a donor liver is attached in piggyback fashion *in-situ* adjacent to, or inside the recipient's diseased liver. The rationale behind this procedure is that destroyed hepatocytes regenerate if given enough time to do so safely. The allograft provides liver function while the native liver regenerates. Once the native liver shows signs of full recovery, immunosuppressives are stopped and the "auxiliary liver" is allowed to involute by slow rejection. The procedure is being increas-ingly accepted as a valid treatment option for ALF, especially in children, but chal-lenges remain for timing of withdrawal.[97–99]

Hepatocyte transplantation: A potential alternative to LT is transplantation of normal mature hepatocytes directly through the portal vein into the recipient's diseased liver. A few children with metabolic diseases have benefited from allogeneic hepatocyte

Table 8
Prognostic markers in ALF

Prognostic Scores	Critical Care Considerations
PELD score $= 4.80[Ln \ serum \ bilirubin \ (mg/dL)] + 18.57 \ [Ln \ INR] - 6.87[Ln \ albumin \ (g/dL)] + 4.36(<1 \ year \ old) + 6.67(growth \ failure)$ Calculator: https://unos.org/resources/allocation-calculators/	Used for children <12 y but does not account for extrahepatic organ failure or comorbidities Plasma transfusions, and extracorporeal liver support can lower INR and bilirubin and can adversely affect the listing status and confound disease severity
Model End Stage Liver Disease (MELD) score $= 3.78 \times Log_e \ serum \ bilirubin \ (mg/dL) + 11.20 \times Log_e \ INR + 9.57 \times Log_e \ serum \ creatinine \ (mg/dL) + 6.43$ Calculator: https://unos.org/resources/allocation-calculators/	Used for children >12 y and adults Does not account for myocardial involvement Need for dialysis allows maximal points on the MELD
Status 1A: Onset of HE within 8 wk of the first symptoms of liver disease in the absence of preexisting liver disease *and* Need for mechanical ventilation *or* Need for CRRT *or* INR>2.0 with need for multiple plasma transfusions	Highest level of allocation based on urgency and presence/absence of HE. Given HE is diagnosed on examination, clinical accuracy is crucial The 3 categories that qualify for status 1A are: primary graft nonfunction following LT (within 7 d), hepatic artery thrombosis, and acute decompensated Wilson disease and autoimmune hepatitis
Kings College Criteria for APAP: Arterial pH < 7.3 *Or* Grade III or IV HE *and* creatinine > 3.4 mg/dL *and* INR>6.5 at time of initial presentation	Adjunct criteria to determine prognosis: Lactate > 3.5 mmol/L after fluid resuscitation (<4 h), or lactate > 3 mmol/L after full fluid resuscitation (12 h); phosphorus > 3.75 mg/dL at 48–96 h Does not account for coingestions, preexisting liver diseases
Kings College Criteria (non-APAP): INR > 6.5 *or* 3/5 of the following: Patient age < than 11 years (or > 40 y) iPALF (indeterminate cause) Drug toxicity, regardless of whether it was the cause of the ALF Serum bilirubin > 17.5 mg/dL (> of >300 μmol/L) jaundice to the development of coma > 7 d INR >3.5	Individual institutions may have their own criteria for listing and delisting based on institutional resources to support a child, experience of the ICU, hepatology, anesthesia, and surgical team and availability of organs based on location
Clichy-Villejuif Criteria HE *and* Factor V < 20% of normal for age less than 30 y Or, Factor V < 30% for age more than 30 y	Designed primarily for viral hepatitis and ALF The positive predictive value of mortality was 82% and the negative predictive value of mortality was 98% in individuals meeting these criteria

(continued on next page)

Table 8 (continued)	
Prognostic Scores	**Critical Care Considerations**
Liver injury units: = (3.507 × peak total bilirubin) + (45.51 × peak INR) + (0.254 × peak ammonia)	Higher score suggests poor prognosis. LIU at admission is more practical and can be used to determine prognosis, as bilirubin, ammonia, and INR can change with interventions

Used to determine disease severity and likelihood of survival while awaiting transplant, as well as chances of surviving without transplant.[84,85].

transplantation, in which the transplanted cells provide the missing/impaired hepatic function once engrafted. Although safety and short-term efficacy have been proven, major hurdles of donor organ shortage, poor cell engraftment, and lack of a long-lasting effect remain, dampening its widespread use.[100,101]

PEDIATRIC ACUTE LIVER FAILURE OUTCOMES

No single criterion can predict outcomes in ALF with absolute certainty or can be universally applicable to all patients with ALF of different causes. Prognosis varies and depends on the cause of the hepatic injury, age, and stage of encephalopathy. Survival without LT is highest in the APAP group (94%), whereas children with non-APAP drug-induced ALF (41%), metabolic disease (44%), or indeterminate ALF (43%) fare less well. In contrast, children with a non-A-E hepatitis or decompensated Wilson disease rarely recover without liver transplantation. Complications of liver failure including sepsis, hemorrhage, or renal failure increase mortality. An INR less than 4 was associated with 73% survival compared with 16.6% in those with an INR greater than 4. In PALF, jaundice for more than 7 days before the onset of encephalopathy, persistent grade 3 or 4 HE, INR greater than 6 (PT > 55 sec), ALT less than 2384 IU/L on admission, and factor V concentration of less than 25% of normal are predictors of poor outcome.[102,103]

SUMMARY

ALF is a multisystem disorder with high mortality and patients should ideally be managed in a multidisciplinary setting with facilities for liver transplant. To date, liver transplant remains the only effective treatment. Liver assist devices and hepatocyte transplant hold a great potential for bridging to LT or maintaining a patient while the native liver regenerates. LT interrupts the natural course of PALF and has proven to be lifesaving when a child fails to respond to targeted therapy. Future studies are required to better predict which patients require LT versus merely to buy time for recovery and to optimize the donor pool and artificial organ systems.

CLINICS CARE POINTS

- Respiratory insufficiency and impending respiratory failure, shock needing vasoactive support, worsening mental status, coagulopathy needing multiple plasma products, and AKI needing dialysis are indications for ICU transfer.

- Although ammonia is a key mediator of HE, ammonia levels do not correlate with degree of brain injury and other protein-bound toxins contribute to the encephalopathy. Hence treatment should be geared to controlling the ammonia and the circulating toxins.

- Judicious use of plasma products is advised in ALF despite elevations in PT/INR because ALF leads to a "rebalanced homeostasis" and spontaneous bleeding risk is low.

- Liver transplantation is life saving and should be considered if etiology-specific therapies fail to reverse liver failure.

ACKNOWLEDGMENTS

The authors acknowledge Anisha Desai for her contribution to generation of figures used in this article.

DISCLOSURE

The authors have nothing to disclose.

REFERENCES

1. Brauer RW. Liver. Annu Rev Physiol 1956;18:253–78.
2. Brauer RW. Liver circulation and function. Physiol Rev 1963;43:115–213.
3. Bernal W, Wendon J. Acute liver failure. N Engl J Med 2013;369(26):2525–34.
4. Desai MS, Lion R, Arikan AA. Critical liver failure:pathophysiological considerations. Curr Concepts Pediatr Crit Care 2016;1:143–64.
5. Miloh T, Desai M. Acute liver failure. In: Kline M, editor. Rudolph's pediatrics. 23rd edition. McGraw Hill Ed; 2018. p. 1876–82.
6. Squires RH Jr, Shneider BL, Bucuvalas J, et al. Acute liver failure in children: the first 348 patients in the pediatric acute liver failure study group. J Pediatr 2006; 148(5):652–8.
7. Squires J.E., Alonso E.M., Ibrahim S.H., et al., North American Society for Pediatric Gastroenterology, Hepatology, and Nutrition Position Paper on the Diagnosis and Management of Pediatric Acute Liver Failure. J Pediatr Gastroenterol Nutr. 2022;74(1):138-158.
8. Squires JE, McKiernan P, Squires RH. Acute liver failure: an update. Clin Liver Dis 2018;22(4):773–805.
9. Acetaminophen toxicity in children. Pediatrics 2001;108(4):1020–4.
10. Rivera-Penera T, Gugig R, Davis J, et al. Outcome of acetaminophen overdose in pediatric patients and factors contributing to hepatotoxicity. J Pediatr 1997; 130(2):300–4.
11. Yan M, Huo Y, Yin S, et al. Mechanisms of acetaminophen-induced liver injury and its implications for therapeutic interventions. Redox Biol 2018;17:274–83.
12. Molleston JP, Fontana RJ, Lopez MJ, et al. Characteristics of idiosyncratic drug-induced liver injury in children: results from the DILIN prospective study. J Pediatr Gastroenterol Nutr 2011;53(2):182–9.
13. DiPaola F, Molleston JP, Gu J, et al. Antimicrobials and antiepileptics are the leading causes of idiosyncratic drug-induced liver injury in american children. J Pediatr Gastroenterol Nutr 2019;69(2):152–9.
14. Stickel F, Patsenker E, Schuppan D. Herbal hepatotoxicity. J Hepatol 2005; 43(5):901–10.
15. Hoofnagle JH, Bjornsson ES. Drug-induced liver injury - types and phenotypes. N Engl J Med 2019;381(3):264–73.

16. Bonacini M, Shetler K, Yu I, et al. Features of patients with severe hepatitis due to mushroom poisoning and factors associated with outcome. Clin Gastroenterol Hepatol 2017;15(5):776–9.
17. Lohse AW, Mieli-Vergani G. Autoimmune hepatitis. J Hepatol 2011;55(1): 171–82.
18. Narkewicz MR, Horslen S, Belle SH, et al. Prevalence and significance of auto-antibodies in children with acute liver failure. J Pediatr Gastroenterol Nutr 2017; 64(2):210–7.
19. Amir AZ, Ling SC, Naqvi A, et al. Liver transplantation for children with acute liver failure associated with secondary hemophagocytic lymphohistiocytosis. Liver Transpl 2016;22(9):1245–53.
20. Canna SW, Marsh RA. Pediatric hemophagocytic lymphohistiocytosis. Blood 2020;135(16):1332–43.
21. Ibrahim SH, Jonas MM, Taylor SA, et al. Liver Diseases in the Perinatal Period: Interactions Between Mother and Infant. Hepatology 2020;71(4):1474–85.
22. Feldman AG, Whitington PF. Neonatal hemochromatosis. J Clin Exp Hepatol 2013;3(4):313–20.
23. Hegarty R, Hadzic N, Gissen P, et al. Inherited metabolic disorders presenting as acute liver failure in newborns and young children: King's College Hospital experience. Eur J Pediatr 2015;174(10):1387–92.
24. Alam S, Lal BB. Metabolic liver diseases presenting as acute liver failure in children. Indian Pediatr 2016;53(8):695–701.
25. Bigot A, Tchan MC, Thoreau B, et al. Liver involvement in urea cycle disorders: a review of the literature. J Inherit Metab Dis 2017;40(6):757–69.
26. Lee WS, Sokol RJ. Mitochondrial hepatopathies: advances in genetics, thera-peutic approaches, and outcomes. J Pediatr 2013;163(4):942–8.
27. McKiernan P, Ball S, Santra S, et al. Incidence of Primary Mitochondrial Disease in Children Younger Than 2 Years Presenting With Acute Liver Failure. J Pediatr Gastroenterol Nutr 2016;63(6):592–7.
28. Molleston JP, Sokol RJ, Karnsakul W, et al. Evaluation of the child with suspected mitochondrial liver disease. J Pediatr Gastroenterol Nutr 2013;57(3):269–76.
29. Korman JD, Volenberg I, Balko J, et al. Screening for Wilson disease in acute liver failure: a comparison of currently available diagnostic tests. Hepatology 2008;48(4):1167–74.
30. Vandriel SM, Ayoub MD, Ricciuto A, et al. Pediatric wilson disease presenting as acute liver failure: an individual patient data meta-analysis. J Pediatr Gastroen-terol Nutr 2020;71(3):e90–6.
31. Pawaria A, Sood V, Lal BB, et al. Ninety days transplant free survival with high volume plasma exchange in Wilson disease presenting as acute liver failure. J Clin Apher 2021;36(1):109–17.
32. Schwarz KB, Dell OD, Lobritto SJ, et al. Analysis of viral testing in nonacetami-nophen pediatric acute liver failure. J Pediatr Gastroenterol Nutr 2014;59(5): 616–23.
33. Di GA, Hartleif S, Warner S, et al. COVID-19 in children with liver disease. Front Pediatr 2021;9:616381.
34. Lightsey JM, Rockey DC. Current concepts in ischemic hepatitis. Curr Opin Gastroenterol 2017;33(3):158–63.
35. Seeto RK, Fenn B, Rockey DC. Ischemic hepatitis: clinical presentation and pathogenesis. Am J Med 2000;109(2):109–13.
36. Alonso EM, Horslen SP, Behrens EM, et al. Pediatric acute liver failure of unde-termined cause: A research workshop. Hepatology 2017;65(3):1026–37.

37. Chapin CA, Burn T, Meijome T, et al. Indeterminate pediatric acute liver failure is uniquely characterized by a CD103(+) CD8(+) T-cell infiltrate. Hepatology 2018;68(3):1087–100.

38. Chapin CA, Taylor SA, Malladi P, et al. Transcriptional analysis of liver tissue identifies distinct phenotypes of indeterminate pediatric acute liver failure. Hepatol Commun 2021;5(8):1373–84.

39. James LP, Alonso EM, Hynan LS, et al. Detection of acetaminophen protein adducts in children with acute liver failure of indeterminate cause. Pediatrics 2006; 118(3):e676–81.

40. Chapin CA, Horslen SP, Squires JE, et al. Corticosteroid Therapy for Indeterminate Pediatric Acute Liver Failure and Aplastic Anemia with Acute Hepatitis. J Pediatr 2019;208:23–9.

41. Squires RH, Alonso EM. Acute liver failure in children. In: Suchy FJ, Sokol RJ, Balistreri WF, editors. Liver disease in children. New York, NY: Cambridge University Press; 2014. p. 32–50.

42. Shawcross DL, Wendon JA. The neurological manifestations of acute liver failure. Neurochem Int 2012;60(7):662–71.

43. Wendon J, Lee W. Encephalopathy and cerebral edema in the setting of acute liver failure: pathogenesis and management. Neurocrit Care 2008;9(1):97–102.

44. Lee WM, Stravitz RT, Larson AM. Introduction to the revised American Association for the study of liver diseases position paper on acute liver failure 2011. Hepatology 2012;55(3):965–7.

45. Wendon JA, Harrison PM, Keays R, et al. Cerebral blood flow and metabolism in fulminant liver failure. Hepatology 1994;19(6):1407–13.

46. Cook AM, Morgan JG, Hawryluk GWJ, et al. Guidelines for the acute treatment of cerebral edema in neurocritical care patients. Neurocrit Care 2020;32(3): 647–66.

47. Kerbert AJ, Engelmann C, Jalan R. Neurocritical care management of hepatic encephalopathy and coma in liver failure. Semin Respir Crit Care Med 2018; 39(5):523–37.

48. Desai MS, Zainuer S, Kennedy C, et al. Cardiac structural and functional alterations in infants and children with biliary atresia, listed for liver transplantation. Gastroenterology 2011;141(4):1264–72.

49. Gorgis N.M., Kennedy C., Lam F., et al., Clinical Consequences of Cardiomyopathy in Children With Biliary Atresia Requiring Liver Transplantation. Hepatology. 2019;69(3):1206-1218.

50. Desai MS. Mechanistic insights into the pathophysiology of cirrhotic cardiomyopathy. Anal Biochem. 2022;636:114388.

51. Parekh NK, Hynan LS, De LJ, et al. Elevated troponin I levels in acute liver failure: is myocardial injury an integral part of acute liver failure? Hepatology 2007; 45(6):1489–95.

52. Moller S, Bernardi M. Interactions of the heart and the liver. Eur Heart J 2013; 34(36):2804–11.

53. Weiss E, Paugam-Burtz C, Jaber S. Shock Etiologies and Fluid Management in Liver Failure. Semin Respir Crit Care Med 2018;39(5):538–45.

54. Wong F. Acute kidney injury in liver cirrhosis: new definition and application. Clin Mol Hepatol 2016;22(4):415–22.

55. Deep A, Stewart CE, Dhawan A, et al. Effect of continuous renal replacement therapy on outcome in pediatric acute liver failure. Crit Care Med 2016; 44(10):1910–9.

56. Deep A., Saxena R. and Jose B., Acute kidney injury in children with chronic liver disease. Pediatr Nephrol. 2019;34(1):45-59.

57. Simonetto DA, Gines P, Kamath PS. Hepatorenal syndrome: pathophysiology, diagnosis, and management. BMJ 2020;370:m2687.

58. Cardoso FS, Gottfried M, Tujios S, et al. Cardoso FS, Gottfried M, Tujios S, Olson JC, Karvellas CJ; US Acute Liver Failure Study Group. Continuous renal replacement therapy is associated with reduced serum ammonia levels and mortality in acute liver failure. Hepatology. 2018;67(2):711-720.

59. Kawada PS, Bruce A, Massicotte P, et al. Coagulopathy in children with liver disease. J Pediatr Gastroenterol Nutr 2017;65(6):603–7.

60. Bulut Y, Sapru A, Roach GD. Hemostatic balance in pediatric acute liver failure: epidemiology of bleeding and thrombosis, physiology, and current strategies. Front Pediatr 2020;8:618119.

61. Stravitz RT, Fontana RJ, Meinzer C, et al. Coagulopathy, bleeding events, and outcome according to rotational thromboelastometry in patients with acute liver injury/failure. Hepatology 2021;74(2):937–49.

62. Lisman T, Stravitz RT. Rebalanced Hemostasis in Patients with Acute Liver Failure. Semin Thromb Hemost 2015;41(5):468–73.

63. Stravitz RT, Lisman T, Luketic VA, et al. Minimal effects of acute liver injury/acute liver failure on hemostasis as assessed by thromboelastography. J Hepatol 2012;56(1):129–36.

64. Nanchal R, Subramanian R, Karvellas CJ, et al. Guidelines for the management of adult acute and acute-on-chronic liver failure in the ICU: cardiovascular, endocrine, hematologic, pulmonary and renal considerations: executive summary. Crit Care Med 2020;48(3):415–9.

65. Stravitz RT, Kramer AH, Davern T, et al. Intensive care of patients with acute liver failure: recommendations of the U.S. Acute Liver Failure Study Group. Crit Care Med 2007;35(11):2498–508.

66. Murphy N, Auzinger G, Bernel W, et al. The effect of hypertonic sodium chloride on intracranial pressure in patients with acute liver failure. Hepatology 2004;39(2):464–70.

67. Kamat P, Kunde S, Vos M, et al. Invasive intracranial pressure monitoring is a useful adjunct in the management of severe hepatic encephalopathy associated with pediatric acute liver failure. Pediatr Crit Care Med 2012;13(1):e33–8.

68. Akcan AA, Srivaths P, Himes RW, et al., Hybrid Extracorporeal Therapies as a Bridge to Pediatric Liver Transplantation. Pediatr Crit Care Med. 2018;19(7):e342-e349.

69. Zoica BS, Deep A. Extracorporeal renal and liver support in pediatric acute liver failure. Pediatr Nephrol 2021;36(5):1119–28.

70. Butterworth RF. Pathogenesis of hepatic encephalopathy and brain edema in acute liver failure. J Clin Exp Hepatol 2015;5(Suppl 1):S96–103.

71. Moller S, Bendtsen F. The pathophysiology of arterial vasodilatation and hyperdynamic circulation in cirrhosis. Liver Int 2018;38(4):570–80.

72. Anastasiadis SN, Giouleme OI, Germanidis GS, et al. Relative adrenal insufficiency in cirrhotic patients. Clin Med Insights Gastroenterol 2015;8:13–7.

73. Maheshwari A, Thuluvath PJ. Endocrine diseases and the liver. Clin Liver Dis 2011;15(1):55–67.

74. Davis AL, Carcillo JA, Aneja RK, et al. American college of critical care medicine clinical practice parameters for hemodynamic support of pediatric and neonatal septic shock. Crit Care Med 2017;45(6):1061–93.

75. Jean S, Chardot C, Oualha M, et al. Extracorporeal membrane oxygenation can save lives in children with heart or lung failure after liver transplantation. Artif Organs 2017;41(9):862–5.
76. Nandhabalan P, Loveridge R, Patel S, et al. Extracorporeal membrane oxygenation and pediatric liver transplantation, "a step too far?": Results of a single-center experience. Liver Transpl 2016;22(12):1727–33.
77. Scott JP, Hong JC, Thompson NE, et al. Central ECMO for circulatory failure following pediatric liver transplantation. Perfusion 2018;33(8):704–6.
78. Lion RP, Tufan PN, Srivaths P, et al. The safety and efficacy of regional citrate anticoagulation in albumin-assisted liver dialysis for extracorporeal liver support in pediatric patients. Blood Purif 2019;47(1–3):23–7.
79. Lion RP, Vega MR., Smith EO, et al, Lion RP, Vega MR, Smith EO, et al. The effect of continuous venovenous hemodiafiltration on amino acid delivery, clearance, and removal in children. Pediatr Nephrol. 2022;37(2):433-441.
80. Rodriguez K, Srivaths PR, Tal L, et al. Regional citrate anticoagulation for continuous renal replacement therapy in pediatric patients with liver failure. PLoS One 2017;12(8):e0182134.
81. Plauth M, Bernal W, Dasarathy S, et al. ESPEN guideline on clinical nutrition in liver disease. Clin Nutr 2019;38(2):485–521.
82. Katarey D, Jalan R. Update on extracorporeal liver support. Curr Opin Crit Care 2020;26(2):180–5.
83. Lee KC, Stadlbauer V, Jalan R. Extracorporeal liver support devices for listed patients. Liver Transpl 2016;22(6):839–48.
84. Squires JE, Rudnick DA, Hardison RM, et al. Liver transplant listing in pediatric acute liver failure: practices and participant characteristics. Hepatology 2018; 68(6):2338–47.
85. Squires RH, Ng V, Romero R, et al. Evaluation of the pediatric patient for liver transplantation: 2014 practice guideline by the American Association for the Study of Liver Diseases, American Society of Transplantation and the North American Society for Pediatric Gastroenterology, Hepatology and Nutrition. Hepatology 2014;60(1):362–98.
86. O'Grady JG, Alexander GJ, Hayllar KM, et al. Early indicators of prognosis in fulminant hepatic failure. Gastroenterology 1989;97(2):439–45.
87. Polson J, Lee WM. AASLD position paper: the management of acute liver failure. Hepatology 2005;41(5):1179–97.
88. Bernuau J, Goudeau A, Poynard T, et al. Multivariate analysis of prognostic factors in fulminant hepatitis B. Hepatology 1986;6(4):648–51.
89. Lu BR, Gralla J, Liu E, et al. Evaluation of a scoring system for assessing prognosis in pediatric acute liver failure. Clin Gastroenterol Hepatol 2008;6(10): 1140–5.
90. Lu BR, Zhang S, Narkewicz MR, et al. Evaluation of the liver injury unit scoring system to predict survival in a multinational study of pediatric acute liver failure. J Pediatr 2013;162(5):1010–6.
91. Nesher E, Island E, Tryphonopoulos P, et al. Split liver transplantation. Transplant Proc 2011;43(5):1736–41.
92. Earl TM, Chari RS. Which types of graft to use in patients with acute liver failure? (A) Auxiliary liver transplant (B) Living donor liver transplantation (C) The whole liver. (C) I take the whole liver only. J Hepatol 2007;46(4):578–82.
93. Firl DJ, Sasaki K, McVey J, et al. Improved survival following living donor liver transplantation for pediatric acute liver failure: analysis of 20 years of us national registry data. Liver Transpl 2019;25(8):1241–50.

94. Lee SG, Ahn CS, Kim KH. Which types of graft to use in patients with acute liver failure? (A) Auxiliary liver transplant (B) Living donor liver transplantation (C) The whole liver. (B) I prefer living donor liver transplantation. J Hepatol 2007;46(4): 574–8.
95. Szymczak M, Kalicinski P, Kowalewski G, et al. Acute liver failure in children-Is living donor liver transplantation justified? PLoS One 2018;13(2)::e0193327.
96. Mysore KR, Himes RW, Rana A, et al. ABO-incompatible deceased donor pediatric liver transplantation: Novel titer-based management protocol and outcomes. Pediatr Transplant. 2018;22(7):e13263.
97. Weiner J, Griesemer A, Island E, et al. Longterm outcomes of auxiliary partial orthotopic liver transplantation in preadolescent children with fulminant hepatic failure. Liver Transpl 2016;22(4):485–94.
98. Rela M, Muiesan P, Andreani P, et al. Auxiliary liver transplantation for metabolic diseases. Transplant Proc 1997;29(1–2):444–5.
99. Jaeck D, Pessaux P, Wolf P. Which types of graft to use in patients with acute liver failure? (A) Auxiliary liver transplant (B) Living donor liver transplantation (C) The whole liver. (A) I prefer auxiliary liver transplant. J Hepatol 2007;46(4): 570–3.
100. Soltys KA, Soto-Gutierrez A, Nagaya M, et al. Barriers to the successful treatment of liver disease by hepatocyte transplantation. J Hepatol 2010;53(4): 769–74.
101. Puppi J, Strom SC, Hughes RD, et al. Improving the techniques for human hepatocyte transplantation: report from a consensus meeting in London. Cell Transplant 2012;21(1):1–10.
102. Lee WS, McKiernan P, Kelly DA. Etiology, outcome and prognostic indicators of childhood fulminant hepatic failure in the United kingdom. J Pediatr Gastroenterol Nutr 2005;40(5):575–81.
103. Ng VL, Li R, Loomes KM, et al. Outcomes of Children With and Without Hepatic Encephalopathy From the Pediatric Acute Liver Failure Study Group. J Pediatr Gastroenterol Nutr 2016;63(3):357–64.

Setting up a Pediatric Intensive Care Unit in a Community/Rural Setting

Marvin B. Mata, MD, MSHS-HCQ, CPHQ, CPPS[a],*,
Alexander Santos, MD[b], Judith Ugale-Wilson, MD[c]

KEYWORDS

- Community PICU • PICU guidelines • ICU design • Staffing • Credentialing
- Care coordination • Telemedicine

KEY POINTS

- A community pediatric intensive care unit (PICU) is a specialized unit for children with life-threatening conditions.
- PICU beds comprise a small proportion of ICU beds in the United States but play a crucial role in bridging health inequities providing access to high-quality care in the rural setting.
- Setting up a PICU in a rural area requires multi-stakeholder collaboration to meet community needs and allocate resources to meet standards for care and expectations.
- The education and training of a dedicated and skilled multidisciplinary team is the most critical investment in delivering high-quality, patient-centered pediatric critical care.
- Creating sustainability involves organizing a high-performance network of pediatric health care systems essential to care coordination and transitions of care.

INTRODUCTION

Following the completion of fellowship, moving into a rural community to practice initially started for us as a requirement for a waiver visa. The opportunity to provide care for critically ill children in an area without a pediatric intensive care unit (PICU) was both interesting and intimidating. Coincidentally it was a welcome reprieve from the fast-paced, busy city lifestyle with the associated higher cost of living. The allure of a spacious home at lower cost is exchanged for fewer amenities. The lack of ethnic food, shopping, and entertainment options meant driving long

a Department of Pediatrics, PICU and Pediatric Hospital Medicine, Rapides Regional Medical Center, 211 4th Street, Alexandria, LA 71303, USA; b Pediatric Critical Care, Children's Healthcare of Atlanta – Scottish Rite, Neonatology Associates of Atlanta, 980 Johnson Ferry Road NE Suite 680, Atlanta, GA 30342, USA; c Department of Pediatrics, Pediatric Critical Care Medicine, East Carolina University Greenville, ECU Brody School of Medicine, 2100 Stantonsburg Road, Greenville, NC 27834, USA
* Corresponding author. Rapides Regional Medical Center, 211 4th St., Alexandria, LA 71301.
E-mail address: Marvin.Mata@hcahealthcare.com

Pediatr Clin N Am 69 (2022) 497–508
https://doi.org/10.1016/j.pcl.2022.01.010
0031-3955/22/© 2022 Elsevier Inc. All rights reserved.

distances for access. Internet access is not always reliable, and cellular service is spotty.

Similarly, setting up a PICU in a rural setting has its challenges. Having trained in a tertiary care hospital, whereby resources are plentiful and readily available, the lack of pediatric subspecialists in the community can be challenging. In addition, the lack of equipment, technology, and financial capacity to invest are limiting factors. However, the biggest challenge is the formation of a dedicated, skilled, and resilient team. It requires hiring and providing hours of staff training to gain proficiency in critical care. All of these challenges add to the prevailing perception of substandard care at rural hospitals. Partnering with families and the community and networking with tertiary organizations improve access and integrate services to keep patients when appropriate and transfer whereby necessary. The reward is overwhelming appreciation, gratitude, and a robust sense of community spirit.

The Value of Setting up a Pediatric Intensive Care Unit in a Community Setting

The most recent levels of PICU care are defined as follows, in ascending order:[1]

1. *Community-based PICUs*, previously categorized as level II, are mainly located in general hospitals and can be rural, suburban, or urban, and academic or nonacademic.
   - *Definitions:* Community hospitals are nonfederal, acute-care hospitals available to the general public. Rural hospitals are those not located within a metropolitan area (as designated by the US Office of Management and Budget and the Census Bureau). Fifty-nine percent of the decline in US community hospitals between 2015 and 2019 were those in rural settings.[2]
2. *Tertiary PICUs*, previously categorized as level I, are units capable of providing advanced care for a wide range of conditions.
3. *Quaternary PICUs* provide comprehensive care to all children with complex conditions, including specialized care, for example, for cardiovascular disease, transplantation, trauma, and cancer.
   - *Why: The need for a PICU in a resource-limited setting*

Between 2001 and 2016, the US pediatric population grew 1.9% to more than 73.6 million children. In 2010, PICU beds (1,917) comprised only 1.8% of all ICU beds (103,900) in the United States.[3] By the end of 2019, the number of PICU beds increased to 5115 or 4.7% of 107,276 ICU beds.[2] Although the PICU bed numbers increased, the number of hospitals with a PICU decreased such that a relatively small percentage (18%) accounted for approximately half of all PICU beds. Moreover, PICUs with 15 beds or more had significant bed growth by 2016, while minimal change was noted in PICUs with fewer than 15 beds.[4] The 2019 American Health Association's hospital statistics system data show that among 107,276 staffed ICU beds in community hospitals in the United States, PICUs still account for only 5115 (4.5%) of all ICU beds in community hospitals.[2]

The availability of community PICUs remains variable across the United States, particularly in rural areas, because resources are not regionalized. This further widens the gap in access to care and influences the community's capacity to handle emergencies such as surges from disasters, mass trauma, and pandemics. As pediatric critical care continues to evolve, the services of community PICUs continue to vary more widely as resources do not allow them to react swiftly. The struggle shrinks the referral base of PICUs as tertiary facilities with better technology attract more patients. Meeting patients' expectations with compassionate care that fits their needs and preferences and being transparent on unit capabilities are crucial to build comfort and trust that will keep patients within the system.

While regionalization will afford multispecialty care under one roof, most specialty centers are concentrated in urban areas. Community PICUs bridge this gap by bringing in high-quality pediatric critical care closer to home.

- *How: Establishing the mission and vision of the Community PICU*

While acutely ill children account for most PICU admissions, children with complex medical problems are also prone to recurrent ICU admissions. They rely on medical technology such as gastrostomy tubes and respiratory support to sustain life or improve function. For families with technology-dependent children, it is an additional burden to live hours away from specialty hospitals. There may be many instances whereby a medical crisis can be addressed in "closer to home" PICUs.

The mission of a community PICU is to help improve the children's health and quality of life by bridging the gaps of care in this setting. With organizational values of service, collaboration, respect, and compassion, the PICU can partner with the community to achieve its vision of delivering an integrated health delivery system and maintaining sustainability.

According to the Society of Critical Care Medicine (SCCM), the overall mortality rate for PICUs ranges from 2% to 6%. This is much lower than in adult ICUs at an average of 10% to 29%.[3] McCrory et al. reported a 2.31% PICU mortality rate in the United States,[5] a significant decrease from a range of 8% to 18% during the early years of pediatric critical care in the 1960s.

High-quality pediatric critical care need not be expensive. A national survey of PICU resources in the United States showed that the smallest units (1–6 beds) had the lowest availability of advanced therapeutic modalities but had higher ratios of nurses and physicians for each bed.[6] Where there is a lack of technology or specialty expertise, it is imperative to build relationships and well-established communication systems with hospitals that can provide higher levels of care for care. It is essential to know conditions that would be better served at a specialty children's hospital.

Minimum Guidelines for Level 1 and 2 Pediatric Intensive Care Units

As health care has increased in complexity, the demand for specialized care has grown exponentially, resulting in the rise of centers of excellence, whereby expertise and resources are centered on specific pediatric disciplines. Limited resources make it difficult for community PICUs to allocate and align available goods and services to meet the evolving expectations and minimum standards of care.

The American Academy of Pediatrics and the SCCM published an updated set of guidelines for appropriate resources and personnel that a community PICU should meet based on the level of care it provides.[7] See Appendices A and B.

Among these guidelines, recruitment and retention of providers to match the expected level of care are some of the most difficult to achieve, but are worth pursuing to minimize turnover, save money and improve the quality of care by delivering services consistently. Administrators need an understanding of the factors contributing to a good fit with the community and the organization to create long-term commitment. There is a misalignment in the weight of essential attributes on why providers choose the rural setting. Although compensation is a compelling incentive, rural physicians prefer the three Cs: connection, comfort, and confidence.[8] Attracting good candidates to the rural setting is challenging due to concerns over a demanding workload, isolation, less time off, lack of flexibility in work hours, and fewer job opportunities for spouses.

As designated Health Professional Shortage Area (HPSA) providers, our initial visits elicited a strong sense of belonging, which can increase comfort and confidence in the decision to stay. This is one of the same values we try to impart to students who express interest in the health care profession. We reach out and help local colleges and medical schools integrate with our system, support their needs, and provide crucial opportunities to deepen their connection to the place they call home.

Pediatric Intensive Care Unit Planning and Design Based on Community Needs and Resources

- Brainstorming - Preliminary planning, data collection, and analysis, budget planning, formulation of aims, and objectives

When setting up a PICU, awareness of community needs and the availability of resources are essential. It requires planning, allocation of resources, and, most importantly, investment in the education and training of health care providers. Collaboration with key stakeholders is essential to establish good communication, gather essential information, and promote engagement in the project.

A needs assessment will identify and analyze strengths, weaknesses, opportunities, availability of resources, and limiting factors. The hospital administration and board of directors are crucial for capital planning and budgeting. The design team (clinical, nonclinical members, and patients and their families) will help define the functionalities needed to create an efficient and safe work environment. The construction team (architect and engineers) oversees the technical aspects of the building process. This multi-stakeholder approach helps overcome multiple barriers and create sustainability.

The 6 domains set by the Institute of Medicine must be met: safe, effective, patient-centered, timely, efficient, and equitable.[9,10] Bridging the gap of inequity in access to high-quality care will help reduce the high burden of morbidity and mortality. The planning and formulation of the unit's goals and objectives are challenging yet crucial in developing an action plan for the organization. A SMART (Simple, Measurable, Achievable, Realistic, and Timely) aim will help define what, who, whereby, when, and why a PICU is vital in a resource-limited setting. The objectives can then be formulated to specify the steps needed to achieve the goals. Short and long-term goals need to be prioritized and matched by specific courses of action.

Slusher and colleagues [11] provided great insights into the fundamental building blocks in developing pediatric critical care services in a resource-limited setting. They adopted lessons from Dr Paul Farmer, who helped strengthen the health system in Liberia by improving training and capacity building during the 2014 Ebola epidemic. He addressed inefficiencies and inequalities through the Four S's:

a) Staff: Properly trained and compensated doctors, nurses, and community health workers
b) Stuff: Medical equipment
c) Space: A clean and sanitary environment to treat patients
d) Systems: Infrastructural and logistical organization

Most community PICUs in a resource-limited setting are in general medical and surgical hospitals. Geographic location generally impacts the four S's, influencing the type of population served, the prevalent diseases, availability of medical providers, capacity for infrastructure, and support services available. Keeping the unit operational entails careful control of fixed and variable costs. This makes acquisition and maintenance of PICU "staff and stuff" equally challenging and the cost per patient more expensive in a lower-volume facility. Networking with tertiary and quaternary facilities will address the gaps not locally available. The collaboration will facilitate care coordination, particularly during transitions of care. This synergistic partnership increases the comfort level of a provider and enables patients with complex, chronic medical conditions to stay locally to mitigate the risk of transfer, and avoid the financial burden of missed work and travel expenses for the family. Furthermore, this same network helps provide coverage for the PICU when necessary.

- Decision making
  - Structural measures

Thompson and colleagues described performance and prescriptive guidelines in determining the optimal requirement in designing an ICU. Performance guidelines refer to the functions that need to be accommodated, while prescriptive guidelines refer to the physical design of the space itself.[12] It must follow local and federal policies and regulatory standards. Optimizing both creates efficiency in the daily workflow processes, promotes safety by reducing medical errors and mitigating patient harm, and, most importantly, improves staff and patient satisfaction by providing a safe and healing environment.

The architecture, layout, size, and design of the PICU can vary widely but it should always be a separate and distinct unit within the hospital. It is a complex, stressful, and high-risk setting which should also promote physiologic, physical, and emotional healing. Understanding human-factors engineering will improve staff performance, enhance patient safety through error reduction, and improve patient comfort. The PICU should have a centralized monitor and workstation to observe the patient from multiple sightlines within the unit. Its layout should allow the staff to access needed equipment and medications and respond to patients with ease. Protection of patient privacy, including any information considered as part of the Health Insurance Portability and Accountability Act (HIPAA), must be prioritized. Optimizing human-system interactions will reduce inefficiencies and burnout and enhance patient-centered care with improved patient–family–provider communication and engagement.

Determining the optimal number of beds be allocated in hospitals is complex and challenging. Ravaghi and colleagues[13] looked into different models but found no specific norms. The models used multiple variables (demand, supply, and external factors) that are patient-related (patient demographics, disease patterns and prevalence, comorbidities) and hospital-related (admission and rate, bed occupancy rate, the average length of stay, patient transfers, technology advances, and funding). Nguyen and colleagues[14] proposed a model for estimating the number of ICU beds needed based on minimizing the mean and variance of three parameters: a. accessibility, the number of days per month with at least one empty bed; b. safety, the number of patient transfers per month due to a full unit; and c. efficiency, the number of days per month with bed underutilization.[14]

To promote cost-effectiveness and efficiency, the number of ICU beds in a hospital should be at least 5% of the total hospital beds. Depending on the hospital size, 6 to 8 beds may be considered for hospitals with fewer than 100 beds, and 8 to 12 beds for hospitals with 100 to 150 beds.[15] Single rooms are preferable to multi-bed rooms and should have optimal space of at least 250 square feet for each patient.[15,16] This accommodates the interdisciplinary team, necessary equipment, procedures, and infection prevention, and enhances privacy.

Most PICU equipment, medications, and other supplies are used to monitor, support respiratory and cardiovascular systems, stabilize, and manage a critically ill child. Medication errors and adverse drug events are serious concerns in the PICU due to their potential for harmful outcomes. Leveraging advances in technology using computerized order entry, clinical decision support tools, clinical pathways, barcoded medication administration, smart IV infusion pumps, electronic prescription, and automated drug-dispensing systems will help reduce errors and improve patient outcomes.

- *Human: organizational and administrative structure, Staffing model, ancillary/support service*
  - i. Organizational structure

    Organizational structure provides guidance and clarity among its individual parts. A clearly defined leadership chain of command and responsibilities for each member will help with communication, decision processes, and promote accountability. It will organize the interaction patterns, link people together, and facilitate critical functions. Promoting a just culture, whereby accountability is balanced at both individual and organizational levels, will empower the staff by creating a partnership for patient safety.

    The pediatric intensivist, who serves as the medical director and leader of the team, should have completed fellowship training and attained board certification. The role includes clinical and administrative duties such as developing and reviewing policies and their implementation, training and performance evaluation of the staff, planning, and budgeting, and oversight of the unit's quality and safety improvement programs.

    A dedicated and skilled multidisciplinary team is the most crucial component to delivering patient-centered care. Members of the PICU team should possess the necessary knowledge, training, and clinical skills to take care of a critically ill child. Defining the duties and responsibilities of each member will determine its success by promoting teamwork, efficiency, and accountability. Working toward a clearly defined goal and standards by which care is delivered will help improve outcomes. Qualified medical providers must always be available to respond to all emergencies within 5 minutes. If they are not physically in the hospital, physicians who provide night coverage should always be available by telephone and be able to respond to emergency issues onsite within 30 minutes.

  - ii. Staffing model

    The PICU care delivery model has continued to evolve from the traditional physician staffing to those supplemented by advanced practice providers (APPs). The evolution of innovative staffing models has played a crucial role in alleviating the stresses of provider shortage in areas of limited resources. Gigli and colleagues[16] did not find increased odds of mortality in PICUs with APP-inclusive staffing.[17] Their integration into the ICU requires adequate planning and thoughtful consideration of multiple factors such as institutional and community expectations and acceptance, organizational governance, financial impact, and recruitment availability. This helps create more consistent coverage, particularly at night when families expect coverage like a larger center. However, the lower patient volumes in this setting with much less third-party insurer reimbursement make consistent coverage more difficult.

    The nursing staff-to-patient ratio should be assessed and adjusted regularly to provide high-quality, efficient, and safe care. Staffing should be evaluated based on acuity and other environmental factors. A 1:1 ratio is needed for critically ill patients requiring frequent interventions such as those with hemodynamic instability, respiratory compromise requiring invasive ventilation, instability following surgery, severe neurologic impairment, and any child with acute decompensation.

Otherwise, a 1 nurse to 2 patient ratio may be sufficient. Some of the environmental factors that may affect staffing ratio include the type of patient-care equipment, immediate availability of support staff, nurse competency, established management protocols, and the layout of the unit. Support services include respiratory therapists, pharmacists, registered dietitians, social workers, case managers, speech-language pathologists, physical and occupational therapists, child life specialists, and patient advocates.

iii. Transport team

The transport team is another essential component of the PICU, allowing the transfer of critically ill children whose needs are not sufficiently met at the local setting. The team comprises the physician, nurse, respiratory therapist, and paramedics equipped with transport skills and annual flight training. The number of members dispatched depends on the patient's needs and the size and configuration of the vehicle. Depending on the location and severity of the medical condition, a patient may be transported via land (ambulance) or air (helicopter or fixed-wing).

The goal is safe patient transport. Initial stabilization is crucial to prevent clinical deterioration because constraints limit the team's ability to assess and perform procedures while enroute.

Expense is a crucial factor that can limit an organization's ability to provide a designated transport team for the community. The budget includes vehicle maintenance and repair, the equipment needed (monitors, defibrillators, portable ventilators, air–oxygen blender, infusion pumps, medications, and so forth), maintenance of a transfer center, personnel benefits, and the education and training of the team. An organization can tap the local emergency services system for help with transports. Communication is key to success as team members from both facilities need to work efficiently to solve issues. Written clinical and operational guidelines are essential for optimal function.

iv. Continuing education and training

Continuing education and training of the staff provide updates on new information and solidify existing knowledge and skills. Simulation courses, online modules, seminars, and competency-based training are some tools that can provide effective programs tailored to meet the unit's specific needs. Employee and patient feedback, performance reviews, and direct observation will help evaluate the program by meeting expected outcome measures. Just-in-time training is another valuable tool to enhance the knowledge and skills of the staff on high-risk but low-volume therapies such as high-frequency oscillatory ventilation, renal replacement therapy, and difficult airway management. When built into the workflow, it can be effectively implemented in the early recognition and immediate management of a clinically deteriorating patient.[18]

- Process measures - Credentialing, privileges, unit policies, clinical pathways, and decision tools

Credentialing, which can take 60 to 90 days, is a crucial process that involves obtaining and verifying the qualifications of health care providers to ensure that they have adequate training and proficiency on specific performance tasks. Organizations can either verify the provider's education and training from the primary source or rely on a credentials-verification organization to obtain accurate information. Diplomas, training certificates, and licenses are the most common sources used to authenticate that an individual meets the minimum competency requirements. This process must be expedited as a provider without credentials cannot perform patient-related care activities and will not be reimbursed by the health plans for such activities.

The Council for Affordable Quality Health Care (CAQH), a not-for-profit organization formed by several of the nation's largest health insurance companies, helps streamline business processes in health care. The CAQH ProView, launched in 2002 and formerly known as the Universal Provider Datasource, expedites the secure collection of a common set of information from health care providers through the CAQH standard database.[19] This eliminates redundancy and errors and reduces credentialing time and resources and consequently administrative cost. With the CAQH standard database, re-attestation can be completed in minutes and is immediately available to any organization authorized by the provider. Organizations can also query the National Practitioner Data Bank, a confidential repository with information regarding medical malpractice and adverse actions related to health care providers.

Privileging is the scope of services an organization grants to individuals based on their credentials and performance evaluation. It ensures that the medical provider has experience and competency in patient management. The Centers for Medicaid and Medicare Services (CMS) requirements for medical staff privileging require that Conditions of Participation (CoPs) be met to ensure the quality of care rendered and protect the health and safety of its beneficiaries. Code of Federal Regulations 482.22 provides specific details regarding standards related to (a) the composition of the medical staff, (b) the medical staff organization and accountability, and (c) the medical staff bylaws. Organizations should review staff privileges every 2 years.[20]

Most general hospitals have emergency-trained medical providers for adult patients. However, care provided for the critically ill child is different from that for the adult. These differences need to be considered when developing admission, consultation, discharge, and transfer of patients. If the resources are not available, the patient will need stabilization and transfer to tertiary care facility.[21,22] This process must adhere to the Emergency Medical Treatment and Labor Act provisions as enforced by the Office of the Inspector General and CMS.

Clinical decision support systems and clinical pathways are interventions that will enhance medical provider decisions and improve patient safety by incorporating validated evidence-based guidelines.

Creating Sustainability through Care Coordination and Networking

Care coordination is defined as a function that helps ensure that patients' needs and preferences for health services and information are met. It involves organizing patient-care activities (**Fig. 1**) and sharing information among all participants concerned with a patient's care to achieve safer and more effective care.[23] While in the PICU, patient needs and preferences are assessed, and care plans are communicated to the health care team to assist during transitions of care. This helps the patients successfully meet their management goals by having a carefully outlined care plan aligned with the available resources in the community. It also establishes better accountability when shared decision-making is involved.

Patient satisfaction in this setting poses a challenge related to meeting subjective expectations. Fewer resources may not adequately meet growing expectations as

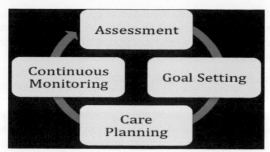

Fig. 1. Delivery of family-centered care coordination services includes[23].

experienced in another health care setting. Clear communication and setting realistic expectations will help improve satisfaction and growth of market share.

An integrated care coordination infrastructure is essential to create and sustain this system. The 4 defining characteristics of care coordination include[24]:

1. Patient and family-centered
2. Proactive, planned, and comprehensive
3. Promotes self-care skills and independence
4. Emphasizes cross-organizational relationships

Bodenheimer identified several barriers to successfully running a care coordination team. These include an overstressed primary-care system, a low number of computerized records, dysfunctional payment systems, and a lack of integrated systems of care. Unfortunately, most of these barriers are present in the rural setting.

The shortage of primary-care physicians and subspecialists and lack of skilled personnel make it challenging to establish care within the community. Care coordinators must be skilled, experienced, and knowledgeable about community agencies, organizations, schools, and early intervention programs. More importantly, care coordinators that can build team relationships with the family, other clinicians, community partners, and other professionals are vital to the functioning of a successful care coordination system.

Electronic health-record systems may not be available or otherwise not interoperable, thus hindering the transfer of information from providers. The great digital divide hinders communication and access to information due to the lack of infrastructure. This is a crucial issue that must be addressed because health-information technology is vital to an efficient care-coordination system. It links systems across care settings.

Tapping community programs is also crucial to help families alleviate some of the stresses related to social determinants of health, impacting their overall well-being and quality of life. This may include assistance with transportation, home health visits, community-based health literacy programs, supplemental nutrition assistance programs, and telemedicine.

- *Transition of care for technology-dependent children*

Building an intermediate care unit/service within a hospital system facilitates the transition of complex technology-dependent children from the PICU to the transitional care service to their home environment by providing a structured education program given to 2 caregivers over a predetermined time frame. This concludes with families staying in the hospital for 24 hours to room-in and assuming the patient's care with nursing supervision. This allows them to simulate the home environment but still have the ability to ask questions and receive additional teaching from staff. The inpatient medical team and the outpatient center provide the resources and a support system that decreases the fragmentation of care. A study by Parker and colleagues showed that a care-coordination program that spans inpatient and outpatient care had been associated with 59% fewer hospitalizations.[25]

- *Role of telemedicine in creating sustainability*

The availability of remote follow-up via telemedicine is critical in rural areas whereby families experience significant transportation barriers to in-person clinic visits.[26] Telemedicine or telehealth allows real-time, audio–video communication between clinicians and members of the care-coordination team and the patient. It also allows remote follow-up and patient monitoring.[27] Pediatric critical care telemedicine consultation increases the accuracy of the provider's assessment, avoids admissions that may be taken care of in a lower level of care setting, and increases the provider comfort level in transporting patients.[27,28]

Organizational and patient-related factors play a role in successfully leveraging technology to provide convenient and easy pediatric critical care access. Some concerns include security and privacy, federal and state policies and regulations, patient and provider attitude and adaptability, the complexity of use, bandwidth or Internet availability, and cost. The American Medical Association provides a detailed guide for telemedicine implementation from getting started to vendor evaluation, selection and contracting, and telehealth workflow.[29]

SUMMARY

Setting up a PICU in the rural setting improves access to high-quality care closer to home. Collaboration between the family, the multidisciplinary PICU team, and the community forms the foundation for better patient care experience and improved outcomes, reducing overall care cost. It requires strategic planning and allocation of available resources to provide safe and effective care in a healing environment. Human-factors engineering will help improve staff performance and patient comfort. Leveraging technology will help create sustainability by facilitating care coordination throughout the continuum of care.

CLINICS CARE POINTS

- Community PICU provides access to care and improves outcomes of children in the rural setting
- Investment in the education and training of the staff is crucial to delivering high-quality pediatric critical care
- The lack of providers and community resources makes care coordination challenging
- Leveraging technology will facilitate networking and help create sustainability

DISCLOSURE

The authors have nothing to disclose.

SUPPLEMENTARY DATA

Supplementary data related to this article can be found online at https://doi.org/10.1016/j.pcl.2022.01.010.

REFERENCES

1. Frankel LR, Hsu BS, Yeh TS, et al. Criteria for Critical Care Infants and Children: PICU Admission, Discharge, and Triage Practice Statement and Levels of Care Guidance. Pediatr Crit Care Med 2019;20(9):847–87. https://doi.org/10.1097/PCC.0000000000001963.
2. Fast Facts on U.S. Hospitals, 2021. American Hospital Association. Available at. https://www.aha.org/statistics/fast-facts-us-hospitals. Accessed September 15, 2021.
3. Critical Care Statistics. Society of Critical Care Medicine. Available at. https://www.sccm.org/Communications/Critical-Care-Statistics. Accessed September 15, 2021.
4. Horak RV, Griffin JF, Brown A-M, et al. Growth and Changing Characteristics of Pediatric Intensive Care 2001–2016. Crit Care Med 2019;47(8):1135–42. https://doi.org/10.1097/CCM.0000000000003863.
5. McCrory MC, Spaeder MC, Gower EW, et al. Time of Admission to the PICU and Mortality. Pediatr Crit Care Med 2017;18(10):915–23. https://doi.org/10.1097/PCC.0000000000001268.
6. Odetola FO, Clark SJ, Freed GL, et al. A National Survey of Pediatric Critical Care Resources in the United States. Pediatrics (Evanston) 2005;115(4):e382–6. https://doi.org/10.1542/peds.2004-1920.
7. Rosenberg D, Moss M. Guidelines and levels of care for pediatric intensive care units. Pediatrics 2004;13. No. 4.
8. Stajduhar T. Rural Physician Recruitment: Results from our rural physician and administrations survey. Jackson Physician Research. 2020. Available at. https://www.jacksonphysiciansearch.com/white-paper-rural-recruitment/. Accessed on October 30, 2021.
9. Relman AS. The Institute of Medicine Report on the Quality of Health Care–Crossing the Quality Chasm: A New Health System for the 21st Century. N Engl J Med 2001;345(9):702.
10. Slonim AD, Pollack MM. Integrating the Institute of Medicine's six quality aims into pediatric critical care: relevance and applications. Pediatr Crit Care Med 2005;6(3):264–9.
11. Slusher TM, Kiragu AW, Day LT, et al. Pediatric Critical Care in Resource-Limited Settings— Overview and Lessons Learned. Front Pediatr 2018;6:49. https://doi.org/10.3389/fped.2018.00049.
12. Thompson DR, Kirk H, Cadenhead C, et al. Guidelines for intensive care unit design. Crit Care Med 2012;40(5):1586–600. https://doi.org/10.1097/CCM.0b013e3182413bb2.
13. Ravaghi H, Alidoost S, Mannion R, et al. Models and methods for determining the optimal number of beds in hospitals and regions: a systematic scoping review. BMC Health Serv Res 2020;20(186). https://doi.org/10.1186/s12913-020-5023-z.
14. Nguyen JM, Six P, Parisot R, et al. A universal method for determining intensive care unit bed requirements. Intensive Care Med 2003;29(5):849–52. https://doi.org/10.1007/s00134-003-1725-z.
15. Rao B, Mittal K, Chaudry D, et al. Indian Society of Critical Care Medicine Experts Committee Consensus Statement on ICU Planning and Designing, 2020. Indian J Crit Care Med 2020;24(Suppl 1):S43–60. https://doi.org/10.5005/jp-journals-10071-G23185.
16. Rosenberg DI, Michele Moss M. Section on Critical Care and Committee on Hospital Care. Pediatrics 2004;114(4):1114–25.

17. Gigli Kristin H, Davis Billie S, Martsolf Grant R, et al. Advanced Practice Provider-inclusive Staffing Models and Patient Outcomes in Pediatric Critical Care. Med Care 2021;59 –(7):597–603. https://doi.org/10.1097/MLR.0000000000001531.

18. Peebles RC, Nicholson IK, Schlieff J, et al. Nurses' just-in-time training for clinical deterioration: Development, implementation and evaluation. Nurse Educ Today 2020;84:104265. https://doi.org/10.1016/j.nedt.2019.104265.

19. Council for Affordable Quality Healthcare (CAQH). Caqh.org. CAQH Proview for Providers and Practice Managers. Available at. https://www.caqh.org/solutions/caqh-proview-providers-and-practice-managers. Accessed July 20, 2021.

20. CMS.gov. State Operations Manual. Appendix A – Survey Protocol, Regulations and Interpretative guidelines for Hospitals. Updated February, 21, 2020. Available at. https://www.cms.gov/Regulations-and-Guidance/Guidance/Manuals/downloads/som107ap_a_hospitals.pdf. Accessed July 15, 2021.

21. Ernst KD. Resources Recommended for the Care of Pediatric Patients in Hospitals. Pediatrics (Evanston) 2020;145(4):e20200204. https://doi.org/10.1542/peds.2020-0204.

22. Bartley J, Streifel AJ. Design of the environment of care for safety of patients and personnel: Does form follow function or vice versa in the intensive care unit? Crit Care Med 2010;38(Suppl). https://doi.org/10.1097/CCM.0b013e3181e6d0c1. Infection Control in the Intensive Care Unit (8 Suppl):S388-S398.

23. Agency for Health Care Research and Quality. Care Coordination and Care Plans for Transitions Across Care Settings. Available at. https://www.ahrq.gov/ncepcr/care/coordination.html. Accessed August 2021.

24. Antonelli R, McAllister J, Popp J. Making Care Coordination A Critical Component of the Pediatric Health System: A Multidisciplinary Framework. 2009. Available at. www.commonwealthfund.org. Accessed August 25, 2021.

25. Parker C, Wall B, Tumin D, et al. Care Coordination Program for Children with Complex Chronic Conditions Discharged from a Rural Tertiary-Care Academic Medical Center. Hosp Pediatr 2020;10(8):1–7.

26. Brown A, Quaile M, Morris H, et al. Outpatient Follow-up Care After Hospital Discharge of Children with Complex Chronic Conditions at a Rural Tertiary Care Hospital. Clin Pediatr 2021;1–8.

27. Kuo D, McAllister J, Rossignol L, et al. Care Coordination for Children with Medical Complexity: Whose Care Is it, Anyway? Pediatrics 2018;141:s224–31, number s3.

28. Harvey JB, Yeager BE, Cramer C, et al. The Impact of Telemedicine on Pediatric Critical Care Triage. Pediatr Crit Care Med 2017;18(11):e555–60. https://doi.org/10.1097/PCC.0000000000001330.

29. AMA Telehealth quick guide. Overview. Practice Implementation. Policy, Coding and Payment. American Medical Association. Available at. https://www.ama-assn.org/practice-management/digital/ama-telehealth-quick-guide.   Accessed August 10, 2021.

PICU Pharmacology

Kevin Valentine, MD[a],*, Janelle Kummick, PharmD, BCPPS[b]

KEYWORDS

- Pharmacology • Critical care pediatrics • Inotropy • Diuretics • Antibiotics
- Extracorporeal membranous oxygenation • Continuous renal replacement therapy

KEY POINTS

- Critically ill children have age-related differences in pharmacokinetics and pharmacodynamics that must be considered when selecting and administering medications.
- Inotropic agents should be selected based on anatomic and physiologic considerations.
- Proper identification of the source and location of respiratory failure dictates therapeutic interventions; lower airway obstructive lesions require different management strategies than the extrathoracic airway obstruction.
- Preservation of renal function is paramount when administering nephrotoxic medications, especially in the presence of acute kidney injury.
- Extracorporeal circuits alter the pharmacokinetics and pharmacodynamics of medications.

PHARMACOLOGY IN PEDIATRIC CRITICAL ILLNESS

Pediatrics does not deal with miniature men and women, with reduced doses and the same class of disease in smaller bodies, but… has its own independent range and horizon...

-Abraham Jacobi, on Pediatrics

Pharmacokinetics and pharmacodynamics are parts of pharmacology related to how drugs move through the body and the response resulting from the drug at the site of action. Critical illness and child development add an additional layer of complexity by altering kinetics and pathophysiology. Pharmacokinetics includes absorption, distribution, metabolism, and excretion/elimination of drugs. In each of these pharmacokinetic phases, there are age-related factors that may change how a drug is affected.[1] Critical illness plays a role and affects each phase differently, resulting in the need to adjust medication dosing, frequency, route of administration, or in the

---

[a] Indiana University School of Medicine, Riley Hospital for Children, 705 Riley Hospital Drive, Suite 4900, Indianapolis, IN 46202, USA; [b] Butler University College of Pharmacy and Health Sciences, Riley Hospital for Children, 705 Riley Hospital Drive, Room W6111, Indianapolis, IN 46202, USA
* Corresponding author.
E-mail address: kmvalent@iu.edu

Pediatr Clin N Am 69 (2022) 509–529
https://doi.org/10.1016/j.pcl.2022.01.011
0031-3955/22/© 2022 Elsevier Inc. All rights reserved.

selection of alternative agents. It is important to understand pediatric pharmacologic principles to increase drug efficacy while limiting adverse and toxic effects.

Absorption

Absorption is the phase that includes the rate and extent to which the drugs move from the administration site into circulation. There are age-related changes in enteral absorption throughout development that should first be considered. The absence of hydrochloric acid in gastric secretions in neonates leads to an increase in the absorption of basic drugs such as penicillin G and a decrease in the absorption of acidic drugs such as phenobarbital. Neonates also have a decreased absorption of lipophilic drugs due to low intraduodenal levels of bile salts. Gastric emptying is decreased during the first 6 months of life and does not reach adult values until approximately 6 to 8 months of life.[2,3] Overall, the rate of absorption is slower in neonates and the effect on age and enteral absorption is not uniform and unpredictable.

The rate and extent to which a drug is absorbed when administered enterally is dependent on drug-specific properties such as particle size, solubility, lipophilicity, ionization, and dissociation rate constant. In addition, patient-specific factors will also influence absorption, and include gastric pH, regional blood flow, surface area, motility, and nutritional intake status. Enteral absorption can be reduced significantly in critical illness. For example, children in a state of shock, or who are on vasopressor therapy may have decreased gastrointestinal perfusion.[3,4] Disease states including trauma, sepsis, and surgery can result in reduced motility and gastric emptying time. Children with heart failure may have impaired drug absorption due to edema and higher drug plasma concentrations due to hepatic dysfunction resulting from congestion.[5] To provide adequate absorption, alternate routes of administration may have to be considered during critical illness.[6] Intravenous drug delivery can provide complete absorption or 100% bioavailability.[7]

Distribution

The distribution phase follows absorption. There are age-dependent changes in body composition throughout development. Infants have greater extracellular and total body water compared with children and adults. In addition, neonates have a higher level of fetal albumin, and both neonates and infants have reduced levels of total plasma proteins.[2,8]

The physiologic factors that affect drug distribution include cardiac output, regional blood flow, capillary permeability, and tissue volume. Drug factors such as protein binding, lipid solubility, changes in acid–base balance, and permeability of cell membranes also affect the extent of drug distribution. The volume of distribution (Vd) is the apparent volume into which the drug is distributed to provide the same concentration as it is in the blood plasma. Disease states that increase Vd includes sepsis, capillary leak, prolonged cardiac bypass time, renal failure, mechanical ventilation, ECMO, and burns.[2,9] Hydrophilic drugs have a small Vd and may therefore require a loading dose for efficacy, compared with lipophilic drugs, which have a large Vd. Drugs with higher protein binding have reduced Vd compared with drugs that are tissue bound.

Metabolism

Metabolism is the phase that results in drug elimination and terminates the pharmacologic activity. The liver is the main organ responsible for drug metabolism. Lipophilic drugs undergo extensive metabolism via phase I to phase III reactions. Phase I reactions are primarily catalyzed by enzymes of the cytochrome P450 system, predominantly CYP3A4.[10] Drugs commonly metabolized by this enzyme include midazolam and methadone. Enzyme activity is substantially reduced in neonates and many of the CYP450 enzymes do not reach adult values until 1 year of life. Disease states that can alter enzyme activity include burns and hypothermia. In addition, alterations in protein binding can result in a larger amount of free drugs available for metabolism.

Elimination

Elimination is the final pharmacokinetic phase resulting in drug removal from the body. The liver and the kidney are the main organs responsible for drug elimination. Glomerular filtration rate has age-related differences in development.[1,11] While the glomerular filtration rate rapidly increases in the first 2 weeks of life, it is lower in a premature neonate compared with a term neonate. Elimination via the hepatic system can be through 2 pathways, active secretion from bile into enterocytes or reabsorption via enterohepatic recycling. In the first few weeks of life, the transport proteins responsible for biliary excretion are decreased.

Drug elimination can be altered in critical illness in a variety of mechanisms. Hepatic and renal dysfunction can slow clearance and drug elimination and increase half-life while renal replacement modalities such as CRRT and ECMO can increase drug clearance.

Antimicrobials

Antimicrobials are one of the most prescribed medication classes in the PICU. Safe administration of antibiotics to critically ill children can be challenging in the presence of changing pharmacokinetic properties resulting from critical illness. Furthermore, inappropriate antibiotic selection and use may occur in the treatment of critically ill children. Decision algorithms can aid in optimizing antibiotic choice, timing as well as de-escalation for critically ill children whereby a diagnosis other than an infection is likely.[12,13]

Characteristics of critically ill children can lead to the increase of the Vd of hydrophilic agents and decrease the concentration of hydrophilic antibiotics. Antimicrobials such as tobramycin are concentration-dependent, and a higher dose may be needed to sustain appropriate concentrations and efficacy. Conversely, acute kidney injury (AKI) decreases the clearance of hydrophilic agents, increases the concentration of hydrophilic antimicrobials, and may require a longer dosing interval. Hepatic injury affects lipophilic agents by decreasing the clearance that leads to increased concentrations of lipophilic antimicrobials. Extracorporeal modalities alter Vd and clearance of antibiotics often leading to subtherapeutic concentrations.[14] **Table 1** shows ECMO and CRRT associated variables to consider when prescribing common PICU antimicrobials.[15,16] When possible, serum levels should be obtained to guide dosing and therapy, and adjustments made with the alteration of extracorporeal parameters.

Cardiovascular

Acute cardiovascular dysfunction is common in critically ill children. Drugs can be used to improve the basic components of cardiac output that include preload, afterload, and contractility. The underlying diagnoses and physical examination findings must be taken into consideration. For example, therapy for dehydration is completely different from that of heart failure although both may present with similar symptoms that include malaise, tachypnea/hyperpnea, hypotension, and tachycardia.

Preload

Augmenting preload with crystalloids such as 0.9% saline or Lactated Ringer's solution is a relatively common intervention for hypovolemia. Colloids, such as 5% albumin

Table 1	
Extracorporeal effects on antimicrobial pharmacokinetics[14–16]	
Drug	**CRRT Effects**
Vancomycin	Clearance t ½ drops after the initiation of CRRT but accumulation can occur. Follow serum levels
Meropenem	Increased clearance yielding need for increased doses/frequency
Cefepime	Increased clearance yielding need for increased doses/frequency
Ambisome	No dose adjustment needed
Micafungin	No dose adjustment needed
Drug	**ECMO Effects**
Acyclovir	No dose adjustment needed
Aminoglycoside	Increased Vd and decreased clearance. Monitor serum levels
Ambisome	No dose adjustment needed
Azithromycin	No dose adjustment needed
Cefepime	Increased Vd, possibly decreased clearance in infants
Fluconazole	Loading dose required and higher doses needed for efficacy
Meropenem	Sequestered with increased clearance. Consider loading dose and continuous infusion
Micafungin	Increased dosing for neonates
Piperacillin/Tazobactam	Decreased AUC in adults
Vancomycin	Increased Vd and decreased clearance. Monitor serum levels

may also be used. Volume administration of 10 to 20 mL/kg should be used and repeated as necessary for intravascular expansion. Other agents as starches and dextrans have been used (more commonly in adults). The benefits of crystalloids versus colloids have not been established.[17]

In conditions of hypervolemia or excess preload such as renal failure or congestive heart failure, diuretic therapy may be appropriate. Loop diuretics and thiazides are commonly used. Furosemide, bumetanide, and torsemide inhibit the Na/K/Cl cotransporter in the loop of Henle. Furosemide at 0.5 to 1 mg/kg every 6 to 8 hours is the diuretic most used in children with hypervolemia. For critically ill children with cardiovascular dysfunction, a continuous infusion of furosemide (0.05–0.2 mg/kg/h) prevents peaks and valleys of drug levels with less hemodynamic instability as compared with intermittent bolus dosing.[18] Of note, appropriate administration of intravenous furosemide (maximum rate of 0.5 mg/kg/min) can reduce/eliminate the risk of hearing loss.[19] Bumetanide (0.015–0.05 mg/kg PO or IV every 12–24 hours) is up to 40 times more potent than furosemide. Torsemide is a loop diuretic with the benefit of higher enteral absorption and is more commonly used in children with heart failure.

Thiazide diuretics inhibit sodium transport in the distal tubule and can be used to provide a synergistic effect with a loop diuretic to augment the distal delivery of sodium and water, resulting in improved diuresis. Chlorothiazide (10–20 mg/kg PO every 12 hours or 2–5 mg/kg IV every 12 hours) and hydrochlorothiazide (0.5–1 mg/kg PO every 12–24 hours) are commonly used in critically ill children. Metolazone is a thiazide-like diuretic that inhibits sodium reabsorption.

Mineralocorticoid receptor antagonists, such as spironolactone (1–3 mg/kg/d PO) have minimal diuretic effects but can be combined with loop or thiazide diuretics for its potassium-sparing effect. The use of diuretics should include the monitoring of serum electrolytes, especially when combination loop-thiazide therapy is used.

Afterload

Vasoactive agents include vasoconstricting and vasodilating agents. Several medications have dose-dependent properties that result in both vasoconstriction and vasodilation. Drugs that induce vasoconstriction of the vessels (vasopressors) increase afterload. Medications with primary vasoconstrictor function should be used with caution in patients with poor myocardial function. Examples of these vasopressors include norepinephrine (NE), vasopressin, and phenylephrine. Medications that induce peripheral vascular vasodilation decrease resistance or afterload to the systemic ventricle. Examples include sodium nitroprusside, calcium channel blockers (CCBs) (such as nicardipine), and ACE inhibitors.

Vasopressors

Norepinephrine (NE) acts primarily on the α-adrenergic receptors and is a potent vasoconstrictor. It is useful in vasodilatory shock states such as septic shock.[20,21] NE also stimulates the beta-adrenergic receptor resulting in inotropic and chronotropic effects and augments blood pressure and coronary blood flow. It is mainly used as a vasopressor in children.

Vasopressin acts on the V1 receptors in the vascular smooth muscles mediating vasoconstriction and has predominant systemic vasoconstrictor effects at the V1 receptor with pulmonary, cerebral, and coronary vasodilation.[22] Vasopressin is used to treat diabetes insipidus and at a lower dose (1–5 milliunits/kg/h) engages V2 receptors in the collecting duct resulting in the insertion of aquaporin channels with the reabsorption of free water and a decrease in urine volume. When administered at a higher dose for shock states (0.5–3 milliunits/kg/min), vasopressin results in an overall increase in cardiac output and increased renal blood flow resulting in a "paradoxic" increase in urine output.[23]

Phenylephrine acts at the alpha-adrenergic receptor as a pure vasoconstrictor. It can be used intravenously at 10 mCg/kg intermittently, or as an infusion of 0.5 to 5 mCg/kg/min in conditions when an immediate increase in systemic blood pressure is needed. Phenylephrine can be used for the management of hypercyanotic spells associated with Tetralogy of Fallot and as secondary pharmacologic support for other clinical states.[24]

Vasodilators

Vasodilators are used in children when a reduction in afterload is required to augment cardiac output by relieving the pressure against which the systemic ventricle must work. Common indications include myocardial dysfunction due to myocarditis or cardiomyopathy, after heart surgery, or in dilated cardiomyopathy and systemic hypertension.

Nitroglycerin and nitroprusside act as venodilators and arterial vasodilators, and increase venous capacitance and decrease vascular afterload. To avoid hypotension, nitroglycerin and nitroprusside dosing should be approached cautiously by starting with the lowest effective dose, and increasing the dose slowly as needed. Nitroprusside causes greater reduction in systemic pressure than nitroglycerin. It has a rapid onset of action and can be used for the treatment of hypertensive emergencies. It is used as a continuous intravenous infusion titrated to effect at 0.5 to 10 mCg/kg/min. Sodium thiosulfate is often reconstituted with nitroprusside during the preparation of the infusion to minimize the potential for cyanide toxicity resulting from nitroprusside metabolism.

CCBs inhibit calcium entry into cells with resultant decreased vascular or myocardial contractility. Nicardipine is used as an infusion (0.5–5 mCg/kg/min) to treat hypertensive emergencies and is useful after cardiac surgery as the dihydropyridine CCBs act mainly on peripheral vasculature.[25–27]

Angiotensin is a potent vasoconstrictor. ACE inhibitors inhibit the conversion to functional angiotensin 2. Captopril is given orally 0.3 to 1.5 mg/kg per day, divided into every 8 hours dosing; enalapril is given orally 0.1 to 0.5 mg/kg per day, as a single dose or divided into 2 doses daily. ACE inhibitors should be started at lower doses to prevent hypotension, hyperkalemia, and renal failure. Special care should be taken when administering ACE inhibitors to neonates who are at an increased risk for nephrotoxicity and AKI.[28,29]

Contractility

Epinephrine has dose-dependent effects at the receptor level. In lower doses of 0.02 to 0.03 mCg/kg/min, epinephrine acts predominantly on beta-adrenergic receptors, increasing contractility and therefore increases oxygen consumption. Epinephrine concomitantly enhances coronary blood flow by improving cardiac output. At lower doses, epinephrine results in vasodilation, but at higher doses (0.05 mCg/kg/min and greater), epinephrine stimulates the alpha-adrenergic receptors resulting in vasoconstriction.

Dopamine has a similar effect profile and dose-dependent receptor engagement as epinephrine. At lower doses (2–5 mCg/kg/min) dopamine affects the β-adrenergic receptors, resulting in an increase in myocardial contractility and chronotropy. At higher doses (5–10 mCg/kg/min), dopamine engages the alpha-adrenergic receptors resulting in peripheral vasoconstriction.

Dobutamine is a synthetic catecholamine delivered by infusion at rates of 2 to 10 mCg/kg/min and is predominantly an inotrope and vasodilator stimulating the beta-receptors, increasing myocardial contractility and afterload reduction.

Epinephrine, dobutamine, and dopamine have relatively short half-lives and duration of action and can therefore be titrated to effect quickly. Neonates have a relatively underdeveloped sympathetic nervous system and higher infusion rates (10–20 mCg/kg/min) of dopamine and dobutamine may be necessary in this population.

Milrinone is a phosphodiesterase 3 (PDE-III) inhibitor that prevents the metabolism of cAMP to AMP. The accumulation of intracellular cAMP leads to improved calcium cycling in the myocardium resulting in increased myocardial contractility and improved myocardial relaxation. In the peripheral vasculature, the increase in intracellular cAMP leads to cellular relaxation and vasodilation.[30] Milrinone administered by continuous infusion (0.25 mCg/kg/min-0.75 mCg/kg/min) is useful for improving cardiovascular system function in patients with cardiomyopathy and has been shown to decrease the risk of low cardiac output syndrome in children after repair of congenital heart disease.[31] Milrinone undergoes renal clearance and therefore should be used with caution in patients with AKI, and premature neonates.[32]

Anti-arrhythmic Agents

Arrhythmias are relatively common in critically ill children and can affect preload and cardiac contractility and limit cardiac output. Supraventricular tachycardia (SVT) is the most common arrhythmia in infants. Management principles should begin with pediatric advanced life support protocol.[33] Adenosine is a rapid-acting medication that interrupts electrical flow through the A-V node causing a transient heart block. It activates the A1 receptor in myocardial cells and can be used to interrupt certain types of SVT or can be used to unmask the underlying etiology for others (eg, atrial flutter). Adenosine has a half-life of 10 seconds due to rapid deamination by adenosine deaminase in the red blood cells. Initial dosing is 0.1 mg/kg by rapid IV push followed by a saline flush to hasten delivery before deamination. The dose can be increased to 0.2 mg/kg up to a maximum of 12 mg in older children and adults.

Esmolol is a selective beta-1 adrenergic blocking agent (class II antiarrhythmic) that slows the A-V node refractory period and can be used for rate control or chemical cardioversion with a bolus of 100 to 500 mCg/kg infused over 1 minute is followed by an infusion of 25 mCg/kg/min. The dose can be increased in increments of 25 to 50 mCg/kg/min depending on the rate response.[34] Side effects include hypotension, negative inotropy, bradycardia, and hypoglycemia in infants and newborns.

Procainamide is a class 1a sodium channel blocking agent with a rapid onset (5–10 minutes) when administered intravenously. It is metabolized in the liver to an active metabolite, N-acetylprocainamide (NAPA). Procainamide dosing should be adjusted using therapeutic drug monitoring, particularly in patients with renal impairment or prematurity who may have abnormal drug accumulation. Loading dose is based on age: neonates 5 to 10 mg/kg; infants and older children 10 to 15 mg/kg over 30 to 60 minutes followed by an infusion of 20 to 80 mCg/kg/min titrated by effect and serum level.[35]

Amiodarone is a versatile agent with effects at multiple levels of the cardiac conduction system.[36] However, it has significant side effects that include hypotension due to myocardial depression, bradycardia, and heart block. Amiodarone has a long half-life and onset of action. It is administered by intravenous infusion of 5 to 15 mCg/kg/min.[36] Bolus dosing should be given as slowly as the clinical situation allows. In ventricular tachycardia, 5 mg/kg can be administered according to PALS guidelines.[33] For tachyarrhythmias that are not immediately life-threatening, a loading dose of 1 to 2 mg/kg over 30 to 60 minutes, up to a total of 5 mg/kg may be considered.

Lidocaine is a class 1b agent that slows conduction in the Purkinje fibers and is used for the treatment of ventricular tachycardia. An IV bolus of 1 mg/kg per dose and an infusion rate of 20 to 50 mCg/kg/min can be used. Lidocaine is metabolized in the liver and may require dose adjustment in patients with hepatic failure.

Magnesium sulfate has a specific role in tachyarrhythmias. Torsade de pointes is a polymorphic ventricular tachycardia that can be treated with IV magnesium sulfate at 25 to 50 mg/kg by IV push. Magnesium sulfate administration can result in hypermagnesemia and hypotension.[37]

CCBs in the nondihydropyridine class (verapamil and diltiazem) affect nodal conduction and can be used in children,[38] but with caution in those under 1 year of age due to the risk of cardiovascular collapse with nondihydropyridine CCBs.[39] The dihydropyridine CCBs have no role in the treatment of tachyarrhythmia. **Table 2** shows suggested strategies for the management of pediatric tachyarrhythmias.[37]

Ductal-dependent Heart Disease

The differential diagnosis of shock in neonates includes ductal-dependent heart disease. Prostaglandin E–1 (PGE-1) maintains ductus arteriosus patency and is important in the treatment of ductal-dependent congenital heart defects. Initiating PGE-1 infusion in a newborn with unexplained shock is imperative. In neonates with ductal-dependent systemic blood flow lesions such as hypoplastic left heart syndrome, interrupted aortic arch, or critical coarctation, patency of ductus arteriosus is necessary to maintain blood flow through the aorta. In neonates with ductal-dependent pulmonary blood flow lesions such as pulmonary atresia, PGE-1 maintains

Table 2
Suggested pharmacotherapy for tachyarrhythmias

Arrhythmia	First-Line Medication	Second-Line Medication
Reentrant SVT	IV: adenosine, esmolol, procainamide Oral: propranolol, digoxin	IV: amiodarone Oral: sotalol, amiodarone, flecainide
Ectopic atrial tachycardia	IV: esmolol, procainamide Oral: propranolol	IV: amiodarone Oral: sotalol, amiodarone, flecainide
Intraatrial reentrant tachycardia	IV: esmolol, procainamide Oral: propranolol, digoxin	IV: amiodarone Oral: metoprolol, atenolol, sotalol
Permanent junctional reciprocating tachycardia	IV: esmolol Oral: propranolol, atenolol, metoprolol	IV: amiodarone Oral: flecainide, sotalol
Junctional ectopic tachycardia	IV: amiodarone	IV: esmolol, digoxin, procainamide
Ventricular tachycardia	IV: esmolol, procainamide, lidocaine	IV: amiodarone Oral: metoprolol, atenolol, sotalol
Ventricular fibrillation	IV: amiodarone, procainamide	IV: lidocaine
Torsades de Pointes	IV: magnesium sulfate	IV: amiodarone, procainamide, lidocaine

Adapted from Moffett B, Salvin J, Kim J. Pediatric Cardiac Intensive Care Society 2014 Consensus Statement: Pharmacotherapies in Cardiac Critical Care Antiarrhythmics. Ped Crit Care Med 2016;3:S49-S58.

blood flow to the lungs. PGE-1 is administered as a continuous intravenous infusion of 0.05 to 0.2 mCg/kg/min. After ductal patency is ensured, the dose can be decreased to 0.03 mCg/kg/min as less drug is required to maintain patency compared with that needed to open a closed ductus arteriosus. Lowering the effective infusion dose mitigates side effects of hypotension, apnea, and fever.

RESPIRATORY
Extrathoracic Airway Obstruction

Viral laryngotracheobronchitis (croup) is a relatively common childhood viral disease. Symptoms include a barky cough but may progress to significant airway compromise requiring intensive care monitoring or intervention. Inhaled racemic epinephrine results in the vasoconstriction of the airway soft tissues and can relieve obstructive symptoms when administered by facemask or high flow devices. If racemic epinephrine is given, children should be monitored for rebound extrathoracic airway obstruction as the effects of the inhaled racemic epinephrine wanes. Steroids may be used depending on the severity of symptoms. Dexamethasone reduces inflammation and edema and is recommended as first-line therapy. It has good bioavailability and can be used in enteral or parenteral form. Budesonide is a form of inhaled corticosteroid and has been shown to have similar effectiveness as dexamethasone. Glucocorticoid treatment reduces hospital length of stay and has been shown to improve symptoms within 2 hours of administration.[40]

Intrathoracic Airway Obstruction

Status asthmaticus is a clinical condition with 3 hallmark processes that include inflammation, bronchospasm, and increased mucous production.[41] It is a common cause of admission to the PICU. Studies suggest that there is a trend toward increasing PICU admission rates for severe asthma potentially related to racial and regional health care disparities, and poor compliance with controller medications in patients with a severe asthma.[42,43] Pharmacotherapy is directed at maintaining adequate oxygenation and reversing airway obstruction, by reducing airway inflammation and bronchospasm. Hypoxemia should be treated with supplemental oxygen to maintain SpO2 more than 92%. Noninvasive modes of ventilation such as bimodal positive airway pressure (BiPAP) and high flow nasal cannula are increasingly being used to avoid more invasive respiratory support such as intubation and mechanical ventilation. However, despite the increasing use of noninvasive support, outcomes such as the need for invasive mechanical ventilation and hospital length of stay remain unchanged.[44–48]

Steroid therapy aimed at reducing inflammation is the main therapy for status asthmaticus. Early corticosteroid therapy is beneficial, and is recommended for children with status asthmaticus, with evidence that early administration minimizes potential time lag to effect.[49] Patients who require PICU admission should be given methylprednisolone IV at a dose of 1 mg/kg every 6 to 12 hours (maximum dose of 60 mg/d) and continued until symptoms are under control.[50] Once symptomatic control of status asthmaticus is achieved, enteral steroids should be started, and continued for 5 to 10 days after symptom onset.

Short-acting, inhaled beta-2 adrenergic agonists such as albuterol are the primary agents used for bronchodilation. Activation of beta-2 adrenergic receptors results in the relaxation of the airway smooth muscle. Continuous nebulization of albuterol may be administered by facemask 0.15 to 0.5 mg/kg/h (maximum 20 mg/h). Beta-2 agonist therapy results in tachycardia and the dose should be decreased as symptoms improve. Using a standardized treatment pathway has been shown to optimize therapy, reduce variation in care and potentially decrease ICU and hospital length of stay.[51–53]

Ipratropium bromide is an inhaled anticholinergic muscarinic antagonist that produces bronchodilation.[54] It is given as adjunctive therapy with inhaled beta-agonists. Studies in critically ill patients are limited, but for those with severe status asthmaticus who present to the emergency department, ipratropium bromide has been shown to decrease the need for hospitalization.[55]

The treatment of status asthmaticus with magnesium sulfate has increased over the last decade.[56] Magnesium antagonizes calcium channels, resulting in smooth muscle relaxation. Studies have suggested the benefits of intravenous administration of magnesium sulfate at a dose of 25 to 50 mg/kg (maximum of 2 g) given over 15 to 20 minutes. Repeated dosing and continuous infusion can result in hypermagnesemia with muscle weakness and respiratory depression; therefore, the measurement of serum magnesium levels is essential.[57]

Parenteral beta-2 agonists may be used in patients with severe bronchoconstriction when delivery of inhaled beta-2 agonists to the intrathoracic airway is difficult. Terbutaline is a selective beta-2 agonist that has the potential advantage of less tachycardia compared with nonselective IV beta-agonists. Initial dose is 5 mCg/kg bolus followed by a continuous infusion of 0.2 to 0.3 mCg/kg/min (maximum of 5 mCg/kg/min). Side effects include tachycardia, jitteriness, and chest pain. There are limited studies comparing the benefits of parenteral versus inhaled beta-agonists.

The most common methylxanthine used for the treatment of asthma is aminophylline. An older medication class with bronchodilator and diuretic properties, aminophylline is administered as a bolus dose of 5 to 6 mg/kg and may be followed by continuous intravenous infusion. Aminophylline is metabolized in the liver and its half-life is prolonged in patients with hepatic dysfunction and heart failure. Side effects include tachycardia, nausea, and seizures. Aminophylline elimination has age-specific properties and should be adjusted accordingly. Initial continuous infusion rates should be at 0.5 to 0.7 mg/kg/h for infants, 1 to 1.2 mg/kg/h for children ages 1 to 9 years, and 0.7 to 0.9 mg/kg/h for older children and adults, adjusted to maintain serum concentrations between 10 and 20 mCg/mL. Monitoring of serum levels is imperative, especially when using more than one bolus dose or with continuous infusions. Due to the narrow therapeutic window of aminophylline, beta-agonists are recommended instead of methylxanthines.[50]

CENTRAL NERVOUS SYSTEM
Intracranial Injury

Children with intracranial pathology are admitted to the ICU with trauma, infection, or hypoxemic/ischemic brain injury. The primary injury can be exacerbated by ongoing intracranial hypertension with progressive secondary injury. Due to the properties of the cranial vault and the blood–brain barrier, certain entities are amenable to therapy to reduce intracranial hypertension, but others are not. Osmotherapeutic agents and medications aimed at reducing brain metabolism can mitigate intracranial pathology.

Osmotherapy can be used for situations whereby cellular edema and cellular fluid can be reduced in the presence of an intact blood–brain barrier. Osmotherapeutic agents include hypertonic saline and mannitol. The use of hypertonic saline has increased relative to mannitol despite few studies supporting the superiority of one therapy over the other.[58] The aim of osmotherapy is to reduce intracranial content without inducing hypovolemia. It is important to monitor serum electrolytes, osmolality, and cardiovascular status. The recommended dose of hypertonic saline is 1 to 3 mL/kg (3% saline), up to a maximum dose of 250 mL.[59] Continuous intravenous infusion of hypertonic saline has also been used for control of ICP. The dose of hypertonic saline should be adjusted to maintain the minimum serum osmolality needed to result in the desired ICP, maintaining serum sodium less than 160 mEq/L, and osmolality less than 360 mOsm/kg.[59]

The effects of mannitol result from the creation of osmotic differences on cerebral tissue and subsequent diuresis. The dose is 0.5 g to 1 g/kg given more than 10 minutes with osmotic effects occurring within 15 to 30 minutes. The dose can be repeated based on clinical response and/or ICP levels, if available. Mannitol is rapidly eliminated and should be given intermittently to achieve maximum osmotic effects and to avoid accumulation and renal injury.

Sedatives are generally indicated in the management of patients with intracranial hypertension. The beneficial effects of barbiturates for refractory intracranial hypertension result from the decrease in cerebral metabolic rate and its antioxidant properties. Pentobarbital can be used to induce an anesthetized state with an IV bolus of 5 mg/kg followed by the continuous infusion of 1 to 2 mg/kg/h. The infusion rate may be titrated to achieve the desired ICP. In refractory intracranial hypertension, or if used concomitantly for the treatment of status epilepticus, a higher infusion rate may be needed to achieve burst suppression or seizure control. The potential for neuronal apoptosis from the use of benzodiazepines and barbiturates warrants more research.[60] Barbiturate therapy is associated with significant hypotension and myocardial depression, and many patients require simultaneous administration of inotropic agents to maintain hemodynamic stability.[61]

Status Epilepticus

Status epilepticus is defined as continuous or repeated convulsive or nonconvulsive seizures lasting 30 minutes or longer. The neuronal hyperactivity leads to an increase in cerebral metabolism which can deprive the brain of oxygen and glucose. Status epilepticus should be considered an emergency that requires the immediate institution of time-based, targeted therapy (**Table 3**).

On the completion of initial evaluation to ascertain the adequacy of airway and circulation, pharmacologic therapy should be started and directed toward the symptoms and underlying etiology. Imaging and testing including lumbar puncture should be considered when the patient's condition allows. Status epilepticus in children is frequently due to subtherapeutic medication levels in those receiving anticonvulsant therapy for underlying seizure disorder, but may also result from infection, trauma, toxic ingestion, hyponatremia, hypoglycemia, and tumors.

Seizures in infants can be due to metabolic derangements that do not respond to antiepileptic medications. Hypoglycemia should be treated with 2 to 4 mL/kg of 10% or 25% dextrose. Hyponatremic seizures can result from the inappropriate preparation of formula or excessive water ingestion. Hyponatremia should be suspected in infants with status epilepticus who are otherwise healthy, and initial assessment should include a detailed history of formula preparation and supplemental water feeds. The goal of treatment with hypertonic saline is not to immediately restore serum sodium levels to normal but to increase serum sodium enough to raise the transmembrane potential to stop seizure activity. Rare causes of status epilepticus, such as pyridoxine deficiency should be considered in the differential diagnosis of refractory infantile seizures.

Benzodiazepines are a family of drugs with good bioavailability regardless of route of administration. These drugs bind to γ-aminobutyric acid (GABA) receptors altering transmembrane potential and reducing neuronal transmission (**Table 2** for first- and second-line medications for the treatment of status epilepticus). Benzodiazepines are recommended for the initial therapy of status epllepticus.[62] Lorazepam is the recommended first-line drug for the treatment of status epilepticus because it can be injected rapidly and has an onset of action of 2 to 3 minutes. Respiratory depression is a potential side effect. Continuous infusion of lorazepam is not recommended due to potential side effects resulting from the accumulation of the diluent propylene glycol.

Intravenous, intramuscular, or transmucosal midazolam is also used as a treatment of status epilepticus. An intravenous infusion of midazolam (0.2–0.6 mg/kg/h) can be used for the treatment of status epilepticus refractory to intermittent dosing. Continuous EEG and cardiovascular monitoring are recommended for continuous infusion therapy.

Diazepam can be administered through the rectal route and is recommended for the treatment of status epilepticus in patients without IV access.

Levetiracetam and fosphenytoin are recommended as second-line therapy for status epilepticus.[63] Levetiracetam is effective and has a good safety profile that includes the absence of respiratory depressive effects often seen with benzodiazepines.

Fosphenytoin is a prodrug of phenytoin. Phenytoin or fosphenytoin should be infused slowly over 20 minutes, as bradycardia and cardiovascular collapse are associated with a rapid infusion. Fosphenytoin can also be administered intramuscularly in patients without IV access. With significant variability in phenytoin metabolism in infants, serum concentrations should be monitored. There are no clear data to support the superiority of fosphenytoin over levetiracetam.

Table 3
Pathway-based management for status epilepticus

Convulsive Status Epilepticus Management Guidelines			
Phase	Time	Management	Notes
Stabilization	0–5 min	1. Evaluate and address ABC's and place on monitors 2. Note time of seizure onset 3. Obtain finger stick glucose A. Treat <60 with 2 mL/kg D25 W 4. Obtain IV access 5. Treat identified reversible causes	*Labs to consider:* • Electrolytes • Infectious work up • Anti-epileptic drug levels • Toxicology

Primary intervention (Benzodiazepine)	5–15 min	• IV Access
		  ○ IV lorazepam (0.1 mg/kg, max 4 mg per dose, up to 2 doses)
		• No IV Access
		  ○ IM midazolam (0.2 mg/kg max 10)
		  ○ Intranasal midazolam (0.2 mg/kg max 10 mg)
		  ○ PR diazepam acceptable if other options not available
			Consider imaging and antibiotics early

Secondary intervention	> 15 min	Choose one: • IV levetiracetam (30–60 mg/kg, max 3000 mg) • IV fosphenytoin (20 mg PE/kg, max 1500 mg). May repeat with 10 mg PE/kg, max 750 mg • Continued seizure despite secondary therapy = admit to ICU and consult neurology	For neonates, may use: • IV phenobarbital (20 mg/kg)
Refractory status epilepticus		Admit to ICU for continuous anti-epileptic drip • Midazolam – load 0.2 mg/kg (max 10 mg), infusion 0.2–0.6 mg/kg/h • Pentobarbital – load 5–15 mg/kg, infusion 1–5 mg/kg/h	Neurotelemetry to be initiated Repeat loading dose with escalations in drip rate to get to steady state quicker

Barbiturates such as phenobarbital or pentobarbital can be used for the treatment of refractory status epilepticus. Adverse effects include respiratory depression and negative inotropy which can result in hypotension. Inotropic support is often required with multiple doses or continuous infusion of barbiturates to counteract the cardiovascular effects. Serum drug levels should be monitored to achieve a level of 20 mCg/mL, but higher levels may sometimes be necessary for the treatment of refractory status epilepticus in neonates whereby clearance is influenced by birth weight and postnatal age.[64] Pentobarbital may be administered by intravenous bolus and continuous infusion for the treatment of status epilepticus unresponsive to first and second lines of therapy.

Table 4 shows first- and second-line medications to treat status epilepticus. Other agents have been used for the management of status epilepticus unresponsive to the drugs listed above. These include: valproic acid, propofol, ketamine, inhaled anesthetics, as well as therapeutic hypothermia.[65]

HEMATOLOGY
Anticoagulation

Pediatric venous thromboembolism can occur in critically ill children and is associated with complications including pulmonary embolism, cerebrovascular events, and death.[66] Early detection, prompt treatment, and prophylaxis can help avoid these complications and to manage long term consequences. Pediatric risk factors for developing venous thrombosis including the presence of an indwelling central venous catheter, surgery, immobilization, dehydration (especially with hyperosmolar-hyperglycemic states), malignancy, infectious and inflammatory conditions. The use of anticoagulants for the treatment of venous thromboembolism is associated with an increased risk of bleeding; therefore, monitoring is recommended. Guidelines for anticoagulation are provided by the American Society of Hematology.[67]

Unfractionated heparin (UFH) is a parenteral anticoagulant that inhibits coagulation factors by binding to antithrombin and augmenting antithrombin activity. Heparin can be used for prophylaxis and treatment. Side effects include potential for bleeding, and in addition, it is associated with heparin-induced thrombocytopenia (HIT), an immune-mediated, prothrombotic state.[68] Benefits of heparin include the ability to monitor drug activity levels by the measurement of activated partial thromboplastin time (aPTT) or anti-Xa levels. In addition, the anticoagulant effects of UFH can be reversed with the administration of protamine.

Low-molecular-weight heparin (LMWH) has similar actions as UFH, and effects can be monitored by the measurement of anti-Xa levels at less frequent intervals than required for UFH. Subcutaneous administration is an added benefit in patients without IV access.

Warfarin is an oral anticoagulant used for prophylaxis and treatment of thromboembolic disease. Warfarin inhibits the synthesis of vitamin K-dependent coagulation factors II, VII, IX, and X and anticoagulant proteins C and S. Warfarin has a narrow therapeutic window and increases the risk of bleeding; therefore the measurement of prothrombin time (PT) and international normalized ratio (INR) are required to monitor effects. To avoid the prothrombotic potential of warfarin during the early stages of administration, therapy should be initiated with concomitant anticoagulation with UFH, which can then be discontinued several days after warfarin therapy is initiated and the INR is at the desired level. Warfarin effects can be reversed by administering vitamin K-dependent factors with fresh frozen plasma, prothrombin concentrates, or with vitamin K.

Argatroban and bivalirudin are parenteral direct thrombin inhibitors (DTIs) often used as alternatives to UFH for anticoagulation, in patients with circulatory devices or those who require anticoagulation but have a history of HIT.[69,70] Bivalirudin is eliminated via nonenzymatic proteolysis and is preferred in patients with hepatic insufficiency. The

Table 4
Status epilepticus medications[a]

Drug	Lorazepam	Midazolam	Diazepam	Fosphenytoin	Levetiracetam
Dosing: Intermittent	0.1 mg/kg/dose IV	0.1–0.2 mg/kg/dose IV/ intranasal/buccal	0.5 mg/kg PR	20 mg PE/kg (max. 1500 mg PE)	30–60 mg/kg IV (max. 3000 mg)
Continuous infusion	NA	0.2–0.6 mg/kg/h	NA	NA	NA
Adverse Effects	Hypotension, respiratory depression			Bradycardia, hypotension	Bone marrow suppression, headache
Pharmacokinetics Onset	15–20 min	1–5 min	15 min	15 min	5–30 min
T ½	6–73 h	2–12 h	30–60 h	12–29 h	6–8 h
Duration	6–8 h	< 2 h	12 h	3 h	
Metabolism	Hepatic via conjugation	CYP450 enzymes	CYP450 enzymes	CYP450 enzymes	Not extensive-enzymatic hydrolysis

Abbreviation: T ½, half-life.
[a] Data from Lexi-Comp Online, Pediatric Lexi-Drugs Online.[74]

Table 5
Anticoagulation

Anticoagulant	Dosing	Goal	Dose Adjustment		
Heparin		aXa 0.3–0.7	Anti-Xa		Rate Change
• Bolus	50–100 units/kg Bolus		<0.1		+5 units/kg/h + 50 units/kg bolus
• Infusion	28 units/kg/h (<1 y)		0.1–0.29		+2.5 units/kg/h
	20 units/kg/h (>1 y)		0.3–0.7		0 units/kg/h
			0.71–0.8		−2.5 units/kg/h
			0.81–1		−2.5 units/kg/h + hold 30 min
			>1		−5 units/kg/h + hold 60 min
Enoxaparin		aXa 0.1–0.5	*Anti-Xa*		*Dose change*
-prophylaxis	0.75 mg/kg SC q 12 h (<2 mo)	aXa 0.5–1	<0.1		Increase 25%
-treatment	0.5 mg/kg SC q 12 h (>2 mo)		0.1–0.5		no change
	1.5 mg/kg SC q 12 h (<2 mo)		0.51–1		decrease 20%
	1 mg/kg SC q 12 h (>2 mo)		>1		decrease 30%
			Anti-Xa		*Dose change*
			<0.35		increase 25%
			0.35–0.49		increase 10%
			0.5–1		no change
			1.1–1.5		Decrease 20%
			1.6–2		Decrease 30%
			>2		Hold until 0.5–1; decrease 40%
DTI		aPTT 50–80 s	*aPTT*		*Rate Change*
Argatroban	0.75 mCg/kg/min		<50 s		Increase dose by 20%
Bivalirudin	0.25 mCg/kg/min		50–80 s		No change
	(hepatic impairment)		81–95 s		aPTT 81–95 Decrease dose by 20%
	0.1–0.3 mg/kg/h		96–120 s		Hold infusion for 1 h then resume at 20% decrease from prior dose
			≥ 121 s		Hold infusion for 2 h then obtain aPTT every 2 h until <95 then resume

(continued on next page)

**Table 5
(continued)**

Anticoagulant	Dosing	Goal	Dose Adjustment	
Warfarin	0.1–0.2 mg/kg PO q 24 h (max 5 mg)	INR 2–3	Dose adjustment after day 3:	
			INR	Dose Change
			1.1–1.4	increase 20%
			1.5–1.9	increase 10%
			2–3	no change
			3.1–3.5	decrease 10%
			>3.5	hold until INR <3.5, decrease 20%

Adapted and modified from Malec L, Young G. Treatment of Venous Thromboembolism in Pediatric Patients. Front Pediatr. 2017 Feb 28;5:26. LMWH, low-molecular-weight heparin; DTI, direct thrombin inhibitor; aPTT, activated partial thromboplastin time; aXa, anti Xa; INR, international normalized ratio; PT, pro-thrombin time.

data for use of these drugs in children are limited and most of the information is extrapolated from studies in adults. Both medications require monitoring to achieve a goal of 1.5 to 2.5 times the baseline aPTT, to maintain aPTT less than 100s.[66] See **Table 5** for anticoagulation medications, monitoring, and adjustment parameters.

Thrombolytic Therapy

The use of recombinant tissue plasminogen activator (rTPA) results in clot lysis with the potential to spare tissues from a devastating injury. Thrombolytic therapy has a role in the treatment of hemodynamically significant PE, and more recently, is considered important in the treatment of pediatric stroke.[67,71,72] A regional stroke team should be involved in the decision to use thrombolytic therapy in this context. rTPA dosing for hemodynamically significant PE is a bolus of 0.5 to 0.7 mg/kg (up to 100 mg) followed by continuous IV infusion of 0.03 to 0.06 (max 2 mg/h) with a continuous heparin infusion of 4 to 10 units/kg/h. For thrombolytic therapy for stroke, the recommended dose is 0.9 mg/kg with the first 0.09 mg/kg given over 5 minutes followed by 0.81 mg/kg over the first hour.[71,73]

Pharmacologic therapy for critically ill children is a complex endeavor that requires knowledge of the developmental stage, drug interactions, end-organ function, and the risk to benefit ratio of a given therapy. While unavoidable, polypharmacy increases the risk of medication errors which account for a large burden of iatrogenic morbidity and mortality that can potentially be avoided with physiologic and laboratory monitoring and clinical assessment.

CLINICS CARE POINTS

• Pediatric dosing/adjustment of medications is frequently weight-dependent; additional care should be taken with certain medications (e.g. cardiovascular) that have differential dose-dependent effects.

DISCLOSURE

The authors have no commercial or financial conflicts of interest or any funding sources.

REFERENCES

1. Alcorn J, McNamara P. Ontogeny of hepatic and renal systemic clearance pathways in infants part I. Clin Pharmacokinet 2002;41:959–98.
2. Kearns G, Abdel-Rahman S, Alander S, et al. Developmental pharmacology – drug disposition, action, and therapy in infants and children. N Engl J Med 2003;349:1157–67.
3. Funk R, Brown J, Abdel-Rahman S. Pediatric pharmacokinetics: human development and drug disposition. Pediatr Clin North Am 2012;59(5):1001–16.
4. Zuppa A, Barrett J. Pharmacokinetics and pharmacodynamics in the critically ill child. Pediatr Clin N Am 2008;55:735–55.
5. Smith B, Yogaratnam D, Levasseur-Franklin K, et al. Introduction to drug pharmacokinetics in the critically III patient. Chest 2012;141:1327–36.
6. Kleinman M, Chameides L, Schexnayder S, et al. Part 14: pediatric advanced life support: 2010 american heart association guidelines for cardiopulmonary resuscitation and emergency cardiovascular care. Circulation 2010;122:S876–908.

7. Cies J, Santos L, Chopra A. IV enoxaparin in pediatric and cardiac ICU patients. Pediatr Crit Care Med 2014;15(2):e95–103.

8. Brodersen R, Honore B. Drug binding properties of neonatal albumin. Acta Paediatr Scand 1989;78(3):342–6.

9. Blot S, Pea F, Lipman J. The effect of pathophysiology on pharmacokinetics in the critically ill patient–concepts appraised by the example of antimicrobial agents. Adv Drug Deliv Rev 2014;77:3–11.

10. Park GR. Molecular mechanisms of drug metabolism in the critically ill. Br J Anaesth 1996;77(1):32–49.

11. Haycock G. Development of glomerular filtration and tubular sodium reabsorption in the human fetus and newborn. Br J Urol 1998;81(Suppl 2):33–8.

12. Karsies T, Sargel C, Marquardt D, et al. An empiric antibiotic protocol using risk stratification improves antibiotic selection and timing in critically ill children. Ann Am Thorac Soc 2014;11(10):1569–75.

13. Battula V, Krupanandan R, Nambi P, et al. Safety and feasibility of antibiotic de-escalation in critically ill children with sepsis – A prospective analytical study from a pediatric ICU. Front Pediatr 2021;9:640857.

14. Sutiman N, Koh J, Watt K, et al. Pharmacokinetics alterations in critically ill pediatric patients on extracorporeal membrane oxygenation: a systematic review. Front Pediatr 2020;8:260.

15. Zuppa AF. Understanding renal replacement therapy and dosing of drugs in pediatric patients with kidney disease. J Clin Pharmacol 2012;52:134S–40S.

16. Sherwin J, Heath T, Watt K. Pharmacokinetics and dosing of anti-infective drugs in patients on extracorporeal membrane oxygenation: a review of current literature. Clin Ther 2016;38(9):1976–94.

17. Lewis SR, Pritchard MW, Evans DJ, et al. Colloids versus crystalloids for fluid resuscitation in critically ill people. Cochrane Database Syst Rev 2018;8(8): CD000567.

18. Luciani G, Nichani S, Chang A, et al. Continuous versus intermittent furosemide infusion in critically ill infants after open heart operations. Ann Thorac Surg 1997; 64(4):1133–9.

19. Robertson C, Bork K, Tawfik G, et al. Avoiding furosemide ototoxicity associated with single-ventricle repair in young infants. Pediatr Crit Care Med 2019;20(4): 350–6.

20. Lampin M, Rousseaux J, Botte A, et al. Noradrenaline use for septic shock in children: doses, routes of administration and complications. Acta Paediatr 2012; 101(9):e426–30.

21. Davis AL, Carcillo JA, Aneja RK, et al. The american college of critical care medicine clinical practice parameters for hemodynamic support of pediatric and neonatal septic shock: executive summary. Pediatr Crit Care Med 2017;18(9): 884–90.

22. Holmes CL, Landry DW, Granton JT. Science review: Vasopressin and the cardiovascular system part 1–receptor physiology. Crit Care 2003;7(6):427–34.

23. Patel BM, Chittock DR, Russell JA, et al. Beneficial effects of short – term vasopressin infusion during severe septic shock. Anesthesiology 2002;96:576–82.

24. Thiele R, Nemergut E, Lynch C. The clinical implications of isolated alpha1 adrenergic stimulation. Anesth Analg 2011;113:297–304.

25. Stone ML, Kelly J, Mistry M, et al. Use of nicardipine after cardiac operations is safe in children regardless of age. Ann Thorac Surg 2018;105(1):181–5.

26. Liviskie CJ, DeAvilla KM, Zeller BN, et al. Nicardipine for the treatment of neonatal hypertension during extracorporeal membrane oxygenation. Pediatr Cardiol 2019;40(5):1041–5.

27. Mastropietro C, Arango Uribe D. Nicardipine for hypertension following aortic coarctectomy or superior cavopulmonary anastomosis. World J Pediatr Congenit Heart Surg 2016;7(1):32–5.

28. Lindle K, Dinh K, Moffett B, et al. Angiotensin-converting enzyme inhibitor nephrotoxicity in neonates with cardiac disease. Pediatr Cardiol 2014;35(3):499–506.

29. Mathur K, Hsu D, Lamour J, et al. Safety of enalapril in infants: data from the pediatric heart network infant single ventricle trial. J Pediatr 2020;227:218–23.

30. Francis GS, Bartos JA, Adatya S. Inotropes. J Am Coll Cardiol 2014;63(20): 2069–78.

31. Hoffman TM, Wernovsky G, Atz AM, et al. Efficacy and safety of milrinone in preventing low cardiac output syndrome in infants and children after corrective surgery for congenital heart disease. Circulation 2003;107(7):996–1002.

32. Paradisis M, Jiang X, McLachlan AJ, et al. Population pharmacokinetics and dosing regimen design of milrinone in preterm infants. Arch Dis Child Fetal Neonatal Ed 2007;92:F204–9.

33. PALS algorithms. 2021. Available at: https://www.acls-pals-bls.com/algorithms/pals/. Accessed November 15, 2021.

34. Cuneo BF, Zales VR, Blahunka PC, et al. Pharmacodynamics and pharmacokinetics of esmolol, a short-acting betablocking agent, in children. Pediatr Cardiol 1994;15:296–301.

35. Moffett BS, Cannon BC, Friedman RA, et al. Therapeutic levels of intravenous procainamide in neonates: a retrospective assessment. Pharmacotherapy 2006;26:1687–93.

36. Saul JP, Scott WA, Brown S, et al. Intravenous amiodarone for incessant tachyarrhythmias in children: a randomized, double-blind, antiarrhythmic drug trial. Circulation 2005;112:3470–7.

37. Moffett B, Salvin J, Kim J. Pediatric cardiac intensive care society 2014 consensus statement: pharmacotherapies in cardiac critical care antiarrhythmics. Ped Crit Care Med 2016;3:S49–58.

38. Porter C, Gillette P, Garson A Jr, et al. Effects of verapamil on supra-ventricular tachycardia in children. Am J Cardiol 1981;48:487–91.

39. Radford D. Side effects of verapamil in infants. Arch Dis Child 1983;58:465–6.

40. Gates A, Gates M, Vandermeer B, et al. Glucocorticoids for croup in children. Cochrane Database Syst Rev 2018;8(8):CD001955.

41. Carroll C, Sala K. Pediatric status asthmaticus. Crit Care Clin 2013;29(2):153–66.

42. Al-Eyadhy A, Temsah M, Alhaboob A, et al. Asthma changes at a pediatric intensive care unit after 10 years: observational study. Ann Thorac Med 2015;10(4): 243–8.

43. Grunwell J, Travers C, Fitzpatrick A. Inflammatory and comorbid features of children admitted to a PICU for status asthmaticus. Pediatr Crit Care Med 2018; 19(11):e585–94.

44. Russi B, Lew A, McKinley S, et al. High-flow nasal cannula and bilevel positive airway pressure for pediatric status asthmaticus: a single center, retrospective descriptive and comparative cohort study. J Asthma 2021;15:1–13.

45. Smith A, Franca U, McManus M. Trends in the use of noninvasive and invasive ventilation for severe asthma. Pediatrics 2020;146(4):e20200534.

46. Craig S, Dalziel S, Graudins A, et al. Interventions for escalation of therapy for acute exacerbations of asthma in children: an overview of Cochrane Reviews. Cochrane Database Syst Rev 2020;8:CD012977.
47. Gates R, Haynes K, Rehder K, et al. High-flow nasal cannula in pediatric critical asthma. Respir Care 2021;66(8):1240–6.
48. Johnson MD. In search of evidence for using noninvasive ventilation for severe acute asthma. Pediatrics 2020;146(4). e2020022103.
49. Agnihotri N, Saltoun C. Acute severe asthma (status asthmaticus). Allergy Asthma Proc 2019;40(6):406–9.
50. National Heart, Lung and Blood Institute. Expert panel report 3: guidelines for the diagnosis and management of asthma (EPR-3 2007). Available from: https://www.nhlbi.nih.gov/health-topics/guidelines-for-diagnosis-management-of-asthma. Accessed November 15, 2021.
51. Brennan S, Lowrie L, Woolridge J. Effects of a PICU Status Asthmaticus de-escalation pathway on length of stay and albuterol use. Pediatr Crit Care Med 2018;19:658–64.
52. Miksa M, Kaushik S, Antovert G, et al. Implementation of a critical care asthma pathway in the PICU. Crit Care Explor 2021;3(2):e0334.
53. Bartman T, Brilli R. Variability reduction - an essential aspect of quality. Pediatr Crit Care Med 2018;19(7):681–2.
54. Gross NJ. Ipratropium bromide. N Engl J Med 1988;319(8):486–94.
55. Qureshi F, Pestian J, Davis P, et al. Effect of nebulized ipratropium on the hospitalization rates of children with asthma. N Engl J Med 1998;339(15):1030–5.
56. Mittal V, Hall M, Antoon J, et al. Trends in intravenous magnesium use and outcomes for status asthmaticus in children's hospitals from 2010 to 2017. J Hosp Med 2020;15(7):403–6.
57. Anderson S, Farrington E. Magnesium treatment in pediatric patients. J Pediatr Health Care 2021;35(5):564–71.
58. Boone M, Oren-Grinberg A, Robinson T, et al. Mannitol or hypertonic saline in the setting of traumatic brain injury: what have we learned? Surg Neurol Int 2015; 23(6):177.
59. Kochanek PM, Tasker RC, Bell MJ, et al. Management of pediatric severe traumatic brain injury: 2019 consensus and guidelines-based algorithm for first and second tier therapies. Pediatr Crit Care Med 2019;20(3):269–79.
60. Thompson KW, Suchomelova L, Wasterlain CG. Treatment of early life status epilepticus: what can we learn from animal models? Epilepsia Open 2018;28(3 S2): 169–79.
61. Tasker R, Goodkin H, Sánchez Fernández I, et al. Pediatric status epilepticus research group. refractory status epilepticus in children: intention to treat with continuous infusions of midazolam and pentobarbital. Pediatr Crit Care Med 2016;17(10):968–75.
62. Glauser T, Shinnar S, Gloss D, et al. Evidence-based guideline: treatment of convulsive status epilepticus in children and adults: report of the guideline committee of the american epilepsy society. Epilepsy Curr 2016;16(1):48–61.
63. Dalziel S, Borland M, Furyk J, et al. PREDICT research network. Levetiracetam versus phenytoin for second-line treatment of convulsive status epilepticus in children (ConSEPT): an open-label, multicentre, randomised controlled trial. Lancet 2019;25(393):2135–45.
64. Völler S, Flint R, Stolk L, et al. DINO study group. Model-based clinical dose optimization for phenobarbital in neonates: an illustration of the importance of data sharing and external validation. Eur J Pharm Sci 2017;15(109S):S90–7.

65. Zimmern V, Korff C. Status epilepticus in children. J Clin Neurophysiol 2020;37(5): 429–33.
66. Polikoff L, Faustino E. Venous thromboembolism in critically ill children. Curr Opin Pediatr 2014;26(3):286–91.
67. Monagle P, Cuello C, Augustine C, et al. American society of hematology 2018 guidelines for management of venous thromboembolism: treatment of pediatric venous thromboembolism. Blood Adv 2018;2(22):3292–316.
68. Aster RH. Heparin-induced thrombocytopenia and thrombosis. N Engl J Med 1995;332(20):1374–6.
69. VanderPluym C, Cantor R, Machado D, et al. Utilization and Outcomes of children treated with direct thrombin inhibitors on paracorporeal ventricular assist device support. ASAIO J 2020;66(8):939–45.
70. O'Brien S, Yee D, Lira J, et al. UNBLOCK: an open-label, dose-finding, pharmacokinetic and safety study of bivalirudin in children with deep vein thrombosis. J Thromb Haemost 2015;13:1615–22.
71. Rivkin M, Bernard T, Dowling M, et al. Guidelines for urgent management of stroke in children. Pediatr Neurol 2016;56:8–17.
72. Henry D. Moving toward a new standard of care for acute pediatric stroke. Pediatr Ann 2021;50(6):e242–4.
73. Mastrangelo M, Giordo L, Ricciardi G, et al. Acute ischemic stroke in childhood: a comprehensive review. Eur J Pediatr 2022;181(1):45–58. Epub ahead of print.
74. Lexi-comp online, pediatric lexi-drugs online. Hudson, OH: Lexi-Comp Inc; Accessed October 19, 2021.

Analgesia, Sedation, Paralytics, Delirium, and Iatrogenic Withdrawal

Kevin Valentine, MD[a],*, Janelle Kummick, PharmD, BCPPS[b]

KEYWORDS

- Sedation • Analgesia • Critical care pediatrics • Paralytics • Delirium • Withdrawal

KEY POINTS

- Critically ill children have age-related differences in pharmacokinetics/pharmacodynamics that must be considered.
- A complex association exists between pain management and sedation in critically ill children.
- Over-sedation has the potential to mask and lead to under-treatment of pain.
- When neuromuscular blocking agents are required, adequate analgosedation must be ensured. Continued use of neuromuscular blockade should be evaluated with the train of 4 monitoring, provision of a paralytic holiday, or both.
- Prolonged pain and sedation management can lead to tolerance and potential withdrawal.
- Tools to measure withdrawal and delirium should be used regularly as part of a protocol to identify at-risk patients and inform appropriate therapies.

PHARMACOLOGIC PRINCIPLES IN CRITICALLY ILL CHILDREN

It is important to distinguish age-related differences in pharmacology for infants and young children compared with older children and adults. In the first year of life, pharmacokinetic changes occur in absorption, distribution, metabolism, and excretion. Neonates and infants have distinct differences in drug metabolism that include[1]: a relative absence of hydrochloric acid in gastric secretions that lead to a decreased absorption of acidic drugs (eg, phenobarbital).[2] increased concentrations of active unbound drug due to decreased plasma protein binding from lower levels of albumin and α1-acid glycoprotein.[3] Immaturity of hepatic (cytochrome P-450) enzymes and low glucuronidation activity,[4] Reduced glomerular filtration and renal tubular secretion

[a] Indiana University School of Medicine, Riley Hospital for Children, 705 Riley Hospital Drive, Suite 4900, Indianapolis, IN 46202, USA; [b] Butler University College of Pharmacy and Health Sciences, Riley Hospital for Children, 705 Riley Hospital Drive, Room W6111, Indianapolis, IN 46202, USA
* Corresponding author.
E-mail address: kmvalent@iu.edu

Pediatr Clin N Am 69 (2022) 531–546
https://doi.org/10.1016/j.pcl.2022.01.012
0031-3955/22/© 2022 Elsevier Inc. All rights reserved.

in the first weeks of life. These differences in renal and hepatic function can lead to prolonged drug elimination. For example, appropriate administration of morphine in this population should include less drug and less frequent dosing intervals to prevent drug accumulation and toxicity.

Analgesia

Pain management in critically ill children is complicated as pain can be multifactorial and subjective. There are 2 distinct types of pain, nociceptive and neuropathic. Nociceptive pain occurs from tissue damage or inflammation, whereas neuropathic pain results from nerve cell dysfunction. Some children may experience a mixed type of pain due to the underlying condition (eg, trauma or burns). Pain is also classified based on duration as acute or chronic. Acute pain is short lived and the goal in treatment is to get the patient through the episode. Chronic pain is continuous or recurrent and the goal in management is to allow function. Appropriate categorization of pain is important to allow for different treatment approaches, of which there are nonpharmacologic and pharmacologic treatments available.

Following categorization, objective measurement tools should be used to assess, document, and provide appropriate treatment of pain. Several pediatric pain assessment tools are available based on the patient's age, clinical condition, and developmental level. The Joint Commission has provided standardization for self-assessment and observational tools for the measurement of pediatric pain.[1] Assessments should occur regularly as pain can change over time and frequent assessments can help determine the efficacy of the intervention/treatment. Common indicators of acute pain may include crying, inconsolability, and facial expressions. Chronic pain can present with behaviors such as abnormal posturing, increased irritability, sleep disruption, and changes in appetite.[2] Documentation of pain can include severity level, location, patient characteristics, onset, and duration. Following a complete pain assessment, the appropriate therapy can be initiated, continued, or modified as applicable.

Pain management should include both nonpharmacological and pharmacologic methods. Nonpharmacologic interventions include a range of diversion techniques appropriate for age. Diversion techniques for infants include pacifiers, swaddling, rocking, and holding. For older children, diversion techniques might differ and can consist of familiar toys, video games, and television. Other nonpharmacologic interventions can include music or art therapy, a calm and low-stimulation environment, and cognitive behavioral therapy. The utilization of nonpharmacologic therapies should always be considered and intertwined with pharmacologic therapy.

Pain management may be different for every child. Patient-specific regimens should be implemented and adapted to meet the needs of each individual. There are 3 pharmacologic analgesic therapies: nonopioid, opioid, and miscellaneous drugs. Nonopioid medications are used for mild to moderate pain and inflammation and include acetaminophen and nonsteroidal anti-inflammatory drugs (NSAIDs). Opioid analgesics are typically used for moderate to severe pain. The intravenous route of administration is preferred for the treatment of acute pain and the enteral route for chronic pain when feasible. Unlike nonopioid medications, opioid analgesics do not have a ceiling dose limit for prolonged or chronic use. Combination therapy with nonopioid and opioid analgesics is beneficial as the utilization of nonopioid analgesics can reduce the requirement for opioids and associated adverse effects. Miscellaneous therapies include medications for adjunct or chronic, cancer, or neuropathic pain. Classes of medications include anti-epileptics, anti-depressants, and skeletal muscle relaxants (Tables 1–3).

Table 1 Nonopioid analgesics[a]				
Drug	**Acetaminophen**	**Ibuprofen**	**Naproxen**	**Ketorolac**
Mechanism of Action	Activation of descending serotonergic inhibitory pathways in the CNS	Reversibly inhibits cyclooxygenase 1 and 2 enzymes; decreased formation of prostaglandin precursors		
Dosing	10–15 mg/kg/dose PO every 4–6 h	4–10 mg/kg/dose PO every 6–8 h	5–6 mg/kg/dose PO every 12 h	0.5 mg/kg/dose IV every 6–8 h
Adverse Effects	Skin rash Ceiling effect	Hepatotoxicity Nephrotoxicity Gastritis		

Abbreviations: IV, intravenous; PO, orals.

[a] Data from Lexi-Comp Online, Pediatric Lexi-Drugs Online.[11]

Nonopioid Analgesics

Acetaminophen
Acetaminophen is the most common nonopioid analgesic used in children. It is primarily used for the treatment of mild to moderate pain alone or in combination with opioid analgesics. The analgesic effects of acetaminophen are due to the activation of serotonergic inhibitory pathways in the CNS but other nociceptive systems (ie, periphery) may be affected. It lacks anti-inflammatory properties. Acetaminophen is available in many dosage forms including tablet, capsule, chewable, suspension, suppository, and parenteral. This drug is unique in that it is metabolized via sulfation in infants and by glucuronidation in adults.[3] Intravenous dosing is 15 mg/kg every 6 hours (max. dose 1 g) for children who are unable to tolerate oral intake. Oral dosing for infants, children, and adolescents is 10 to 15 mg/kg/dose every 4 to 6 hours. To avoid the risk of hepatotoxicity, dosing limits should not be exceeded. The daily dose should be limited to 75 mg/kg/d, not to exceed 4000 mg per day regardless of route of administration.

Nonsteroidal Anti-inflammatory Drugs
NSAIDs are used for the treatment of mild to moderate pain alone, or in combination with opioid analgesics for moderate to severe pain. One of the biggest differences between NSAIDs and acetaminophen is the additional anti-inflammatory effect provided by NSAIDs, but studies evaluating the analgesic effects of NSAIDs compared with acetaminophen show conflicting results as to whether NSAIDs provide a greater analgesic response.[4–6] The mechanism of action of NSAIDS is reversible inhibition of cyclooxygenase-1 and 2 enzymes that result in the inhibition of prostaglandin synthesis. NSAIDs are available in many dosage forms including tablets, capsules, suspension, and parenteral. Common oral forms of NSAIDs used in children include ibuprofen and naproxen. Ketorolac is an NSAID that is primarily administered in parenteral form. An important distinction is that intravenous NSAIDs do not provide more analgesia compared with enteral options.[7] The utilization of NSAIDs may be limited due to adverse effects such as gastrointestinal bleeding and increased platelet aggregation. This class of medications should also be used with caution in the neonatal population due to limited safety data.[8] In addition, caution should be used in patients with decreased intravascular volume, renal or hepatic insufficiency.

Table 2
Opioid analgesics [a]

IV Drug	Fentanyl	Hydromorphone	Methadone	Morphine
Dosing INT	1–2 mCg/kg/dose IV every 1–2 h	0.005–0.015 mg/kg/dose IV every 3–6 h	0.025–0.1 mg/kg/dose IV every 4–8 h	0.05 mg/kg/dose IV every 2–4 h
CI	1–5 mCg/kg/h	0.003–0.05 mg/kg/h	NA	0.01–0.2 mg/kg/h
Adverse Effects	Tachyphylaxis Chest wall rigidity	Histamine release	QTc prolongation	Histamine release
Pharmacokinetics Onset	Immediate	5 min	10–20 min	5–10 min
T ½	2–36 h	2–3 h	4–62 h	2–10 h
Duration	0.5–1 h	3–4 h	22–48 h (repeat doses)	3–5 h
Metabolism	CYP3A4	Glucuronidation	CYP3A4, CYP2B6, CYP2C19, CYP2C9, and CYP2D6	

PO Drug	Hydrocodone/ Acetaminophen	Methadone	Morphine	Oxycodone
Dosing	0.1–0.2 mg/kg/dose PO every 4–6 h	0.1–0.2 mg/kg/dose PO every 6–8 h	0.1–0.2 mg/kg/dose PO every 3–4 h	0.025–0.1 mg/kg/dose PO every 4–6 h
Adverse Effects	Bradycardia Nephrotoxicity	QTc prolongation	Drowsiness Headache Nausea Constipation	
Pharmacokinetics Onset	10–20 min	0.5–1 h	30 min	10–15 min
T ½	4 h	4–62 h	4–13 h	3–4 h
Duration	4–8 h	22–48 h (repeat doses)	3–5 h	3–6 h
Metabolism	CYP2D6, CYP3A4	CYP3A4, CYP2B6, CYP2C19, CYP2C9, and CYP2D6	Hepatic via conjugation	CYP3A4, CYP2D6

Abbreviations: CI, continuous infusion; INT, intermittent; IV, intravenous; NA, not applicable; PO, oral; T ½, half-life.
[a] Data from Lexi-Comp Online, Pediatric Lexi-Drugs Online.[11]

Table 3
Miscellaneous analgesics [a]

Drug	Gabapentin	Pregabalin	Amitriptyline	Duloxetine
Dosing	5 mg/kg/dose PO every 8 h	3–5 mg/kg/dose PO every 12 h	0.1–0.5 mg/kg/dose PO every 24 h	30 mg PO every 24 h
Adverse Effects	Drowsiness Fatigue Peripheral edema	Weight gain, peripheral edema	Fatigue, cardiac arrhythmia	Weight loss, abdominal pain, nausea and vomiting, and drowsiness
Pharmacokinetics T ½	4–5 h	3–6 h	13–36 h	10–12 h
Metabolism	Not metabolized and excreted as unchanged drug	Excreted as 90% unchanged drug	Hepatic demethylation to active metabolite	CYP1A2, CYP2D6

Abbreviations: PO, oral; T ½, half-life.

[a] Data from Lexi-Comp Online, Pediatric Lexi-Drugs Online.[11]

Opioid Analgesics

Opioid analgesics should be reserved for moderate to severe pain. Opioids bind to G-protein-coupled receptors, mu, delta, or kappa, located in the brain and spinal cord to modulate nociception. These medications can be used intermittently or by continuous infusion. Intermittent dosing is useful for the treatment of acute pain while continuous infusion may be indicated for other conditions such as postoperative pain, providing consistent and sustained analgesia that is especially helpful for patients on mechanical ventilation. The utilization of opioid analgesics in children should be individualized. There are pharmacokinetic differences based on age that should influence the choice of opioid and dosage. Neonates and infants have immature hepatic and renal systems that can result in inadequate metabolism and slower elimination. Many of the opioid analgesics are available in a variety of intravenous and enteral dosage forms suitable for various ages (see **Table 2**). The most used opioid analgesics in critically ill children for intermittent and continuous infusion are fentanyl, morphine, and hydromorphone.

Fentanyl

The pharmacokinetics of fentanyl (see **Table 2**) make this agent ideal for short procedures such as intubation. Fentanyl is a lipophilic drug, and the pharmacokinetics may be altered in patients on extracorporeal support such as extracorporeal membrane oxygenation (ECMO) or continuous renal replacement therapy (CRRT). Approximately 70% of the drug is lost in the circuit, reducing efficacy that leads to higher drug requirements.[9] Fentanyl differs from the other opioids in that it can cause tachyphylaxis within approximately 5 days of use. In addition, a major adverse effect of fentanyl is chest wall rigidity, occurring when given rapidly in less than 3 minutes and with higher doses of 3 to 5 mCg/kg[10] for the induction phase of intubation or line placement. Accepted treatments for chest wall rigidity are reversal with naloxone or neuromuscular blockade with mechanical ventilatory support.

Morphine

Morphine is a commonly used opioid in pediatrics as intermittent dosing or continuous infusion. It should be used with caution in patients with renal dysfunction as morphine is eliminated by the kidneys and can accumulate, causing toxic effects. Morphine undergoes hepatic metabolism to morphine 6- and 3-glucuronide. Morphine-6-glucuronide is the active metabolite responsible for the analgesic effects of the drug but both metabolites undergo renal excretion. Dosing should be individualized as the half-life is variable based on age.[11] Hypotension can be common in patients who have hemodynamic instability and results from a combination of mechanisms including histamine-mediated vasodilation, direct inhibition of sympathetic nerve activity leading to negative chronotropic and inotropic effects, and reduction in baroreceptor mediated reflex responses.

Hydromorphone

Hydromorphone is an opioid that should be considered in patients that require a longer duration of analgesia and as an alternative to morphine in patients with renal failure. Although hydromorphone is like morphine, it is important to note that hydromorphone is 5 times more potent than morphine.

While maintaining appropriate pain control is crucial for patient care, the utilization of opioids can result in several adverse effects. The most common include respiratory depression, constipation, nausea and vomiting, sedation, and pruritis. Adverse effects such as respiratory depression or sedation can be minimized by reducing the dose when possible. Other adverse effects such as constipation and pruritis may require additional treatment or a change in opioids to mitigate the effect. Patients may have a higher opioid dosing requirement following prolonged use and those who develop tolerance or a reduction in sensitivity to the opioid, may require higher doses to sustain the same response. A strategy to alleviate tolerance is to provide opioid rotation, using different opioids to prevent associated adverse effects from dose escalation, particularly in patients requiring long-term pain control.

Some opioid analgesics have fallen out of favor due to the lack of efficacy and significant adverse effect profile. Meperidine can have severe adverse effects including cardiac arrest and seizures especially with multiple dosing. Codeine and tramadol have an FDA warning that the use in children is contraindicated due to the serious risk of respiratory depression and death.[12,13]

If pain is not adequately controlled with a nonopioid, with or without an opioid, there are other pharmacologic classes that can be used as an adjunct therapy. These include anti-epileptics, anti-depressants, and skeletal muscle relaxants (see **Table 3**). Pain management is not a one size fits all and may need to be modified throughout the course of treatment.

Sedation

Historically, sedation practices used sedative medications alone, but subsequently, analgesics were added as needed as we believed that children required both sedation and analgesia to facilitate critical care. Sedation needs often occur concurrently with pain management in critically ill children. Analgosedation is the process of treating pain and leveraging the properties of analgesics with the intent of mitigating exposure to multiple drug classes and avoiding the side effects of polypharmacy. Sedative agents should be carefully selected and used only when needed. Over-sedation can result in the inability to accurately measure pain potentially resulting in inadequate analgesia and nonrestorative sleep patterns.[14] In addition to neurodevelopmental concerns of using sedative agents in newborns,[15,16] literature supports an association between benzodiazepines and pediatric delirium.[17] Standardized sedation scales should be used to provide an objective assessment of the patient and determine appropriate pharmacotherapy regardless of medication regimen. There are several pharmacologic therapies for children based on the indication for sedation and patient clinical status (**Table 4**).

Alpha-2 Adrenergic Agonists

Dexmedetomidine is an alpha-2 adrenergic receptor agonist with 100 times the potency at central receptors when compared with clonidine. Continuous intravenous infusion results in sedative effects and mild analgesic properties with minimal respiratory depression. Ninety-three percent of dexmedetomidine is protein bound and it has a long half-life. Dexmedetomidine was marketed for sedation in patients 24 to 48 hours before extubation, but studies have reported longer use for sedation in children of up to several weeks, with minimal adverse effects.[18] Dexmedetomidine has been shown to decrease postoperative opioid requirements for up to 7 days without dose-dependent analgesic effect. It has been shown to provide short term neuroprotection in neonates exposed to anesthetics; however, further studies are required to evaluate long-term outcomes.[19]

Clonidine is also an alpha-2 adrenergic agonist administered as intermittent enteral doses or a transdermal patch for the prevention of dexmedetomidine withdrawal. The use of clonidine is limited by the side effects that include bradycardia and rebound hypertension if the drug is discontinued too quickly after prolonged use.

Table 4
Sedation medications [a]

Drug	Dexmedetomidine	Midazolam	Lorazepam	Propofol	Clonidine	Ketamine
Dosing INT	NA	0.025–0.1 mg/kg/dose IV once	0.025–0.1 mg/kg/dose IV once	1–2 mg/kg/dose IV once	1–5 mCg/kg/dose PO every 6–8 h	0.5–2 mg/kg/dose IV once
CI	0.2–1 mCg/kg/h	0.03–0.12 mg/kg/h	NA	20–100 mCg/kg/min	NA	0.3–1 mg/kg/h
Adverse Effects	Bradycardia, hypotension	Hypotension, respiratory depression		Bradycardia, hypotension, propofol infusion syndrome	Bradycardia, hypotension	Hypertension, tachycardia, emergence delirium
Pharmacokinetics Onset	5–10 min	1–5 min	15–20 min	30 s	Unknown	30 s
T ½	2–10 h	2–12 h	6–73 h	Initial 40 min	6 h	10–15 min
Duration	60–120 min	< 2 h	6–8 h	3–10 min	6–8 h	5–10 min
Metabolism	Glucuronidation	CYP450 enzymes	Hepatic via conjugation	Glucuronidation	Hepatic via enterohepatic recirculation	Hepatic via several pathways

Abbreviations: CI, continuous infusion; INT, intermittent; IV, intravenous; NA, not applicable; PO, oral; T ½, half-life.
[a] Data from Lexi-Comp Online, Pediatric Lexi-Drugs Online.[11]

Benzodiazepines

Benzodiazepines are sedative agents that do not have analgesic activity and are used intermittently for procedural sedation or as a continuous infusion when more constant sedation is needed. Preparations include intravenous and enteral dosage forms. For critically ill patients requiring a continuous infusion, midazolam is the benzodiazepine of choice. Of note, midazolam is a lipophilic agent, therefore, higher doses may be required, or an alternative sedative should be selected for patients on ECMO or CRRT. The relatively large surface area of the extracorporeal circuit tubing and filters leads to drug sequestration and decreased availability of lipophilic medications over time.

Lorazepam is a benzodiazepine with a longer half-life compared with midazolam and can, therefore, be administered intermittently. Respiratory depression is an adverse effect especially when used in conjunction with opioid analgesics. Patients on lorazepam require close monitoring, and the lowest effective dose is used whenever possible.

Propofol

Propofol is an agent that has sedative and amnestic effects. It is a general anesthetic that acts as a GABA agonist and blocks the NMDA receptor causing total CNS depression. This medication has a short half-life and can be used for procedural sedation or by continuous intravenous infusion if longer period of sedation is required. The drug is in a lipid emulsion and prolonged use requires monitoring of nutrition and total fat intake. In addition, propofol can result in propofol-related infusion syndrome (PRIS), with metabolic acidosis, hypotension, rhabdomyolysis, cardiac and renal failure, and death. Due to the risk of PRIS, propofol is not desirable for prolonged use in children.

Ketamine

Ketamine is a sedative agent that has analgesic properties with opioid-sparing effects. It differs from other sedatives in that it is not associated with respiratory depression and hypotension, and therefore may be used as an alternative to benzodiazepines. The mechanism of action of ketamine is NMDA antagonism with direct action on the cortex and limbic system creating a state of dissociation of surroundings.[20] With its analgesic and sedative effects, ketamine is commonly used for procedural sedation and the lack of respiratory depression makes it especially useful in the emergency department. Lower doses of ketamine produce analgesic effects and aid in hyperalgesia and opioid tolerance. Adverse effects include tachycardia, hypertension, excessive salivation, hallucinations, and emergence delirium.

Analgesia and sedation can be a challenge in critically ill child. It is important to assess and monitor every patient with standardized, individualized assessment tools to determine their need for analgosedation according to clinical status. Careful drug selection and considerations for dosing should include age, weight, pharmacokinetic changes, renal and hepatic function.

NEUROMUSCULAR BLOCKING AGENTS

Critically ill patients may require NMBAs to facilitate mechanical ventilation, invasive procedures, and to minimize movements in patients with unstable airways or craniofacial/thoracic trauma or surgery. The addition of NMBAs can improve respiratory system compliance by reducing patient-ventilator dyssynchrony, but analgosedation must be optimized to avoid ongoing paralysis of a patient who is awake and in pain.

Nondepolarizing Agents

The nondepolarizing class of NMBAs includes vecuronium, pancuronium, rocuronium, atracurium, and cis-atracurium (**Table 5**). These drugs are competitive antagonists

Table 5 Neuromuscular blocking agents[a]			
Drug	Rocuronium	Vecuronium	Cisatracurium
Intermittent	0.6–1.2 mg/kg IV	0.1 mg/kg IV	0.1–0.15 mg/kg IV
Continuous infusion	0.4–0.7 mg/kg/h	0.05–0.15 mg/kg/h	0.06–0.24 mg/kg/h
Onset	30–60 s	1–3 min	2–3 min
Duration	30–40 min	30–60 min	30–45 min
Adverse Effects	Hypertension Hypotension Tachycardia	Hypertension Hypotension Tachycardia	Bradycardia Bronchospasm Hypotension
Uses	Intubation Skeletal muscle relaxation		

[a] Data from Lexi-Comp Online, Pediatric Lexi-Drugs Online.[11]

and block acetylcholine binding to receptors on the motor endplate, thereby inhibiting depolarization. Neuromuscular blocking agents (NMBAs) have differing elimination and characteristics. For example, cis-atracurium is eliminated by Hoffman degradation and not dependent on renal or hepatic function.[21]

Depolarizing Agents

Succinylcholine is a membrane depolarizing agent that has a rapid onset of action and a short half-life.[22] It acts as a molecular receptor analog to acetylcholine and induces membrane depolarization. Administration of succinylcholine results in initial fasciculations resulting from active membrane depolarization, followed by flaccid paralysis. The recommended dose in children is 1 mg/kg/dose IV. The onset of paralysis occurs within 1 minute after injection and dissipates within 4 to 6 minutes as the drug is rapidly metabolized by plasma pseudocholinesterase. Succinylcholine is contraindicated in patients with increased intracranial pressure, spinal cord injuries, muscular dystrophy, concurrent hyperkalemia, rhabdomyolysis, or an individual or family history of malignant hyperthermia.

In patients requiring continuous neuromuscular blockade, the train of 4 (TOF) is useful in judging the effect of continuous neuromuscular blockade.[23] Monitoring the TOF in patients who are receiving a continuous infusion or numerous intermittent doses of NMBAs helps prevent overexposure to the paralytic. A paralytic "holiday" whereby the NMBA infusion is interrupted at a predetermined time to evaluate the degree of the neuromuscular blockade can be used concomitantly with TOF monitoring. This allows neuromuscular junction function recovery before the reinstitution of NMBAs. **Fig. 1** shows an example of a paralytic holiday schedule.

REVERSAL AGENTS

Rapid reversal of neuromuscular blockade is sometimes necessary for patients in the ICU who have received nondepolarizing agents. Acetylcholine esterase inhibitors provide an increase in acetylcholine and can overcome the competitive antagonism of the nondepolarizing NMBAs. Neostigmine, 0.05 to 0.07 mg/kg IV (maximum of 5 mg) has a peak action within 5 to 8 minutes and can be used for this purpose. Atropine may have to be administered with neostigmine to counteract excessive muscarinic effects that include bradycardia, increased secretions, and bronchospasm. Sugammadex is a newer medication that encapsulates aminosteroid, nondepolarizing NMBAs (rocuronium and vecuronium), directly reversing their pharmacologic actions.[24]

Daily holiday timing: 8:00am or after shift-change (whichever is sooner) for patients receiving
continuously infused neuromuscular blocking agents (rocuronium, vecuronium , or cisatricurium)

1. Patient assessment
   - Unsafe movement/severe hemodynamic instability: **do not proceed with holiday and skip to
     step #5**
   - Safe movement/immobility and hemodynamically stable: proceed with holiday (step #2)
2. Have available IV push paralytic/sedation/analgesia vials at bedside
3. Stop continuous paralytic infusion
4. Patient reassessment
   - Unsafe movement/hemodynamic instability
     o Give IV push paralytic/analgesic/sedative prior to restarting paralytic infusion
     o Restart continuous neuromuscular blockade infusion (follow infusion restart guideline
        below)
   - Safe movement and hemodynamically stable: OK to continue to hold continuous infusion and
     manage sedation/analgesia with PRN orders
5. Report back to rounding team; discuss ongoing need for paralytic infusion

Neuromuscular blockade infusion restart guideline

Timing of return to spontaneous movement	Resume dose at:	Calculation
<15 min	100% of previous dose	Resume previous dose
15 – 30 min	75% of previous dose	=previous dose x 0.75
31 – 60 min	50% of previous dose	=previous dose x 0.5
61 – 120 min	25% of previous dose	=previous dose x 0.25
>2 hr	Consult MD prior to restart	

Fig. 1. Paralytic holiday schedule.

There are several drugs frequently used in critically ill children that can potentiate
the effects of NMBAs and result in prolonged paralysis or myopathy. These include
aminoglycosides, beta-blocking agents, furosemide, and steroids. Electrolyte abnormalities and hypothermia can also result in prolonged paralysis from NMBAs. A persistent neuromyopathy can occur with prolonged use of NMBAs, especially when used in
combination with corticosteroids, though the association may not be as strong as was
once thought.[25] Regardless of the cause, critical illness neuromyopathy is associated
with undesirable outcomes such as prolonged duration of mechanical ventilation, and
prolonged ICU and hospital stay.[26]

DELIRIUM

The recognition of delirium is evolving. It was previously thought of as a phenomenon
limited to adult patients but is increasingly recognized to also be a problem affecting
children. Studies show that delirium occurs in 20% to 60% of critically ill children and
is associated with prolonged ICU length of stay.[27–29] Routine use of validated
screening tools for prompt recognition of delirium is supported by position statements
since 2014.[30–33] Additionally, screening is an inexpensive intervention that raises
awareness for the diagnosis of delirium which is often mistakenly thought to be agitation, pain, and other forms of cognitive disorders associated with critical illness.[29,34]
The clinical diagnosis should be confirmed by clinicians with specific training in the

Table 6
Anti-psychotic agents[a]

Drug	Risperidone	Quetiapine	Olanzapine	Haloperidol
Dosing	0.01–0.04 mg/kg PO every 24 h	0.5 mg/kg/dose PO every 8 h	0.1 mg/kg PO Q24	0.025 mg/kg IV
Adverse Effects	Hypotension, EPS, NMS	EPS, NMS, QTc prolongation, hypotension	NMS, EPS, diabetes mellitus, hypotension	EPS, TD, dystonia, QTc prolongation, NMS
Pharmacokinetics T ½	20 h	6–7 h	21–54 h	21–24 h
Metabolism	CYP2D6, CYP3A4	CYP3A4	CYP1A2, CYP2D6; glucuronidation	CYP1A2, CYP2D6

Abbreviations: EPS, extrapyramidal symptoms; NMS neuroleptic malignant syndrome; PO, oral; T ½
, half-life; TD, tardive dyskinesia.
[a]Data from Lexi-Comp Online, Pediatric Lexi-Drugs Online.[11]

recognition of the 3 main subtypes: hyperactive, hypoactive, and mixed-type delirium. Minimization and avoidance/removal of agents that are associated with the development of delirium remain the best intervention. Despite the potential benefits of sedation, the least number of sedative agents needed to achieve sedative effects should be used to allow more accurate treatment of pain and mitigate factors that lead to delirium.

While recognition and appropriate diagnosis of delirium are important, prevention is paramount. Nonpharmacologic means of reducing delirium risk, such as maintaining a normal day–night circadian rhythm with exposure to sunlight and promotion of normal sleep, are low-cost methods available to everyone. The optimal prevention and management solutions for delirium in children remain unclear though some protocols are in use.[35] Pharmacologic management of delirium is often institution dependent and there are no widely accepted guidelines. Meta-analyses to evaluate antipsychotic medication use in adults with delirium have mixed results with respect to treatment of symptoms of hyperactive delirium and has not been shown to improve outcomes.[36–38]

There are presently no data supporting antipsychotic drug use for the prevention or treatment of delirium in children, or for the specific treatment of children with hypoactive delirium. The data are mixed with respect to patient outcomes but there are some studies that support the use of second-generation antipsychotic drugs for the pharmacologic reduction of hyperactive delirium symptoms in children.[39–43] See **Table 6** for antipsychotic medication dosing. There are currently no FDA-approved medications for the treatment of pediatric delirium. Use of these agents should be accompanied by monitoring for adverse drug events that include QTc prolongation, hypotension, over-sedation, extrapyramidal symptoms, and neuroleptic malignant syndrome.

WITHDRAWAL

Iatrogenic withdrawal syndrome (IWS) refers to a range of symptoms that occur after abrupt discontinuation or sudden reduction of the dose of sedative and analgesic medications in a health care environment. IWS results from prolonged use of sedative/analgesic medications and follows the spectrum of increased drug needs/

tolerance and dependence. Iatrogenic withdrawal can be prevented/mitigated by understanding the complex relationship between the duration of drug exposure and dosage. It is rare for patients to develop dependence and withdrawal when a sedative or analgesic has been given for less than 4 days, but treatment of more than 7 days significantly increases risk.[44-47] To avoid IWS, screening should be performed using validated scoring tools for pediatrics such as the Withdrawal Assessment Tool −1 or WAT-1.[48]

The prevention and/or treatment of IWS should be with a drug selected from the same family as the medication that led to withdrawal. For opioid dependence/IWS, methadone, morphine, and hydromorphone in tapering dosage are reasonable choices (see **Table 2** for opioid dosing). For benzodiazepine dependence/IWS, lorazepam is a reasonable choice (see **Table 4** for dosing). The duration of dose tapering should follow a standardized pathway but may need to be adjusted according to patient characteristics. A standardized approach to screening improves the ability to apply defined criteria and a protocol reduces the potential for unnecessary medication exposure. Studies show that using a weaning protocol reduces the duration and total dose of opioid administration.[49,50]

Comfort care for critically ill children must take into account the pharmacologic differences between children and adults. Adequate provision of analgesia is a key principle. With adequate pain control, the need for sedation can be better assessed. Clinicians should minimize or avoid medications that mask pain and promote delirium. Tools to measure withdrawal and delirium should be used to identify at-risk patients and inform appropriate, evidence-based therapies.

CLINICS CARE POINTS

- Analgosedation should be employed for patient comfort as needed with a focus on pain management and lighter sedation to lessen the potential for delirium generation and iatrogenic withdrawal.
- Each ICU patient should be screened for delirium each day with a focus on prevention.

DISCLOSURE

The authors have nothing to disclose.

REFERENCES

1. Pain assessment and management standards. Available at: https://www.jointcommission.org/resources/patient-safety-topics/pain-management-standards-for-accredited-organizations/. Accessed November 15, 2021.
2. WHO guidelines on the pharmacological treatment of persisting pain in children with medical illnesses. Geneva: World Health Organization; 2012.
3. Kearns GL, Abdel-Rahman SM, Alander SW, et al. Development pharmacology - drug disposition, action, and therapy in infants and children. N Engl J Med 2003; 349:1157–67.
4. Berde CB, Sethna NF. Analgesics for the treatment of pain in children. N Engl J Med 2002;347:1094–103.
5. Rusy LM, Houck CS, Sullivan LJ, et al. A double-blind evaluation of ketorolac tromethamine versus acetaminophen in pediatric tonsillectomy: analgesia and bleeding. Anesth Analg 1995;80:226–9.

6. Baer GA, Rorarius MG, Kolehmainen S, et al. The effect of paracetamol or diclofenac administered before operation on postoperative pain and behaviour after adenoidectomy in small children. Anaesthesia 1992;47:1078–80.
7. Tramer MR, Williams JE, Carroll D, et al. Comparing analgesic efficacy of non-steroidal anti-inflammatory drugs given by different routes in acute and chronic pain: a qualitative systematic review. Acta Anaesthesiol Scand 1998;42:71–9.
8. Morris JL, Rosen DA, Rosen KR. Nonsteroidal anti-inflammatory agents in neonates. Pediatri Drugs 2003;5(6):386–400.
9. Buck ML. Pharmacokinetic changes during extracorporeal membrane oxygenation. Clin Pharmacokinet 2003;42:403–17.
10. Johnson PN, Miller JL, Hagemann TM. Sedation and analgesia in critically ill children. AACN Adv Crit Care 2012;23:415–34.
11. Online Lexi-Comp. Pediatric Lexi-drugs online. Hudson, OH: Lexi-Comp Inc; 2021.
12. FDA requires labeling changes for prescription opioid cough and cold medicines to limit their use to adults 18 years and older. Available at: https://www.fda.gov/files/drugs/published/Drug-Safety-Communication–Opioid-Cough-and-Cold-Meds.pdf. Accessed November 15, 2021.
13. FDA restricts use of prescription codeine pain and cough medicines and tramadol pain medicines in children' recommends against use in breastfeeding women. Available at: https://www.fda.gov/drugs/drug-safety-and-availability/2017-drug-safety-communications. Accessed November 15, 2021.
14. Kudchadkar SR, Aljohani OA, Punjabi NM. Sleep of critically ill children in the pediatric intensive care unit: a systematic review. Sleep Med Rev 2014;18(2):103–10.
15. Duerden EG, Guo T, Dodbiba L, et al. Midazolam dose correlates with abnormal hippocampal growth and neurodevelopmental outcome in preterm infants. Ann Neurol 2016;79(4):548–59.
16. Ng E, Taddio A, Ohlsson A. Intravenous midazolam infusion for sedation of infants in the neonatal intensive care unit. Cochrane Database Syst Rev. 2012 Jun 13;(6):CD002052. Update in. Cochrane Database Syst Rev 2017;CD002052.
17. Alvarez RV, Palmer C, Czaja AS, et al. Delirium is a common and early finding in patients in the pediatric cardiac intensive care unit. J Pediatr 2018;195:206–12.
18. Carroll CL, Krieger D, Campbell M, et al. Use of dexmedetomidine for sedation of children hospitalized in the intensive care unit. J Hosp Med 2008;3:142–7.
19. Mason KP, Lerman J. Review article: Dexmedetomidine in children: current knowledge and future applications. Anesth Analg 2011;113(5):1129–42.
20. Dolansky G, Shah A, Mosdossy G, et al. What is the evidence for the safety and efficacy of using ketamine in children. Paediatr Child Health 2008;13(4):307–8.
21. Kisor DF, Schmith VD. Clinical pharmacokinetics of cisatracurium besilate. Clin Pharmacokinet 1999;36:27–40.
22. Zuppa AF, Curley MAQ. Sedation analgesia and neuromuscular blockade in pediatric critical care: Overview and current landscape. Pediatr Clin North Am 2017;64(5):1103–16.
23. deBacker J. Hart N, Fan E. Neuromuscular blockade in the 21st century management of the critically ill patient. Chest 2017;151(3):697–706.
24. Akha AS, Rosa J 3rd, Jahr JS, et al. Sugammadex: cyclodextrins, development of selective binding agents, pharmacology, clinical development, and future directions. Anesthesiol Clin 2010;28(4):691–708. Erratum in: Anesthesiol Clin. 2011 Mar;29(1):1.

25. Wilcox SR. Corticosteroids and neuromuscular blockers in development of critical illness neuromuscular abnormalities: A historical review. J Crit Care 2017;37: 149–55.

26. Field-Ridley A, Dharmar M, Steinhorn D, et al. ICU-acquired weakness is associated with differences in clinical outcomes in critically ill children. Pediatr Crit Care Med 2016;17(1):53–7.

27. Traube C, Silver G, Reeder RW, et al. Delirium in critically ill children: an international point prevalence study. Crit Care Med 2017;45(4):584–90.

28. Staveski SL, Pickler RH, Khoury PR, et al. Prevalence of ICU delirium in postoperative pediatric cardiac surgery patients. Pediatr Crit Care Med 2021;22(1): 68–78.

29. Traube C, Silver G, Gerber LM, et al. Delirium and mortality in critically ill children: epidemiology and outcomes of pediatric delirium. Crit Care Med 2017;45(5): 891–8.

30. Harris J, Ramelet AS, van Dijk M, et al. Clinical recommendations for pain, sedation, withdrawal and delirium assessment in critically ill infants and children: an ESPNIC position statement for healthcare professionals. Intensive Care Med 2016;42(6):972–86.

31. Traube C, Silver G, Kearney J, et al. Cornell Assessment of Pediatric Delirium: a valid, rapid, observational tool for screening delirium in the PICU*. Crit Care Med 2014;42(3):656–63.

32. Smith HA, Boyd J, Fuchs DC, et al. Diagnosing delirium in critically ill children: Validity and reliability of the Pediatric Confusion Assessment Method for the Intensive Care Unit. Crit Care Med 2011;39(1):150–7.

33. Smith HAB, Gangopadhyay M, Goben C, et al. The Preschool Confusion Assessment Method for the ICU: Valid and reliable delirium monitoring for critically ill infants and children. Crit Care Med 2016;44(3):592–600.

34. Tobias JD. Monitoring the depth of sedation in the pediatric ICU patient: where are we, or more importantly, where are our patients? Pediatr Crit Care Med 2005;6(6):715–8.

35. CICU, PCU, and PICU Clinical Pathway for Screening/Treatment of Children with Delirium. Available at: https://www.chop.edu/clinical-pathway/picu-pcu-delirium-clinical-pathway. Accessed November 15, 2021.

36. Neufeld KJ, Yue J, Robinson TN, et al. Antipsychotic medication for prevention and treatment of delirium in hospitalized adults: A systematic review and meta-analysis. J Am Geriatr Soc 2016;64(10):2171–3, 705-714.

37. Nikooie R, Neufeld KJ, Oh ES, et al. Antipsychotics for treating delirium in hospitalized adults: A systematic review. Ann Intern Med 2019;171(7):485–95.

38. Oh ES, Needham DM, Nikooie R, et al. Antipsychotics for preventing delirium in hospitalized adults: A systematic review. Ann Intern Med 2019;171(7):474–84.

39. Traube C, Witcher R, Mendez-Rico E, et al. Quetiapine as treatment for delirium in critically ill children: A case series. J Pediatr Intensive Care 2013;2(3):121–6.

40. Capino AC, Thomas AN, Baylor S, et al. Antipsychotic use in the prevention and treatment of intensive care unit delirium in pediatric patients. J Pediatr Pharmacol Ther 2020;25(2):81–95.

41. Cronin MT, Di Gennaro JL, Watson RS, et al. Haloperidol and quetiapine for the treatment of ICU-associated delirium in a tertiary pediatric ICU: A propensity score-matched cohort study. Paediatr Drugs 2021;23(2):159–69.

42. Joyce C, Witcher R, Herrup E, et al. Evaluation of the safety of quetiapine in treating delirium in critically ill children: A retrospective review. J Child Adolesc Psychopharmacol 2015;25(9):666–70.

43. Sassano-Higgins S, Freudenberg N, Jacobson J, et al. Olanzapine reduces delirium symptoms in the critically ill pediatric patient. J Pediatr Intensive Care 2013;2(2):49–54.
44. Katz R, Kelly HW, Hsi A. Prospective study on the occurrence of withdrawal in critically ill children who receive fentanyl by continuous infusion. Crit Care Med 1994;22(5):763–7.
45. Franck LS, Vilardi J, Durand D, et al. Opioid withdrawal in neonates after continuous infusions of morphine or fentanyl during extracorporeal membrane oxygenation. Am J Crit Care 1998;7(5):364–9.
46. Tobias JD. Tolerance, withdrawal, and physical dependency after long-term sedation and analgesia of children in the pediatric intensive care unit. Crit Care Med 2000;28(6):2122–32.
47. Best KM, Boullata JI, Curley MA. Risk factors associated with iatrogenic opioid and benzodiazepine withdrawal in critically ill pediatric patients: a systematic review and conceptual model. Pediatr Crit Care Med 2015;16(2):175–83.
48. Franck LS, Scoppettuolo LA, Wypij D, et al. Validity and generalizability of the Withdrawal Assessment Tool-1 (WAT-1) for monitoring iatrogenic withdrawal syndrome in pediatric patients. Pain 2012;153(1):142–8.
49. Amirnovin R, Sanchez-Pinto LN, Okuhara C, et al. Implementation of a risk-stratified opioid and benzodiazepine weaning protocol in a pediatric cardiac ICU. Pediatr Crit Care Med 2018;19(11):1024–32.
50. Walters RA, Izquierdo M, Rodriguez JC, et al. Iatrogenic opiate withdrawal in pediatric patients: Implementation of a standardized methadone weaning protocol and withdrawal assessment tool. J Pharm Pract 2021;34(3):417–22.

COVID-19 in Children

Meena Kalyanaraman, MD[a],*, Michael R. Anderson, MD MBA[b,1]

KEYWORDS

- SARS-CoV-2 • COVID-19 • ARDS • MIS-C • Pediatric COVID • Risk factors
- Epidemiology

KEY POINTS

- Although children are less affected than adults with coronavirus disease 2019 (COVID-19), more than 5 million children in the United States have been infected and the overall public health implications of the pandemic on children are severe.
- Certain high-risk conditions make children more prone to severe disease.
- Children are admitted to the pediatric intensive care unit for severe acute COVID-19, which is severe acute respiratory syndrome coronavirus-2 (SARS-CoV-2) infection associated with 1 or more organ system involvement or multisystem inflammatory syndrome in children (MIS-C).
- Pediatric critical care physicians should be cognizant of complications from hyperinflammation in SARS-CoV-2 infections, management of COVID-19-associated acute respiratory failure, and special precautions to be taken during aerosol-generating procedures.
- Presentations of MIS-C can be like other diseases and might be especially hard to differentiate from Kawasaki disease.
- Diagnosis and treatment of MIS-C using available guidelines can result in favorable outcomes in critically ill children.

INTRODUCTION

The coronavirus disease 2019 (COVID-19) pandemic has wreaked havoc across the world, with an estimated 242,688,319 human infections and 4,932,928 deaths worldwide as of November of 2021.[1]

Children were first thought to be immune from infection, but the truth is a much more sobering tale of infections, hospitalizations, deaths, and long-term (long-haul) symptoms. This article outlines what is known about the epidemiology of COVID-19 infection in children to date. In addition, it discusses severe COVID-19 disease in children

---

[a] Pediatric Critical Care Medicine, Children's Hospital of New Jersey at Newark Beth Israel Medical Center, C-5, 201 Lyons Avenue, Newark, NJ 07112, USA; [b] Children's National Hospital, George Washington University School of Medicine and Health Sciences
[1] Present address: 1331 Maryland Ave SW, Washington DC 20021.
* Corresponding author.
E-mail address: Meena.Kalyanaraman@rwjbh.org

Pediatr Clin N Am 69 (2022) 547–571
https://doi.org/10.1016/j.pcl.2022.01.013
0031-3955/22/© 2022 Elsevier Inc. All rights reserved.

and addresses the public health toll the pandemic has exerted on children and issues that must be addressed with lessons learned to help prepare for the next pandemic.

Epidemiology and Early Pandemic Reports

Unlike many pediatric illnesses in which knowledge of epidemiology, clinical course, and outcomes are gathered over a long time, the COVID-19 pandemic saw a shift to fast-track publication of case reports, meta-analysis, and essential updates from both the private sector and government (eg, Centers for Disease Control and Prevention [CDC]/Morbidity and Mortality Weekly Report [MMWR]). At a time of a public health emergency, rapid publication of domestic and international experience must be balanced with academic and scientific rigor.

The first reports of pediatric COVID-19 illness emerged from the Shanghai Children's Medical Center in China in March 2020 with data from 2135 children with COVID-19 reported to the Chinese Center for Disease Control and Prevention.[2] The median age of children with COVID-19 was 7 years, and 56% were male. Although 51% of the patients were said to have mild symptoms, 38% had moderate symptoms (pneumonia and wheezing), and 6% had severe or critical clinical findings such as hypoxia and respiratory failure. Lu and colleagues[3] published a cohort analysis of 171 COVID-19–positive children from Wuhan Children's Hospital in April 2020. Seventy had fever, 12 had pneumonia, 3 required mechanical ventilation, and 1 died. Although these early reports showed that children had a less severe clinical course than adults, a small but concerning percentage of children progressed to respiratory failure.

The University of Texas–San Antonio and Texas Children's Hospital published a meta-analysis/case summary of children with COVID-19,[4] with 131 studies from 26 countries and 7780 children from January to May 2020 (**Table 1**). The median age was 8.9 years, and 75.6% were exposed to an adult with COVID-19. Need for intensive care unit (ICU) care was 3.3%, and length of hospital stay was 11.6 days. Approximately 35% had underlying medical conditions, with immunodeficiency being the most common at 30.5% (**Table 2**).

Table 1
Characteristics of children with COVID-19.

	# Studies	# Patients	N (%)
Male gender	113	4640	2582 (55.6)
Mean age (years)	116	4517	8.9 ± 0.5
Exposure from family member	94	1360	1028 (75.6)
Travel to/lived-in high-risk area	84	962	689(71.6)
Np/th roat SARS-CoV-2 detection	89	787	681(86.5)
Positive fecal viral shedding	31	321	67(20.9)
Positive urine viral shedding	22	54	2(3.7)
Length of hospital stay (days)	68	652	11.6 ± 0.3
Intensive care unit admission	88	3564	116(3.3)

Continuous data presented as Mean ± SD. NP-nasopharyngeal.

(Hoang, A., Chorath, K., Moreira, A., Evans, M., Burmeister-Morton, F., Burmeister, F., Naqvi, R., Petershack, M., & Moreira, A. (2020). COVID-19 in 7780 pediatric patients: A systematic review. EClinicalMedicine, 24, 100433. https://doi.org/10.1016/j.eclinm.2020.100433)

Table 2
Characteristics of children with COVID-19

	# Studies	# Patients	N (%)
Underlying conditions	*20*	*665*	*233(35.6)*
Immunosuppression			71(30.5)
Respiratory			49(21.0)
Cardiovascular			32(13.7)
Medically complex/congenital malformations			25(10.7)
Not reported			17(7.3)
Hematologic			8(3.8)
Neurologic			8(3.4)
Obesity			8(3.4)
Prematurity			5(3.4)
Endocrine/metabolic			5(2.1)
Renal			4(1.7)
Gastrointestinal			5(3.4)
Co-infections	*35*	*1183*	*72(5.6)*
Bacterial			
Mycoplasma pneumoniae			42(58.3)
Enterobacter sepsis			2(2.8)
Streptococcus pneumoniae Viral			1(1.4)
Influenza virus A/B			8(11.1)
Respiratory syncytial virus			7(9.7)
Cytomegalovirus			3(4.2)
Epstein-Barr virus			3(4.2)
Adenovirus			2(2.8)
Human metapneumovirus			2(2.8)
Human parainfluenza virus			2(2.8)

Children and Susceptibility to Severe Acute Respiratory Syndrome Coronavirus-2

Viner and colleagues[5] performed a meta-analysis on 13,926 published articles and summarized 32 studies with data from 41,460 children. Compared with data from 14 studies on adults with COVID-19, children had lower susceptibility to SARS-CoV-2 with a pooled odds ratio (OR) of 0.56 (95% confidence interval [CI], 0.37–0.85). Data regarding transmission of COVID-19 by children were inconclusive. Gaythorpe and colleagues[6] reviewed 128 studies to examine COVID-19 susceptibility and transmissibility in children and showed the OR of an asymptomatic child having an infection was 21.1% (95% CI, 14.0%–28.1%), and the proportion of children with severe disease was 3.8% (95% CI, 1.5%–6.0%). The investigators were not able to determine a child's ability to spread COVID-19.

UNITED STATES EXPERIENCE

An analysis of 12,306 children from the United States infected with COVID-19 from April to October 2020 examined symptoms and clinical course.[7] Symptoms included respiratory (16%), gastrointestinal (13.9%), rash (8.1%), and neurologic (4.8%).

Eighteen percent had nonspecific findings such as fever and malaise. Five percent required hospitalization, of whom 17.6% needed mechanical ventilation. Male and female children are equally affected, and risk of hospitalization is greater among non-Hispanic black and Hispanic children compared with non-Hispanic whites. Among hospitalized children, the rate of ICU admissions is similar to adults.[8]

PROGRESSION AND SEVERITY OF DISEASE

Graff and colleagues[9] reported on which children are at most significant risk for severe complications from COVID-19 infection. At the time, there were up to 1.3 million children infected with COVID-19 in the United States. This group examined the clinical course of children with the diagnosis of COVID-19 at their institutions from March to July 2020, where 454 children tested positive for SARS-CoV-2. The most frequent risk factor for COVID-19 exposure was a family member testing positive for SARS-CoV-2. Participation in social gatherings of 10 or more was a significant risk factor as well. Forty-five percent of the children with COVID-19 were identified with at least 1 comorbid condition: pulmonary (16%), gastrointestinal (11%), and neurologic (11%). Among the comorbid conditions, asthma, diabetes, and obesity were predictors of severe COVID-19 in children. Eighty-five were hospitalized, of whom 66 were symptomatic (the remaining 19 patients were admitted for other reasons and never had COVID symptoms). Of the 66 symptomatic patients, 55% required respiratory support, and 17% required critical care (**Fig. 1**). The need for hospitalization was associated with

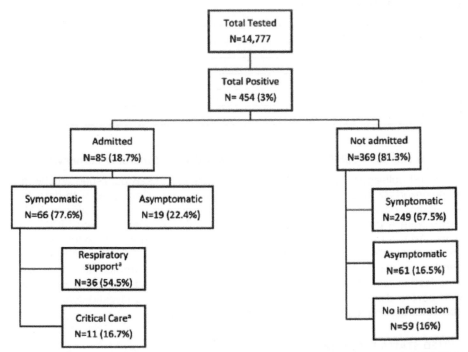

Fig. 1. Summary of children with positive COVID-19 test (Graff, K., Smith, C., Silveira, L., Jung, S., Curran-Hays, S., Jarjour, J., Carpenter, L., Pickard, K., Mattiucci, M., Fresia, J., McFarland, E. J., Dominguez, S. R., & Abuogi, L. (2021). Risk Factors for Severe COVID-19 in Children. Pediat)

younger age (0–3 months) and the presence of comorbidities. Requirement for respiratory support was associated with Hispanic ethnicity, age 0 to 3 months, obesity, and asthma. The need for critical care was associated with obstructive sleep apnea and increased C-reactive protein (CRP) level at the time of admission.

Investigators from the CDC examined disease severity in children admitted with COVID-19 from March to October 2020 using the Premier Health Care Database and identified 20,714 children with COVID-19, 2430 of whom were hospitalized.[10] Severe COVID-19 disease was associated with boys younger than 1 year, and the presence of comorbidity. There was no association between race/ethnicity and severe COVID-19.

THE DELTA VARIANT SURGE AND CHILDREN

The American Academy of Pediatrics and the Children's Hospital Association began publishing pediatric data weekly starting in the fall of 2020, indicating increasing numbers of children (<17 years old) with COVID-19 and hospitalization rates, especially during the Delta surge of 2021.[11]

As of October 2021, 5,899,148 children were reported to have COVID-19, representing 16.2% of US cases with an overall rate of 7838 cases per 100,000 children.

Compared with adults, the hospitalization rate for children with COVID-19 remained low until a spike in September 2021. Pediatric hospitalization rates varied between 1.3 and 3.2 per 100,000 children for ages 0 to 4 years and 0.8 to 1.4 for children 5 to 17 years.

Per Centers for Disease Control and Prevention Data

During a subsequent 6-week period after the Delta variant became predominant, COVID infection rates increased each week to 1.4 during the week ending August 14, 2021, which was 4.7 times the rate during the week ending June 26, 2021, and approached the peak hospitalization rate of 1.5 observed during the week ending January 9, 2021. Weekly rates increased among all age groups; the sharpest increase occurred among children aged 0 to 4 years, for whom the rate during the week ending August 14, 2021, (1.9) was nearly 10 times that during the week ending June 26, 2021 (0.2).

Although overall hospitalization rates remained lower in children compared with adults, 20% to 26.4% of hospitalized children required ICU care, and 9% to 12% of children required mechanical ventilation. The mortality from COVID-19 is low (for states reporting, 0%–0.26% of total COVID deaths were children.)

EFFECT OF COMMUNITY VACCINATION ON PEDIATRIC CORONAVIRUS DISEASE 2019

However, because of areas in the United States with low vaccination rates in adults, the Delta variant emerged in 2021 as the predominant strain of COVID-19 causing infection in children. In addition, because children less than 12 years were ineligible to receive any of the emergency use approval (EUA) vaccines in early 2021, and the refusal to wear masks and adhere to social distancing recommendations, the number of children with COVID-19 infections increased, and they were 1.5 to 3 times more likely to require emergency care for COVID-19.[12]

Clinics Care Points

- Despite lower overall hospitalization rates for COVID-19 in children, the rate of ICU admissions among hospitalized children is similar to adults.

- Intensivists should be aware of underlying conditions that can put children at risk for severe COVID-19.
- Hospitalization rates for children have increased since the start of the pandemic, especially during the Delta surge of 2021.
- Efficacy studies for vaccines in children and vaccination recommendations for children are underway.

PATHOGENESIS

Transmission of SARS-CoV-2 is primarily through airborne droplets and to a lesser extent from contaminated surfaces, and rarely through body fluids. The virus can transmit over long distances, especially when indoors. Incubation period is 3 to 6 days. The entry into host cells is mediated by its spike glycoprotein (S-glycoprotein) binding to the ACE2 cellular receptor in the upper respiratory tract to begin primary replication.[13] Patients can be asymptomatic carriers or have mild symptoms at this stage. Viral load is increased in the first week, followed by a progressive decline in 7 to 10 days with increase in immunoglobulin (Ig) M and IgG antibodies against viral antigens. The persistence of high viral load leads to migration of virus in the airway with entry into alveolar epithelial cells, where it replicates, causing localized inflammation and pneumonia. Cell apoptosis occurs, with increased capillary permeability and release of proinflammatory proteins. Cytokine storm can ensue with release of inflammatory markers such as interleukin (IL)-2/6/7/10, granulocyte colony-stimulating factor, interferon gamma-induced protein 10 (IP-10), macrophage chemoattractant protein-1 (MCP-1), macrophage inflammatory protein-1 (MIP-1), and tumor necrosis factor-α (TNF-α), which can cause acute respiratory distress syndrome (ARDS), septic shock, and multiorgan dysfunction.[14]

CORONAVIRUS DISEASE 2019 IN CRITICALLY ILL CHILDREN

Children with COVID-19 are admitted to the PICU because of severe acute COVID-19 illness, which is SARS-CoV-2 infection with 1 or more organ system involvement or COVID-19-associated multisystem inflammatory syndrome in children (MIS-C).

SEVERE ACUTE CORONAVIRUS DISEASE 2019

Children with severe acute COVID-19 are admitted to the PICU for respiratory problems such as pneumonia and ARDS. Cardiovascular, gastrointestinal, neurologic, hematologic, and acute kidney injury (AKI) complications can result from severe acute COVID-19. Risk factors for severe acute COVID-19 are the presence of 1 or more underlying conditions such as obesity, chronic pulmonary disease, neurologic disease, cardiovascular disease, medical complexity and technology dependence, sickle cell disease, or immunosuppresion.[15–19] Underlying chronic respiratory diseases such as asthma and cystic fibrosis were not significantly exacerbated by SARS-CoV-2.[19] Younger age, obesity, hypoxia on admission, increased white blood cell count, and bilateral infiltrates on chest radiograph are predictors of severe respiratory disease.[20]

DIAGNOSIS
Laboratory Tests

Detection of SARS-CoV-2 nucleic acid using real-time reverse transcriptase-polymerase chain reaction (RT-PCR) is considered the gold-standard for the diagnosis of COVID-19.[21] The virus can be detected in the upper airway (nasopharynx swab) or lower airway secretions (tracheal aspirates, bronchoalveolar lavage), blood, urine, and stool. Leukocytosis or leukopenia, lymphocytosis or lymphopenia, and increases of CRP, serum ferritin, lactate dehydrogenase (LDH), D-dimers, procalcitonin, erythrocyte sedimentation rate (ESR), serum aminotransferases, and creatine kinase-myocardial bands (CK-MB) have been observed.[22,23] Increases of CRP, procalcitonin, pro–B-type natriuretic peptide (BNP) and platelet count are more common in children requiring PICU admission compared with other hospitalized patients.[24] Organ dysfunction was associated with increased CRP, increased white blood cell count, and thrombocytopenia.[25]

Hyperinflammation associated with increased LDH, D-dimer, IL-6, CRP, and ferritin, and decreased lymphocyte count, platelet count, and albumin level were associated with worse outcomes in adult patients with COVID-19.[26]

Imaging Studies

Chest radiography is routinely performed in most children hospitalized for acute respiratory failure from COVID-19. Although chest radiographs do not have high sensitivity and specificity for the diagnosis of COVID-19, they are useful to monitor disease progression. Bilateral distribution with presence of peripheral or subpleural ground-glass opacifications and consolidation are common findings in COVID-19 pneumonia or ARDS (**Fig. 2**). Typical features of viral respiratory infections in children, such as increased perihilar markings and hyperinflation, were not reported in children with COVID-19.[27,28]

Computed tomography (CT) scans are considered the gold standard for imaging with COVID-19 respiratory disease.[29] CT scans are highly sensitive and specific and can detect infection before the appearance of clinical signs.[29,30] Three phases of evolution have been observed in children with COVID-19 disease. These phases are the halo sign, defined as nodules or masses surrounded by ground-glass opacifications seen in the early phase of the disease; widespread ground-glass opacifications in the progressive phase; and consolidative opacities in the developed phase. Peribronchial thickening and inflammation along the bronchovascular bundle are observed more frequently in children than adults.[31] Fine mesh reticulations and so-called crazy-paving sign have been reported. Pleural effusion and lymphadenopathy are rare.[31] Compared with adults, children were found to have less positive CT findings, lower number of pulmonary lobes involved, and lower overall semiquantitative lung

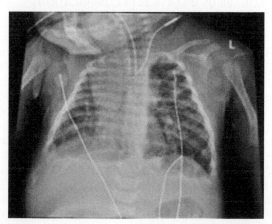

Fig. 2. Chest radiograph of infant with bronchopulmonary dysplasia who developed COVID-19 ARDS showing bilateral ground-glass opacities.

score, which measures the extent of lung involvement.[31] Because of these findings and concerns for radiation exposure, transport of unstable patients to CT suites, and infection control issues, chest CT is not recommended as the initial diagnostic test in children suspected of having COVID-19. However, it may be considered to answer specific clinical questions such as presence of pulmonary embolism, for assessment of those not responding to treatment, and to track evolution of fibrotic disease. Lung ultrasonography is a useful imaging modality because semiquantitative scores in lung ultrasonography have been shown to be consistent with those in lung CT scans in adults who are critically ill with COVID-19, and should be considered in children.[30,32]

Recommendations for Diagnostic Tests in Severe Acute Coronavirus Disease 2019

Laboratory tests: SARS-CoV-2 RT-PCR, COVID-19 IgG, complete blood count (CBC), complete metabolic panel (CMP), LDH, CRP, procalcitonin, ESR, prothrombin time (PT), partial thromboplastin time (PTT), D-dimer, troponin, and BNP. Ferritin, and cytokine panel when available, provide additional information about the hyperinflammatory state.

Cardiac evaluation: baseline electrocardiogram (ECG) should be obtained in all patients, and those with abnormal troponin should undergo echocardiography.

Imaging studies: chest radiograph in all patients, and CT scan if pulmonary embolism is suspected.

Clinics Care Points

- Severe acute COVID-19, which is SARS-CoV-2 infection with 1 or more organ system involvement, requires PICU admission.
- Pediatric intensivists should be familiar with MIS-C and its complications.
- The gold standard for diagnosis of COVID-19 is detection of SARS-CoV-2 nucleic acid using RT-PCR.
- Hyperinflammation plays a major role in pathogenesis of SARS-CoV-2 and complications of severe acute COVID-19.
- Intensivists should be familiar with chest radiograph changes in severe acute COVID-19, and chest CT should be considered only in those patients in whom pulmonary embolism is a concern.

SEVERE ACUTE CORONAVIRUS DISEASE 2019 COMPLICATIONS
Acute Respiratory Failure

Clinical features: SARS-CoV-2 pneumonia can cause acute respiratory failure and progress to ARDS. Diagnostic criteria for COVID-19 ARDS are the same as for pediatric ARDS (PARDS) from other causes. Patients typically have worsening respiratory symptoms 1 week after disease onset, new opacities on chest imaging that are not caused by cardiac failure or volume overload, partial pressure of oxygen (Pao_2) to fraction of inspired oxygen (Fio_2) ratio less than or equal to 300 mm Hg or oxygen saturation by pulse oximetry/Fio_2 less than or equal to 264 during noninvasive ventilation, oxygenation index (OI) greater than or equal to 4, or oxygen saturation index (OSI) greater than or equal to 5 during invasive mechanical ventilation. Mild, moderate, and severe PARDS are defined as OI/OSI of 4 to 8 or 5 to 7.5, 8 to 16 or 7.5 to 12.3, and greater than 16 or greater than 12.3 respectively.[33]

Pathologic changes in these patients are like PARDS from other causes with initial diffuse alveolar damage and fibrosis with disease progression. Differences have been noted in adults between ARDS from COVID-19 compared with ARDS from other causes, including phenotypic subtypes such as type L, characterized by low elastance with preserved compliance, and type H, characterized by high elastance with low compliance, and increased association with thrombosis.[34] Studies in children have not shown significant differences in compliance between PARDS from COVID-19 and other causes.

Management

General principles of management

Management of COVID-19–associated acute respiratory failure is outlined in **Fig. 3**. The principles of management and end goals of respiratory therapy are the same as for other causes of acute respiratory failure in children.[33,35,36] Patients who have SpO_2 less than 90% need supplemental oxygen, noninvasive ventilation, or intubation and mechanical ventilation based on severity. Intubation protocols with special precautions for patients with COVID-19 should be developed based on resources available.[37,38] Ventilator strategies as outlined in **Fig. 3** help in the management of COVID-19 PARDS, and ARDSNet protocols for positive end-expiratory pressure (PEEP)/Fio_2 may be followed. In a retrospective study in children before the COVID-19 pandemic, use of lower PEEP relative to Fio_2 than what is recommended by the ARDSNet model resulted in higher mortality.[38–40] In addition to recommendations in **Fig. 3**, intravascular volume expansion should be avoided in patients without hypotension. Adequate mean arterial pressure should be maintained, and inotropic support provided as

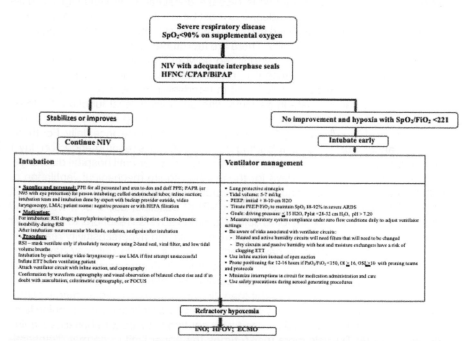

Fig. 3. Management of acute respiratory failure in severe COVID-19. BiPAP, bilevel positive airway pressure; CPAP, continuous positive airway pressure; ETT, endotracheal tube; HEPA, high-efficiency particulate air filter; HFNC, high-flow nasal cannula; LMA, laryngeal mask airway; NIV, noninvasive ventilation; PAPR, powered air purifying respirator; PEEP, positive end-expiratory pressure; POCUS, point-of-care ultrasonography; PPE, personal protective equipment; Pplat, plateau pressure; RSI, rapid sequence intubation; Spo_2, oxygen saturation by pulse oximetry.

needed, and nutritional support must be adequate.[38,41] Patients who have refractory hypoxemia may need treatment such as inhaled nitric oxide, high-frequency oscillatory ventilation, or extracorporeal membrane oxygenation (ECMO) as recommended in the management of PARDS from other causes.

COVID-19–specific management

1. Rapid spread of infection from SARS-CoV-2 can occur during various aerosol-generating procedures (AGPs). Appropriate personal protection equipment (PPE) should be used by all staff and visitors. Special precautions should be taken to minimize spread during AGP, such as coughing and sneezing, use of noninvasive ventilation including high-flow nasal cannula, bag-mask ventilation, intubation, tracheal suction, planned or accidental extubation, chest physiotherapy, cardiopulmonary resuscitation, and use of nebulized medications outside of a closed circuit.[38]

2. Antiviral therapy: remdesivir is an antiviral medication that is an inhibitor of the SARS-CoV-2 RNA-dependent RNA polymerase (RdRp), which is essential for viral replication. Remdesivir is approved by the US Food and Drug Administration (FDA) for treatment of patients greater than or equal to 12 year old hospitalized with COVID-19 who weigh greater than or equal to 40 kg, and is FDA authorized via EUA for use in hospitalized patients less than 12 years of age or weighing from 3.5 to less than 40 kg.[42,43] In neonates less than 3.5 kg, use should be directed by recommendations from infectious disease consultants on weighing the risks versus benefits. Intravenous remdesivir is most beneficial if used early in the course of illness (<10 days) and has been shown to reduce symptom duration in adults but does not seem to reduce mortality. There are few studies in children, but remdesivir seems to be well tolerated.[44,45] Lyophilized powder formulation should be used in children less than 40 kg because it contains half the amount of sulfobutylether-β-cyclodextrin sodium salt, an excipient in remdesivir that is cleared through the kidneys and can accumulate in patients with decreased renal function. Children weighing greater than or equal to 3.5 kg and less than 40 kg should receive a loading dose of 5 mg/kg on day 1 followed by 2.5 mg/kg/dose once daily. For those greater than or equal to 40 kg, a loading dose of 200 mg is recommended on day 1 followed by 100 mg daily. Duration of therapy is 5 days or until hospital discharge, whichever is earlier, and 10 days for those who require mechanical ventilation or ECMO. Laboratory monitoring during remdesivir therapy should include CBC, CMP, PT/International Normalized Ratio (INR) at baseline, day 5 of therapy, and more often if there is concern for toxicity. Common adverse reactions to remdesivir include reversible increases of transaminase levels and hypersensitivity reactions. Bradycardia and hypotension have been reported in adults but may have been related to concomitant use of other medications.[46] Contraindications to its use are hypersensitivity to remdesivir or any component of the formulation. Remdesivir is not recommended in children older than 28 days with estimated glomerular filtration rate less than 30 mL/min, and in full-term neonates with serum creatinine level 1 mg/dL or greater and should be used with caution in those with baseline alanine transaminase (ALT) levels more than 5 times the upper limit of normal. Transaminase levels might be increased because of COVID-19 and, if remdesivir is used, it should be discontinued if ALT levels increase to more than 10 times the upper limit of normal or if ALT increase is accompanied by signs or symptoms of liver inflammation. Dose adjustments are needed for those on ECMO or renal replacement therapy (RRT) because of interactions between remdesivir and the circuits, which can cause significant changes in the pharmacokinetics of the drug.

3. Antiinflammatory therapy: dexamethasone is recommended for hospitalized children with COVID-19 who require high-flow oxygen, noninvasive ventilation, invasive mechanical ventilation, or ECMO.[47] The dexamethasone dosing regimen for children is 0.15 mg/kg/dose (maximum dose, 6 mg) once daily for up to 10 days. Steroids should be used with caution because there are reports of increased mortality and decreased viral clearance with certain viral infections and development of neuropathy and myopathy in critically ill patients. However, dexamethasone significantly reduces mortality in adult patients with COVID-19 who require mechanical ventilation and is recommended for treatment of children with severe acute COVID-19 disease.[48–50] Patients with exacerbation of asthma with COVID-19 should receive methylprednisolone and those with adrenal insufficiency and catecholamine-resistant refractory shock should receive hydrocortisone in doses recommended for such conditions.

4. Immunomodulator therapy: IL-1 receptor antagonist such as anakinra should be considered in children for whom corticosteroids is contraindicated, who are refractory to corticosteroids, or who have severe acute COVID-19 causing ARDS, shock, or signs of significant hyperinflammation.[50] Dosing guidelines as mentioned in relation to MIS-C treatment may be followed.

5. Other specific treatments, such as monoclonal antibodies, convalescent plasma, and IL-6 inhibitors, are not recommended in critically ill children.[50]

Sepsis and Septic Shock

Manifestations are like those resulting from other infections, and recommendations of the 2020 Surviving Sepsis Campaign should be followed.[51]

Acute Kidney Injury

Presentation and management are the same as for any critically ill patient developing AKI. The hypercoagulable state in COVID-19 can cause clotting of filters used in RRT and can be prevented with the addition of prefilter heparin and/or citrate.[52]

Neurologic Complications

Meningitis, encephalitis, acute disseminated encephalomyelitis, Guillain-Barré syndrome, myositis, acute necrotizing hemorrhagic encephalopathy, seizures, and cerebrovascular disease from hypercoagulable state have all been reported in severe acute COVID-19.[53] Diagnosis and management are the same as when these complications arise from other causes.

Hypercoagulable State

COVID-19 induces a prothrombotic state from hyperactivation of the inflammatory and hemostatic pathways.[54] Thrombotic complications in adults with COVID-19 is well recognized but are rare in children with COVID-19 and, when they occur, are usually in the lungs.[55] Serum D-dimer levels are used to assess for hypercoagulation, and a daily screen of D-dimer, PT, and platelet count is recommended.[38] When not contraindicated, pharmacologic thromboprophylaxis combined with mechanical thromboprophylaxis with sequential compression devices is recommended. Anticoagulant thromboprophylaxis with low-molecular-weight heparin is recommended in patients who have increased D-dimer levels or clinical risk factors for venous thromboembolism. Children who are at high risk for venous thromboembolism include those who are critically ill, with a history of thromboembolism, or those who have increased inflammatory markers (CRP>150 mg/L, D-dimer>1500 ng/mL, IL-6>100pg/mL, ferritin>500 ng/mL), and should be treated with subcutaneous low-molecular weight-heparin (<2 months, 1.5 mg/kg/dose every 12 hours; ≥2 months, 1 mg/kg/dose every 12 hours) to achieve anti-Xa factor levels of 0.5 to 1 IU/mL.[56] Children who are clinically unstable or have severe renal impairment should receive continuous intravenous infusion of unfractionated heparin as anticoagulant thromboprophylaxis using pediatric heparin nomogram to guide therapy.[57,58]

Myocarditis

Patients with MIS-C commonly have myocarditis, and, occasionally, in severe acute COVID-19. Presentation and management are the same as for myocarditis from other infections.

Clinics Care Points

- Pathophysiology and diagnosis of PARDS from COVID-19 is the same as for PARDS from other causes.
- Intensivists must be familiar with additional precautions to be taken during intubation and AGPs.
- Intensivists should know ventilator strategies and therapies used specifically in COVID-19 acute respiratory failure, including antiviral, antiinflammatory, and immunomodulator therapies.
- Multiorgan dysfunction and failure from severe acute COVID-19 should be recognized and treated.
- COVID-19 induces a prothrombotic state, and thrombotic complications in severe acute COVID-19 should be diagnosed and treated and thromboprophylaxis instituted in children at high risk for venous thromboembolism.
- A multidisciplinary approach should be instituted to minimize spread of the virus within critical care units while still providing excellent patient care.

Coronavirus Disease 2019-associated Multisystem Inflammatory Syndrome in Children

The diagnosis of MIS-C is usually made weeks after a child is infected with SARS-CoV-2, and almost all patients are positive for SARS-CoV-2 either by RT-PCR, SARS-CoV-2 antibody testing, or both, whereas the rest have a history of contact with someone with COVID-19.[59–61] The CDC, World Health Organization, and Royal College of Pediatrics and Child Health provided definitions of MIS-C from SARS-CoV-2 infection.[62–64] All 3 definitions have many similarities but the CDC definition is the most widely used in North America.

DEFINITION
Centers for Disease Control and Prevention Definition of Multisystem Inflammatory Syndrome in Children

- An individual less than 21 years old presenting with fever, laboratory evidence of inflammation, and evidence of clinically severe illness requiring hospitalization, with multisystem (≥2) organ involvement (cardiac, renal, respiratory, hematologic, gastrointestinal, dermatologic, or neurologic); and
- No alternative plausible diagnoses; and
- Positive for current or recent SARS-CoV-2 infection by RT-PCR, serology, or antigen test; or exposure to a suspected or confirmed COVID-19 case within the 4 weeks before the onset of symptoms.

Fever here is defined as greater than or equal to 38.0°C for greater than or equal to 24 hours, or report of subjective fever lasting greater than or equal to 24 hours.

Evidence of inflammation includes, but is not limited to, 1 or more of the following: increased CRP, fibrinogen, procalcitonin, D-dimer, ferritin, LDH, IL-6, or neutrophil levels; increased ESR; reduced lymphocyte levels; and low albumin levels.

The CDC suggests that some individuals may fulfill full or partial criteria for Kawasaki disease (KD) but should be reported if they meet the case definition for MIS-C, and to consider MIS-C in any child who dies with evidence of SARS-CoV-2 infection.

CLINICAL FEATURES

Patients with MIS-C usually present with persistent fever, cardiorespiratory and gastrointestinal symptoms, mucocutaneous lesions, and, in severe cases, hypotension, and shock. Cardiac, cardiorespiratory, and gastrointestinal complications are the most common reasons for PICU admission. Belay and colleagues[60] reported illness involving at least 4 organ systems in almost 90% of cases in a cohort of 1733 patients. Children with MIS-C have required intensive care more than those with severe acute COVID-19, and intensivists should be cognizant of the similarities and differences between MIS-C and severe acute COVID-19.[20,60,61] Children with MIS-C are often male and previously healthy, whereas severe acute COVID-19 is more common in children with existing risk factors with no gender predilection. Large studies from United States and United Kingdom have shown that MIS-C and severe acute COVID-19 are both more common in African American, Hispanic, and Asian children compared with white children. Mortality in hospitalized children is less than 2%.[60,61,65,66] Differences have been observed between the occurrence of MIS-C and severe acute COVID-19 among various age groups. Severe acute COVID-19 rates are higher in children 0 to 5 years and 13 to 20 years of age, whereas MIS-C is higher in the 6- year to 12-year age group.[61] MIS-C has been associated with more severe outcomes in children older than 5 years, whereas severe acute COVID-19 is associated with worse outcomes in children less than 1 year of age.[67,68] Higher values of D-dimer, CRP, and ferritin, and lower platelet and absolute lymphocyte count have been shown to be predictive of severe MIS-C. Higher neutrophil to lymphocyte ratio, higher CRP, and lower platelet count have been observed in MIS-C compared with COVID-19.[61] Mucocutaneous signs and symptoms on presentation are seen in almost two-thirds of patients with MIS-C, but only in 10% of patients with COVID-19.[61]

Abdominal pain and vomiting can occur in 60% of patients with MIS-C and can be of such severity as to be mistaken for acute appendicitis.[60] The possibility of MIS-C coexisting with acute appendicitis should be considered.[69,70] Patients with severe acute COVID-19 can present with gastrointestinal symptoms but these are usually not as severe as those seen in patients with MIS-C. Feldstein and colleagues[61] reported gastrointestinal symptoms on presentation in 90% of patients with MIS-C compared with 58% of patients with severe acute COVID-19. Abdominal imaging in patients with MIS-C have demonstrated inflammation, including mesenteric adenopathy, mesenteric edema, ascites, bowel wall thickening, and gallbladder wall thickening (Fig. 4).

Cardiorespiratory involvement and the need for vasoactive agents were observed in 56%, 67%, and 45% respectively in patients with MIS-C compared with 9%, 12%, and 9% respectively in patients with severe acute COVID-19 in a case series of 1116 patients studied by Feldstein and colleagues.[61] Belay and colleagues[60] reported hypotension (51%), shock (37%), cardiac dysfunction (31%), and myocarditis (17%) in the largest cohort of patients with MIS-C reported thus far. Mucocutaneous lesions and conjunctival injection and laboratory markers of BNP and IL-6 were associated with coronary artery abnormalities.[61,67] The incidence of coronary artery dilatation

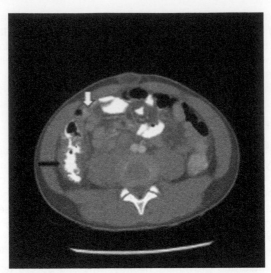

Fig. 4. Abdominal CT of 11-year-old African-American male with MIS-C who presented with fever, mucocutaneous symptoms, severe abdominal pain, vomiting, and CoV-2 antibody (Ab) IgG+. Bowel wall thickening of ascending colon (*black arrow*) with several enlarged lymph nodes (*white arrow*).

and aneurysms (CAA) in MIS-C is 4% to 24%.[60,61,71–73] In patients with KD, the risk of coronary artery thrombosis is directly related to size of CAA and increases exponentially at z-scores of more than 10.[74,75] Depressed left ventricular (LV) function has been noted in a third of patients.[60,61] Similar to patients with other causes of poor cardiac function, children with MIS-C or severe acute COVID-19 with LV dysfunction are at risk for intracardiac thrombosis.[76] Knowledge of duration of persistence of abnormalities in inflammatory markers, troponin, D-dimer, LV dysfunction, and CAA is limited because of lack of consistent follow-up protocols and patient compliance. In the small number of children seen in follow-up so far, most of the abnormalities return to normal.[61,77]

Respiratory complications in MIS-C can be like those seen in severe acute COVID-19 with some differences. Lower respiratory infection was reported in 17% of patients with MIS-C compared with 36% of patients with severe acute COVID-19. Severe respiratory disease without cardiovascular involvement was observed in 24% of MIS-C compared with 71% of patients with severe acute COVID-19 in the study by Feldstein and colleagues.[61] However, patients with MIS-C had a greater need for noninvasive and invasive ventilation (36% and 18%) compared with those with severe acute COVID-19 (33% and 15%). This finding may be related to higher prevalence of cardiorespiratory complications in patients with MIS-C. Radiographic abnormalities in MIS-C with cardiorespiratory complications include pleural effusions and bilateral pulmonary consolidation with lower zone predominance (**Figs. 5** and **6**). Pleural effusions are rarely reported in patients with severe acute COVID-19.[78] Depressed myocardial function, shock, need for aggressive intravascular volume expansion, severe systemic inflammation, and hypoalbuminemia are seen more often in patients with MIS-C compared with those with severe acute COVID-19, likely contributing to third spacing and pleural effusion in patients with MIS-C.

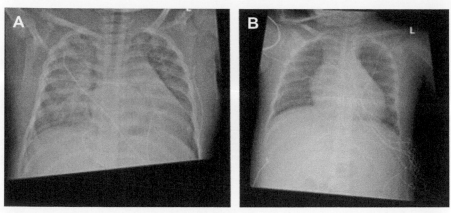

Fig. 5. Chest radiographs of a 5-year-old Hispanic male with MIS-C who presented with fever; cardiorespiratory, mucocutaneous, and abdominal symptoms; hypoalbuminemia; positive for SARS-CoV-2 RT-PCR and CoV-2 IgG Ab. (*A*) On presentation, when he had moderately decreased LV systolic function and required BiPAP. (*B*) Three days after presentation, with normal biventricular systolic function and resolution of respiratory symptoms, hypoalbuminemia, and fever.

DIAGNOSIS

The diagnostic pathway for MIS-C recommended by the American College of Rheumatology is a clinically useful tool.[50] The tier 1 and tier 2 evaluations shown in **Fig. 7** are a comprehensive list of tests for evaluation of MIS-C. Recommendations for laboratory studies for patients in the ICU include daily CBC, basic metabolic panel, and D-dimer; troponin every 6 hours; and BNP every 48 hours, and are adjusted in frequency based on clinical condition. Recommendations for monitoring of cardiac complications in MIS-C in addition to those listed in tier 2 include the following: (1) ECG every 48 hours in hospitalized patients or more frequently for those with conduction abnormalities and again at follow-up. (2) Echocardiogram repeated at 1 to 2 weeks

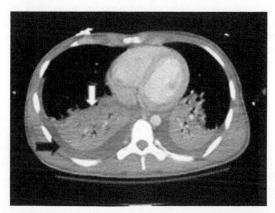

Fig. 6. Chest CT of an 18-year-old African-American male with MIS-C who presented with fever, shock with LV dysfunction requiring inotropic/vasoactive medication, pneumonia, mucocutaneous symptoms, hypoalbuminemia, CoV-2 Ab IgG+, requiring BiPAP with pleural effusion (*black arrow*) and bilateral lower lobe consolidation (*white arrow*).

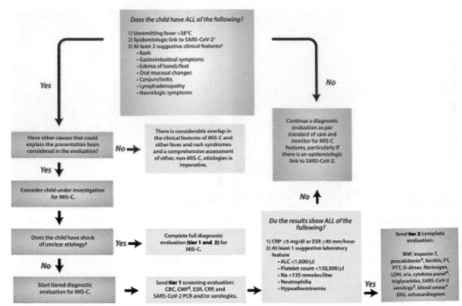

Fig. 7. Diagnostic pathway for MIS-C. Moderate to high consensus was reached by the task force in the development of this diagnostic pathway for MIS-C associated with SARS-CoV-2. [a]An epidemiologic link to SARS-CoV-2 infection is defined as a child with any of the following criteria: positive for SARS-CoV-2 by polymerase chain reaction (PCR), positive for SARS-CoV-2 by serology, preceding illness resembling COVID-19, or close contact with an individual with confirmed or suspected COVID-19 in the past 4 weeks. [b]Suggestive clinical features include rash (polymorphic, maculopapular, or petechial, but not vesicular), gastrointestinal symptoms (diarrhea, abdominal pain, or vomiting), oral mucosal changes (red and/or cracked lips, strawberry tongue, or erythema of the oropharyngeal mucosa), conjunctivitis (bilateral conjunctival infection without exudate), and neurologic symptoms (altered mental status, encephalopathy, focal neurologic deficits, meningismus, or papilledema). [c]The CMP includes measurement of sodium, potassium, carbon dioxide, chloride, blood urea nitrogen, creatinine, glucose, calcium, albumin, total protein, aspartate aminotransferase, alanine aminotransferase, alkaline phosphatase, and bilirubin. [d]Procalcitonin, cytokine panel, and blood smear test results should be sent, if available. [e]Serologic test results should be sent if not sent in tier 1 evaluation, and if possible, SARS-CoV-2 IgG, IgM, and IgA test results should be sent. ALC, absolute lymphocyte count; u/a, urinalysis. (*With permission* from Henderson LA, et al. Arthritis & Rheumatology, Volume: 73, Issue: 4, Pages: e13-e29, First published: 05 December 2020, DOI: (10.1002/art.41616).

and 4 to 6 weeks after initial presentation. Patients with LV dysfunction and coronary artery aneurysm require more frequent echocardiography. (3) Cardiac MRI 2 to 6 months after the acute illness to assess for myocardial fibrosis and scarring.

Patients who do not meet all the criteria for diagnosis of MIS-C should be evaluated for diseases with similar presentations, such as KD, toxic shock syndrome, or hemophagocytic lymphohistiocytosis.

MANAGEMENT

Treatment should be directed at supportive care of multiorgan dysfunction and mitigation of the underlying inflammatory process. The treatment of MIS-C as recommended by the American College of Rheumatology is outlined in **Fig. 8**.[50]

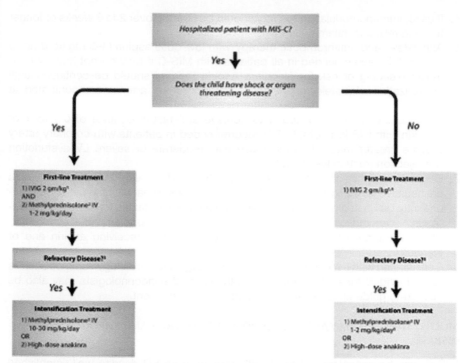

Fig. 8. Algorithm for initial immunomodulatory treatment of MIS-C. Moderate to high consensus was reached by the task force in the development of this treatment algorithm for MIS-C associated with SARS-CoV-2. [a]Intravenous immunoglobulin (IVIG) dosing is 2 g/kg based on ideal body weight. Cardiac function and fluid status should be assessed before IVIG is given. In some patients with cardiac dysfunction, IVIG may be given in divided doses (1 g/kg daily over 2 days). [b]Methylprednisolone or another steroid at equivalent dosing may be used. [c]Refractory disease is defined as persistent fevers and/or ongoing and significant end-organ involvement. [d]Low-dose to moderate-dose glucocorticoids (methylprednisolone 1–2 mg/kg/d) may be considered for first-line therapy in some MIS-C patients with concerning features (ill appearance, highly increased B-type natriuretic peptide levels, unexplained tachycardia) who have not yet developed shock or organ-threatening disease. [e]If the patient was given low-dose to moderate-dose glucocorticoids as first-line therapy, methylprednisolone IV dosing should be 10 to 30 mg/kg/d for intensification treatment. (*With permission* from Henderson LA, et al. Arthritis & Rheumatology, Volume: 73, Issue: 4, Pages: e13-e29, First published: 05 December 2020, DOI: (10.1002/art.41616).

Additional treatment guidelines:

1. Initial treatment with intravenous immunoglobulin (IVIG) and glucocorticoids is associated with lower risk of LV dysfunction and shock, and decreased need for adjunctive therapy compared with IVIG alone.[79]
2. Anakinra 1 to 2 mg/kg/d should be considered in patients in whom corticosteroids are contraindicated.
3. High-dose anakinra, greater than 4 mg/kg/d, is recommended for those refractory to treatment with IVIG with or without steroids. In some cases, anakinra as high as 10 mg/kg/d (maximum 100 mg/dose) through subcutaneous or intravenous routes divided every 6 to 12 hours may be needed. If the patient does not show improvement with this regimen, the diagnosis of MIS-C should be reconsidered.

4. If used, immunomodulation therapy should be tapered over 2 to 3 weeks or longer to avoid rebound inflammation.
5. Antiplatelet and antithrombotic therapy with low-dose aspirin (3–5 mg/kg/d up to 81 mg/d) is recommended in all patients with MIS-C if they do not have uncontrolled bleeding or risk for bleeding. Aspirin therapy should be continued until normalization of platelet count and normal coronary arteries are confirmed at greater than or equal to 4 weeks after diagnosis.
6. Anticoagulation with enoxaparin to achieve anti–factor Xa level of 0.5 to 1 or warfarin with INR level of 2 to 3 is recommended in patients with coronary artery Z-score greater than 10 and in those with moderate or severe LV dysfunction with ejection fraction less than 35%.
7. Empiric antibiotics should be used in all patients with severe MIS-C until cultures are negative for 48 hours or as directed by infectious disease consultants. Ceftriaxone may be used alone or in combination with metronidazole for possible appendicitis or vancomycin/clindamycin for those with possible toxic shock syndrome.
8. Stress ulcer prophylaxis is recommended in patients receiving aspirin and or steroids.
9. Consultation with infectious disease, immunology, and cardiology subspecialists is recommended for all patients. Hematologists and endocrinologists may also be needed to guide anticoagulation and steroid management.

MULTISYSTEM INFLAMMATORY SYNDROME IN CHILDREN AND KAWASAKI DISEASE

MIS-C may be especially difficult to differentiate from KD despite well-established diagnostic criteria.[62,80] The following are differences between MIS-C and KD:

1. MIS-C is common among black and Hispanic children, whereas incidence of KD is highest in children of Asian descent.
2. MIS-C is reported in children aged from 3 months to 20 years, with those older than 5 years more severely affected, whereas KD is usually seen in children less than 5 years of age.
3. Patients with MIS-C frequently need PICU admission, whereas patients with KD rarely do.
4. Increased serum ferritin, leukopenia, lymphopenia, and thrombocytopenia are common in MIS-C. Thrombocytosis is a characteristic feature of KD.
5. Myocarditis, LV cardiac dysfunction, shock, the need for intravascular fluid expansion, and vasopressor/inotropic support is more common in MIS-C.
6. Coronary artery dilatations and aneurysms are reported in 4% to 24% of children with MIS-C. The progression and long-term sequelae are not known at this time. In the pre-IVIG era, CAA occurred in 20% to 25% of children with KD.[81] With IVIG therapy, persistent CAAs are much less common, but are still noted in 4% to 6% of patients, with approximately 1% developing giant CAA despite treatment.[82,83]
7. Respiratory and cardiorespiratory complications requiring noninvasive or invasive ventilation are more common in children with MIS-C.
8. Gastrointestinal and neurologic complications and coagulopathy are more common in MIS-C.
9. IVIG and moderate-dose to high-dose aspirin are the established recommended treatment of KD.[84] In addition to IVIG and aspirin, steroids and biologic drugs are frequently used in patients with MIS-C.[50]
10. Most children with KD have a good prognosis, whereas the long-term clinical outcomes of MIS-C are not clear.

Clinics Care Points

- Intensivists should be familiar with the CDC definition of MIS-C and various clinical presentations of MIS-C.
- Intensivists should know the differences in clinical manifestations of severe acute COVID-19 and MIS-C.
- Algorithms for diagnosis and management of MIS-C should be followed.
- Intensivists should be aware of the cardiorespiratory, cardiac, and gastrointestinal complications of MIS-C, their presentation, and management.
- Intensivists should be familiar with the differential diagnosis for MIS-C and especially its differentiation from KD.

UNIQUE PEDIATRIC INTENSIVE CARE UNIT CARE ISSUES RELATED TO THE PANDEMIC

The SARS-CoV-2 pandemic has demanded unprecedented and rapid adaptation of all personnel involved in the care of critically ill children. Surges of this pandemic, which caused acute shortage of ICU beds worldwide, resulted in many PICU teams providing care for adults with COVID-19 in addition to children with severe acute COVID-19.[85,86] Hospitals must develop protocols for implementation in their critical care units based on their needs and resources, with emphasis on minimizing the spread of virus while still providing excellent patient care.

The following recommendations can help PICUs during the current pandemic and future infection outbreaks:[87]

1. Monitoring: monitoring patients from outside the room while having a direct line of sight might require installation of windows or glass doors.
2. Nursing care: moving intravenous pumps outside of patient rooms while paying attention to the possibilities of inadvertent dislodgement of catheters, increased risk of central line–associated bloodstream infection, and inability of nurses to hear pump alarms when they are inside the patient rooms with PPE. Reduction, or grouping, of blood sampling as much as possible.
3. Respiratory care: coordination of team members to minimize entry into rooms, address measures to decrease aerosol generation, set appropriate ventilator alarm limits, change ventilator circuits or filters as needed rather than by protocol, and use of metered-dose inhalers instead of nebulizers when possible. Consider vibrating mesh nebulizer rather than in-line gas-driven nebulizer when nebulized medication must be given. Prone positioning teams and protocols should be in place to safely place patients in the prone position while addressing possible dislodgement of tubes and catheters and development of pressure ulcers.
4. Pharmacy: critical care pharmacists can help with development of specific management guidelines as treatments evolve during the pandemic and help with measures to reduce the number of times nurses must enter patient rooms for medication administration.
5. Structure related: zones and protocols should be developed for donning and doffing PPE. A protocol should be developed for room cleaning and disinfection with approved disinfectants while ensuring safety of environmental service workers.
6. Patient communication: social workers, child-life specialists, patient representatives, and pastoral care providers can be enlisted, along with the use of audio or video communication to help facilitate communication with family members during pandemic-induced restricted visiting.

7. Mental health issues of all team members should be addressed. Posttraumatic stress (PTS) has been noted to be high among pediatric critical care physicians in association with various COVID-19 patient care experiences. These observations, along with association of PTS with thoughts of quitting the profession because of the pandemic, could have implications for the workforce in the future.[88]

PUBLIC HEALTH CONCERNS FOR CHILDREN

1. Mental health: the mental health crisis facing children was substantial even before the pandemic. The significant pressures on families, schools, and communities resulting from the pandemic have made the situation worse. Children's hospitals are feeling the considerable burden of this crisis every day. Emergency rooms are filled to capacity, and staff are at the breaking point. According to the Kaiser Family Foundation, there have been marked increases in suicidal ideations, anxiety disorders, obsessive-compulsive disorder diagnosis, and substance abuse in children.[89] Significant efforts and resources are needed to address the mental health crisis in children.
2. The fragility of the medical home and health system: children are best served in a coordinated, fully staffed medical home. Care is coordinated, and the most medically fragile children receive timely and coordinated care. However, the pandemic has had a negative impact on America's pediatric practices. In a recent survey by the American Academy of Pediatrics, two-thirds of practices have experienced a significant decrease in visits.[90] This decrease has both public health impacts (delays in vaccines, late diagnosis) and a negative fiscal impact on the long-term survival of the medical home.

Tags for SEO: severe acute COVID-19, MIS-C, hyperinflammation, KD.

CLINICS CARE POINTS

- Mental health issues of critical care teams and children affected during this pandemic should be addressed.

ACKNOWLEDGMENT

The authors thank Dr. Tej Phatak, MD, MBA, Chief of Pediatric Radiology at Children's Hospital of New Jersey at Newark Beth Israel Medical Center, for providing us with the radiology images used in this review article.

DISCLOSURE

The authors have nothing to disclose.

REFERENCES

1. Centers for Disease Control and Prevention. Laboratory-confirmed COVID-19-associated hospitalizations 2021. https://gis.cdc.gov/grasp/COVIDNet/COVID19_5.html#virusTypeDiv.
2. Dong Y, Mo X, Hu Y, et al. Epidemiology of COVID-19 among children in China. Pediatrics 2020;145(6):e20200702.

3. Lu X, Zhang L, Du H, et al. SARS-CoV-2 Infection in Children. N Engl J Med 2020; 382(17):1663–5. https://doi.org/10.1056/NEJMc2005073.

4. Hoang A, Chorath K, Moreira A, et al. COVID-19 in 7780 pediatric patients: a systematic review. EClinicalMedicine 2020;24:100433.

5. Viner RM, Ward JL, Hudson LD, et al. Systematic review of reviews of symptoms and signs of COVID-19 in children and adolescents. Arch Dis Child 2020. https://doi.org/10.1136/archdischild-2020-320972.

6. Gaythorpe KAM, Bhatia S, Mangal T, et al. Children's role in the COVID-19 pandemic: a systematic review of early surveillance data on susceptibility, severity, and transmissibility. Sci Rep 2021;11(1):13903.

7. Parcha V, Booker KS, Kalra R, et al. A retrospective cohort study of 12,306 pediatric COVID-19 patients in the United States. Sci Rep 2021;11(1):10231.

8. Delahoy MJ, Ujamaa D, Whitaker M, et al. Hospitalizations associated with COVID-10 among children and adolescents-COVID-NET, 14 states, March 1, 2020-August 14, 2021. MMWR Morb Mortal Wkly Rep 2021;70:1255–60.

9. Graff K, Smith C, Silveira L, et al. Risk factors for severe cOVID-19 in children. Pediatr Infect Dis J 2021;40(4):e137–45.

10. Preston LE, Chevinsky JR, Kompaniyets L, et al. Characteristics and disease severity of US children and adolescents diagnosed With COVID-19. JAMA Netw Open 2021;4(4):e215298.

11. Children's Hospital Association and the American Academy of Pediatrics. Children and COVID-19: state-level data report. Available at. https://www.aap.org/en/pages/2019-novel-coronavirus-covid-19-infections/children-and-covid-19-state-level-data-report.

12. Siegel DA, Reses HE, Cool AJ, et al. Trends in COVID-19 cases, emergency department visits, and hospital admissions among children and adolescents aged 0-17 years - United States, August 2020-August 2021. MMWR Morb Mortal Wkly Rep 2021;70(36):1249–54.

13. Cevik M, Kuppalli K, Kindrachuk J, et al. Virology, transmission, and pathogenesis of SARS-CoV-2. BMJ 2020;371:m3862.

14. Mangalmurti N, Hunter CA. Cytokine storms: understanding COVID-19. Immunity 2020;53(1):19–25.

15. Bixler D, Miller AD, Mattison CP, et al. SARS-CoV-2-associated deaths among persons aged <21 years – United States, February 12-July 31, 2020. MMWR Morb Mortal Wkly Rep 2020;69:1324.

16. Gonzalez-Dambrauskas S, Vasquez-Hoyos P, Camporesi A, et al. Pediatric critical care and COVID-19. Pediatrics 2020;146(3):e20201766.

17. Shekerdemian LS, Mahmood NR, Wolfe KK, et al. Characteristics and outcomes of children with coronavirus disease 2019 (COVID-19) infection admitted to US and Canadian pediatric intensive care units. JAMA Pediatr 2020;174(9):868–73.

18. Kalyanaraman M, McQueen D, Morparia K, et al. ARDS in an ex-premature infant with bronchopulmonary dysplasia and COVID-19. Pediatr Pulmonology 2020; 55(10):2506–7.

19. Moeller A, Thanikkel L, Duijts L, et al. COVID-19 in children with underlying chronic respiratory diseases: survey results from 174 centres. ERJ Open Res 2020;6(4):00409–2020.

20. Fernandes DM, Oliveira CR, Guerguis S, et al. Severe acute respiratory syndrome Coronavirus 2 clinical syndromes and predictors of disease severity in hospitalized children and youth. J Pediatr 2021;230:23–31.

21. Corman VM, Landt O, Kaiser M, et al. Detection of 2019 novel coronavirus (2019-nCoV) by real-time RT-PCR. Euro Surveill 2020;25:2000045.

22. Chen Z, Fu J, Shu O, et al. Diagnosis and treatment recommendations for pediatric respiratory infection caused by the 2019 novel coronavirus. World J Pediatr 2020;16(3):240–6.
23. Lu X, Zhang L, Hui D, et al. SARS-CoV-2 infection in children. N Engl J Med 2020; 382:1663–5.
24. Chao JY, Derespina KR, Herold BC, et al. Clinical characteristics and outcomes of hospitalized and critically ill children and adolescents with coronavirus disease 2019 (COVID-19) at a tertiary care medical center in New York City. J Pediatr 2020;223:14–9.e2.
25. Fisler G, Izard SM, Shah S, et al. Characteristics and risk factors associated with critical illness in pediatric COVID-19. Annals Intensive Care 2020;10(1):171.
26. Hariyanto TI, Japar KV, Kwenandar F, et al. Inflammatory and hematologic markers as predictors of severe outcomes in COVID-19 infection: a systematic review and meta-analysis. Am J Emerg Med 2021;41:110–9.
27. Foust AM, Phillips GS, Chu WC, et al. International expert consensus statement on chest imaging in pediatric COVID-19 patient management: imaging findings, imaging study reporting, and imaging study recommendations. Radiol Cardiothorac Imaging 2020;2(2):e200214.
28. Nino G, Zember J, Sanchez-Jacob R, et al. Pediatric lung imaging features of COIVD-19: a systematic review and meta-analysis. Pediatr Pulmonol 2021; 56(1):252–63.
29. Chung M, Bernheim A, Mei X. CT imaging features of 2019 novel coronavirus (2019-nCoV). Radiology 2020;295:202–7.
30. Kumar J, Meena J, Yadav A, et al. Radiological findings of COVID-19 in children: a systematic review and meta-analysis. J Trop Pediatr 2021;67(3):fmaa045.
31. Chen A, Huang J, Liao Y, et al. Differences in clinical and imaging presentation of pediatric patients with COVID-19 in comparison with adults. Radiol Cardiothorac Imaging 2020;2(2):e200117.
32. Denina M, Scolfaro C, Silvestro E, et al. Lung ultrasound in children with COVID-19. Pediatrics 2020;146(1):e20201157.
33. Pediatric acute respiratory distress syndrome: consensus recommendations from the pediatric acute lung injury consensus conference. Pediatr Crit Care Med 2015;16(5):428–39.
34. Gattinoni L, Chiumello D, Caironi P, et al. COVID-19 pneumonia: different respiratory treatments for different phenotypes? Intensive Care Med 2020;46:1099–102.
35. Kneyber MCJ, de Luca D, Calderini E, et al. Section respiratory failure of the European Society for Paediatric and Neonatal Intensive Care. Recommendations for mechanical ventilation of critically ill children from the paediatric mechanical ventilation consensus conference (PEMVECC). Intensive Care Med 2017;43: 1764–80.
36. Rimensberger PC, Cheifetz IM, Pediatric Acute Lung Injury Consensus Conference Group. Ventilatory support in children with pediatric acute respiratory syndrome: proceedings from the Pediatric Acute Lung Injury Consensus Conference. Pediatr Crit Care Med 2015;16:S51–60.
37. Matava CT, Kovatsis PG, Lee JK, et al. Pediatric airway management in COVID-19 patients: consensus guidelines from the Society for Pediatric Anesthesia's Pediatric Difficult Intubation Collaborative and the Canadian Pediatric Anesthesia Society. Anesth Analg 2020;131(1):61–73.
38. Rimensberger PC, Kneyber MCJ, Deep A, et al. Caring for critically ill children with suspected or proven coronavirus disease 2019 infection: recommendations

by the scientific sections' collaborative of the European Society of Pediatric and Neonatal Intensive Care. Pediatr Crit Care Med 2021;22(1):56–67.

39. Brower RG, Matthay MA, Morris A, et al. Acute Respiratory Distress Syndrome Network. Ventilation with lower tidal volumes as compared with traditional tidal volumes for acute lung injury and the acute respiratory distress syndrome. N Engl J Med 2000;342:1301–8.

40. Khemani RG, Parvathaneni K, Yehya N, et al. Positive end-expiratory pressure lower than the ARDS network protocol is associated with higher pediatric acute respiratory distress syndrome mortality. Am J Respir Crit Care Med 2018; 198(1):77–89.

41. Kache S, Chisti MJ, Gumbo F, et al. COVID-19 PICU guidelines: for high- and limited-resource settings. Pediatr Res 2020;88(5):705–16.

42. Available at: https://www.accessdata.fda.gov/drugsatfda_docs/label/2020/ 214787Orig1s000lbl.pdf

43. Available at: https://www.fda.gov/media/137564/download

44. Goldman DL, Aldrich ML, Hagmann SHF, et al. Compassionate use of remdesivir in children with severe acute COVID-19. Pediatrics 2021;147(5). e2020047803.

45. Chiotos K, Hayes M, Kimberlin DW, et al. Multicenter interim guidance on use of antivirals for children with coronavirus disease 2019/severe acute respiratory syndrome coronavirus 2. J Pediatr Infect Dis Soc 2021;10(1):34–48.

46. Jacinto JP, Patel M, Goh J, et al. Remdesivir-induced symptomatic bradycardia in the treatment of COVID-19 disease. Heart Rhythm Case Rep 2021;7(8):514–7.

47. COVID-19 Treatment Guidelines Panel. Coronavirus Disease 2019 (COVID-19) treatment guidelines. National Institutes of Health. Available at. https://www. covid19treatmentguidelines.nih.gov/. [Accessed 20 October 2021]. Accessed.

48. Horby P, Lim WS, Emberson J, et al. Dexamethasone in hospitalized patients with COVID-19. N Engl J Med 2021;384(8):693–704.

49. Sterne JA, Murthy S, Diaz JV, et al. Association between administration of systemic corticosteroids and mortality among critically ill patients with COVID-19: a meta-analysis. JAMA 2020;324(13):1330–41.

50. Henderson LA, Canna SW, Friedman KG, et al. American College of Rheumatology clinical guidance for multisystem inflammatory syndrome in children associated with SARS-CoV-2 and hyperinflammation in pediatric COVID-19: version 2. Arthritis Rheumatol 2021;73(4):e13–29.

51. Weiss SL, Peters MJ, Alhazzani W, et al. Surviving Sepsis campaign international guidelines for the management of septic shock and sepsis-associated organ dysfunction in children. Pediatr Crit Care Med 2020;21(2):e52–106.

52. Khwaja A. KDIGO clinical practice guidelines for acute kidney injury. Nephron Clin Pract 2012;120:c179–84.

53. Siracusa L, Cascio A, Giordano S, et al. Neurological complications in pediatric patients with SARS-CoV-2 infection: a systematic review of the literature. Ital J Pediatr 2021;47:123. https://doi.org/10.1186/s13052-021-01066-9.

54. Levi M, Thachil J, Iba T, et al. Coagulation abnormalities and thrombosis in patients with COVID-19. Lancet Haematol 2020;7(6):e438–40.

55. Zaffanello M, Piacentini G, Nosetti L, et al. Thrombotic risk in children with COVID-19 infection: a systematic review of the literature. Thromb Res 2021;205:92–8.

56. Loi M, Branchford B, Kim J, et al. COVID-19 anticoagulation recommendations in children. Pediatr Blood Cancer 2020;67(9):e28485.

57. Goldenberg NA, Sochet A, Albisetti M, et al. Consensus-based clinical recommendations and research priorities for anticoagulant thromboprophylaxis in

children hospitalized for COVID-19-related illness. J Thromb Haemost 2020; 18(11):3099–105.

58. Monagle P, Chan A, Goldenberg N, et al. Antithrombotic therapy in neonates and children: antithrombotic therapy and prevention of thrombosis 9th edition: American College of Chest Physicians evidence based clinical practice guidelines. Chest 2012;141(2 Suppl):e737S–801S.

59. Hospitalizations associated with COVID-19 among children and adolescents — COVID-NET, 14 states, March 1, 2020–August 14, 2021. Weekly/September 10, 2021/70(36);1255- 1260. https://www.cdc.gov/mmwr/volumes/70/wr/mm7036e2.htm.

60. Belay ED, Abrams J, Oster ME, et al. Trends in geographic and temporal distribution of US children with multisystem inflammatory syndrome during the COVID-19 pandemic. JAMA Pediatr 2021;175(8):837–45.

61. Feldstein LR, Tenforde MW, Friedman KG, et al. Characteristics and outcomes of US children and adolescents with multisystem inflammatory syndrome in children (MIS-C) compared with severe acute COVID-19. JAMA 2021;323(11):1074–87.

62. Information for healthcare providers about multisystem inflammatory syndrome in children (MIS-C). Available at: https://www.cdc.gov/mis/mis-c/hcp/index.html.

63. Royal College of Paediatrics and Child Health. Guidance: paediatric multisystem inflammatory syndrome temporally associated with COVID-19 2020. Available at. https://www.rcpch.ac.uk/resources/guidance-paediatric-multisystem-inflammatory-syndrome-temporally-associated-covid-19-pims.

64. World Health Organization. Multisystem inflammatory syndrome in children and adolescents with COVID-19 2020. Available at. https://www.who.int/publications/i/item/multisystem-inflammatory-syndrome-in-children-and-adolescents-with-covid-19.

65. Saatci D, Ranger TA, Garriga C, et al. Association between race and COVID-19 outcomes among 2.6 million children in England. JAMA Pediatr 2021;175(9): 928–38.

66. Payne AB, Gilani Z, Godfred-Cato S, et al. Incidence of multisystem inflammatory syndrome in children among US persons infected with SARS-CoV-2. JAMA Netw Open 2021;4(6):e2116420.

67. Abrams JY, Oster ME, Godfred-Cato SE, et al. Factors linked to severe outcomes in multisystem inflammatory syndrome in children (MIS-C) in the USA: a retrospective surveillance study. Lancet Child Adolesc Health 2021;5(5):323–31.

68. Bellino S, Punzo O, Rota MC, et al. COVID-19 disease severity risk factors for pediatric patients in Italy. Pediatrics 2020;146(4). e2020009399.

69. Anderson JE, Campbell JA, Durowoju L, et al. COVID-19-associated multisystem inflammatory syndrome in children (MIS-C) presenting as appendicitis with shock. J Pediatr Surg Case Rep 2021;71:101913.

70. Meyer JS, Robinson G, Moonah S, et al. Acute appendicitis in four children with SARS-CoV-2 infection. J Pediatr Surg Case Rep 2021;64:101734.

71. Dufort EM, Koumans EH, Chow EJ, et al. Multisystem inflammatory syndrome in children in New York State. N Engl J Med 2020;383:347–58.

72. Kavurt AV, Bağrul D, Gül AEK, et al. Echocardiographic findings and correlation with laboratory values in multisystem inflammatory syndrome in children (MIS-C) associated with COVID-19. Pediatr Cardiol 2021;1–13.

73. Valverde I, Singh Y, Sanchez-de-Toledo J, et al. Acute cardiovascular manifestations in 286 children with multisystem inflammatory syndrome associated with COVID-19 infection in Europe. Circulation 2021;143(1):21–32.

74. McCrindle BW, Rowley AH, Newburger JW, et al. Diagnosis, treatment, and long-term management of Kawasaki disease: a scientific statement for health

professionals from the American Heart Association [review]. Circulation 2017; 135(17):e927–99.

75. Tsuda E, Tsujii N, Hayama Y. Stenotic lesions and the maximum diameter of coronary artery aneurysms in Kawasaki disease. J Pediatr 2018;194:165–70.

76. Giglia TM, Massicotte MP, Tweddell JS, et al. Prevention and treatment of thrombosis in pediatric and congenital heart disease: a scientific statement from the American Heart Association. Circulation 2013;128(24):2622–703.

77. Davies P, du Pré P, Lillie J, et al. One-year outcomes of critical care patients post-COVID-19 multisystem inflammatory syndrome in children. JAMA Pediatr 2021; 30:e212993.

78. Rostad BS, Shah JH, Rostad CA, et al. Chest radiograph features of multisystem inflammatory syndrome in children (MIS-C) compared to pediatric COVID-19. Pediatr Radiol 2021;51(2):231–8.

79. Son MBF, Murray N, Friedman K, et al. Multisystem inflammatory syndrome in children - Initial therapy and outcomes. N Engl J Med 2021;385(1):23–34.

80. Zhang QY, Xu BW, Du JB. Similarities and differences between multiple inflammatory syndrome in children associated with COVID-19 and Kawasaki disease: clinical presentations, diagnosis, and treatment. World J Pediatr 2021;17(4):335–40.

81. Kato H, Sugimura T, Akagi T, et al. Long-term consequences of Kawasaki disease. A 10- to 21-year follow-up study of 594 patients. Circulation 1996;94(6): 1379–85.

82. Newburger JW. Treatment of Kawasaki disease. Lancet 1996;347(9009):1128.

83. Ogata S, Tremoulet AH, Sato Y, et al. Coronary artery outcomes among children with Kawasaki disease in the United States and Japan. Int J Cardiol 2013;168(4): 3825–8.

84. Newburger JW, Takahashi M, Burns JC, et al. The treatment of Kawasaki syndrome with intravenous gamma globulin. N Engl J Med 1986;315(6):341–7.

85. Yager PH, Whalen KA, Cummings BM. Repurposing a pediatric ICU for adults. N Engl J Med 2020;382(22):e80.

86. Wasserman E, Toal M, Nellis M, et al. Rapid transition of a PICU space and staff to adult coronavirus disease 2019 ICU care. Pediatr Crit Care Med 2021;22(1):50–5.

87. Halpern NA, Kaplan LJ, Rausen M, et al. Configuring ICUs in the COVID-19 era. 2020. https://www.sccm.org/COVID19RapidResources/Resources/Configuring-ICUs-in-the-COVID-19-Era-A-Collection.

88. Kalyanaraman M, Sankar A, Timpo E, et al. Posttraumatic stress among pediatric critical care physicians in the United States in association with coronavirus disease 2019 patient care experiences. J Intensive Care Med 2021.

89. Kaiser Family Foundation. Available at: www.kff.org/coronavirus-covid-19/issue-brief/mental-health-and-substance-use-considerations-among-children-during-the-covid-19-pandemic/.

90. American Academy of Pediatrics: PLACES Survey. 2020. Available at: https://publications.aap.org/aapnews/news/14172/Survey-Pediatricians-reeling-from-pandemic-s?searchresult=1.

Clinical Informatics and Quality Improvement in the Pediatric Intensive Care Unit

Kshama Daphtary, MD, MBI*, Orkun Baloglu, MD

KEYWORDS

- Pediatric intensive care unit • Clinical informatics • Clinical decision support
- Quality improvement • Artificial intelligence • Machine learning

KEY POINTS

- The concept of a learning health system was first described by the Institute of Medicine in 2007 as a model that integrates science, informatics, incentives, and culture to achieve continuous improvement and improve value in health care.
- Data, analytics, and knowledge are keys to decision-making, not only at the bedside but also to drive innovation and sustain improvement as part of the continuous improvement cycle.
- Knowledge of clinical informatics, the application of informatics and information technology to deliver health care services, is essential to achieve quality, safety, and value.
- The explosion of big data and artificial intelligence (AI) has opened the doors to new CDS systems, especially in predictive analytics; intensivists should be familiar with the opportunities, challenges, and limitations.

INTRODUCTION

Since the 1999 publication of the Institute of Medicine (IOM) report, "To Err is Human: Building a Safer Health System," there has been growing awareness about the importance of ensuring quality and safety in the health care setting. In 1991, the IOM advocated for the prompt development and implementation of computer-based patient records. They envisioned that these records would not merely be a replacement of paper records but had the potential to improve the care of individual patients and populations.[1,2] In 2004, President George W. Bush created the Office of the National Coordinator for Health Information Technology, which outlined a plan to ensure that

Department of Pediatric Critical Care Medicine, Cleveland Clinic Lerner College of Medicine of Case Western Reserve University, 9500 Euclid Avenue, M-14, Cleveland, OH 44195, USA
* Corresponding author.
E-mail address: daphtak@ccf.org

Pediatr Clin N Am 69 (2022) 573–586
https://doi.org/10.1016/j.pcl.2022.01.014
0031-3955/22/© 2022 Elsevier Inc. All rights reserved.
pediatric.theclinics.com

most Americans had electronic health records (EHRs) within the next 10 years. There was widespread adoption of EHRs following the passage of the Health Information Technology for Economic and Clinical Health (HITECH) Act that provided fiscal incentives to implement EHRs that were "certified" as meeting minimal standards and that demonstrated "meaningful use" of the EHRs. The concept of a learning health system was first described by the IOM in 2007 as a model that integrates science, informatics, incentives, and culture to achieve continuous improvement and improve value in health care.[3] Data, analytics, and knowledge are keys to decision-making, not only at the bedside but also to drive innovation and sustain improvement as part of the continuous improvement cycle. Knowledge of clinical informatics, the application of informatics and information technology to deliver health care services, is essential to achieve quality, safety, and value. In this article, we discuss the role of clinical informatics in quality improvement and patient safety in the pediatric intensive care unit (PICU).

The PICU is a data-rich environment. Patients admitted to the PICU are cared for by many providers. Data obtained from multiple sources are integrated into the EHR, allowing access by multiple health care providers within the hospital system simultaneously. The EHR thus serves as a repository of information and a means of communication between health care providers. EHR data can be integrated into an enterprise data warehouse that organizes and standardizes data that exist in separate silos within or across organizations, enabling analysis and reporting. Data warehouses can be used to develop multiple data marts and internal registries. Health Information Exchanges (HIEs) address interoperability issues and enable the bidirectional exchange of data either through a centralized data repository or through a federated network of sites. EHR-linked data can be exported to external registries for different purposes such as public health reporting, population health management, reporting of quality measures. These concepts are illustrated in **Fig. 1**.

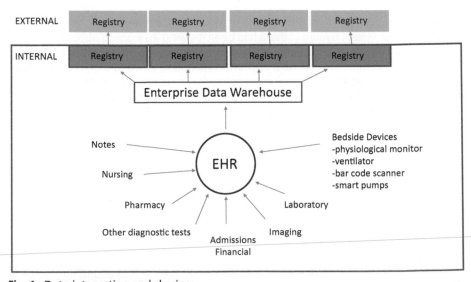

Fig. 1. Data integration and sharing.

THE ELECTRONIC HEALTH RECORD AND CLINICAL DECISION SUPPORT

The EHR is now ubiquitous, and its widespread adoption has resulted in health care safety and quality benefits related to information accessibility, clinical decision support (CDS), medication safety, test result management, and other areas.

CDS provides clinicians, staff, patients, and other individuals with knowledge and person-specific information, intelligently filtered, or presented at appropriate times, to enhance health and health care.[4] CDS integrated with EHR often makes use of web-based applications. Early randomized controlled clinical studies showed that computerized CDS systems reduce costs and improve quality compared with usual care supported with a paper medical record.[5,6] CDS systems encompass a multitude of tools. The simplest uses information about the current clinical context to retrieve highly relevant documents (eg, infobuttons). Other CDS systems organize and present information in a way that facilitates problem-solving and decision making (eg, dashboards and visual displays). Intelligent systems provide patient-specific and situation-specific alerts, advice, reminders, order sets, or other recommendations for direct action. They may follow simple algorithms or rule-based logics, or they may use probabilistic approaches or derive their conclusions based on machine learning (ML) from large amounts of data.

In the following sections, we elaborate on some of the functions and features that potentially improve patient safety and quality in the PICU; due to the paucity of published literature on health information technology applications in the PICU, we describe their use in adult ICUs.

Device Integration and Data Acquisition

EHRs are real-time patient-centered records that make information available instantly and securely to authorized users. Early hospital information systems included integration with laboratory information systems and radiology information systems. Picture archiving and communication system (PACS) made it possible to view images within the EHR. Electronic nursing documentation has replaced folded paper flowsheets. Advances in device integration technology have made it possible to access data not previously available and reduce error attributable to manual entry. Although it is possible to view the patient monitor in real-time and record low-resolution, discrete data in the EHR, existing EHRs do not capture physiologic waveforms. Multimodality monitoring refers to standard ICU monitoring supplemented with neurophysiologic parameters. Collection of waveform resolution data, integration, and time synchronization of these data with other contextual data provide valuable information. Commercial systems have been developed to integrate data from multiple devices, but these do not integrate seamlessly with existing EHRs. Apart from device connectivity, there is a need for standard terminology for data and metadata. Despite the challenges in the collection, transfer, display, archiving, and analysis of high-resolution physiologic data, multimodal monitoring provides exciting opportunities, especially with the availability of cloud-based storage and advancements in big data analytics.

Data Visualization and Dashboards

The plethora of information generated from a single patient in the PICU can be overwhelming and lead to cognitive overload. Providers must access, integrate, and analyze these data to make critical decisions, often with time constraints. Data visualization, the graphical representation of information and data using charts, graphs, maps, and other visuals, makes it easier to process the data and gain insights about the information represented. It allows for the effective and efficient processing of data and has the potential to lower cognitive overload. A dashboard is an information visualization tool capable of querying multiple databases and conveying real-time information concisely. An interactive dashboard makes it easy to sort, filter, or drill into different types of data as needed. Features such as alerts and reminders can be built into the dashboard to help clinicians improve compliance with best practices or organizational standards. Implementing user-centered design processes for innovative information displays can improve accuracy and efficiency in diagnoses and treatment by the integration and organization of information, representation of trends, and implementing graphical approaches to make relationships between data visible.[7]

Visualization displays and dashboards have been used successfully in the ICU and acute care units in a variety of ways, depending on the intention and design. Commercial EHRs can present patient data in different formats such as timeline flowsheets and graphs, summaries, and snapshots; these may be customizable for different users. Novel formats and systems customized for ICU use have been designed and implemented; some have demonstrated improved outcomes.[8] Dashboards can be incorporated into daily workflow and can increase situational awareness and potentially improve patient safety.[9] An ICU-specific patient viewer and monitoring system, the Ambient Warning and Response Evaluation (AWARE) developed as a superstructure for the existing EHR, based on the information needs of clinicians, reduced the time spent on preround data collection and reduced cognitive load and errors of cognition.[10,11] This sophisticated tool has several components including dashboards that prioritize and organize data (multipatient and single patient), and CDS including automated surveillance algorithms (or sniffers) and alerts for several conditions. In addition, tools such as task-list and readiness for discharge facilitate communication between team members and during transitions of care. Checklists/rounding tools assist clinicians in developing and executing a coordinated daily plan of care. And an administrative dashboard with feedback and reporting tools allows easy access to quality improvement metrics. Shaw and colleagues evaluated a dynamic unit-based dashboard that displayed real-time compliance with specific PICU safety bundles. They demonstrated the use of a dashboard was associated with a decrease in the number of patient urinary catheter hours, a reduction in catheter-associated urinary tract infection rate, and an improvement in patient medication reconciliation but had no impact on restraint orders, deep vein thrombosis prophylaxis or pressure ulcer rates.[12] An experimental study compared the impact of a graphical information display on the diagnosis of circulatory shock. The use of an integrated display was associated with higher performances and more accurate identification of etiology compared with conventional information displays when used by novice physicians.[13]

Real-time dashboards built in an adult ICU for patients admitted with COVID-19 provided opportunities to review treatment regimens and clinical outcomes and amend protocols quickly based on local data. The dashboard, rapidly built for frontline clinicians to monitor patient status in multiple wards and proactively intervene as clinically necessary and transfer patients to the appropriate level of care resulted in a significant reduction in urgent intubations and cardiac resuscitations on the general wards and enabled physicians to efficiently assess patient volumes and case severity to prioritize clinical care and appropriately allocate scarce resources.[14]

Checklists

The use of checklists has become an essential part of PICU workflow. Checklists have been integrated within EHRs and incorporated into daily rounds and have impacted outcomes. Use of an EHR-enhanced checklist along with a unit-wide dashboard in a PICU to improve compliance with an evidence-based care bundle resulted in a reduction in central line-associated bloodstream infection rates.[15] As compared with a static checklist with limited EHR data, a sophisticated dynamic checklist providing CDS prompts with the display of relevant data automatically pulled from the EHR was integrated efficiently into daily rounds and well-received by users.[16] This application pulled in accurate and relevant data from the EHR regarding key QI areas including sedation, dosing adjustment of medications in renal dysfunction, early discontinuation of central venous and urinary catheters, and stress ulcer prophylaxis. A previous iteration of the application incorporated CDS to display best practices; the newer version highlighted best practice potential indications for the condition alongside data from the EHR showing if the patient was meeting recommendations. Use of this checklist application increased adherence to best practices around stress ulcer prophylaxis usage, VTE prophylaxis prescribing, adjustment of medications for renal dysfunction, and frequency of updating weight and height measurements.

Medication Safety

Medication errors occur frequently in children admitted to the PICU and may cause harm. Computerized prescriber order entry (CPOE) and CDS, have been shown to reduce prescription medication errors and ICU mortality.[17] CDS encompasses a variety of tools to enhance decision-making in the clinical workflow; these can manifest as alerts and reminders, clinical guidelines, order sets, focused patient data reports and summaries, documentation templates, diagnostic support, and contextually relevant reference information. Early CDS for medication safety included drug-allergy and drug–drug interaction alerts, drug-age and drug-dose support, and safeguards for duplication; these reduce prescription errors. Strategies recommended to minimize dispensing errors and improve efficiency include robotic automated dispensing systems and bar-coded medication administration (BCMA) systems.[18] Processes and technologies targeted to reduce medication errors during the administration phase include BCMA and smart infusion pumps. Smart pumps are equipped with predetermined clinical guidelines, hospital-defined drug libraries with dosing parameters, and dose error reduction systems. They can generate alerts when there is a risk of an adverse drug interaction or when the pump's parameters are set outside of specified safety limits for the medication being administered. Closed-loop electronic medication management systems include these technologies implemented together and integrated with the EHR. Benefits include support for prescribing, dispensing, and medication administration, and enable the tracking of medications across the workflow from CPOE. In addition, it allows checking, dispensing, administration, and documentation in the eMAR. These have been shown to reduce medication errors and allow the analysis of the most error-prone phase of the medication cycle.[19,20]

Early Detection of Deterioration or Acute Conditions and Risk Prediction

Recently, proactive approaches have been taken to recognize patient deterioration or conditions such as sepsis to provide timely intervention to reduce morbidity and mortality. Physiologic and device monitors incorporate parameter-specific alarms to improve patient safety. Unfortunately, these alarms occur frequently, and few are of clinical significance. EHRs contain detailed, dynamic data and can facilitate early detection of acute and potentially catastrophic conditions. Using simple algorithms and rule-based logic, alerts can be set up as triggers when predetermined thresholds for a combination of set parameters are met. In addition to the broad range of patient data collected from various sources, the EHR also collects rich metadata about the timing, frequency, and location of actions and observations that affect the patient. This enables predictive modeling. Predictive analytics is usually defined as the branch of advanced analytics that deals with predictions about future events (eg, will a patient develop an acute event of interest such as septic shock). Most existing clinical applications were derived from ML algorithms using static population-wide prediction models. Newer models allow for real-time time processing and continuous learning at the patient level providing more personalized predictions (prescriptive analytics - for example, will a patient with shock benefit from a certain type of inotropic agent, such as epinephrine or norepinephrine).

Constant surveillance of data in the EHR for conditions with established criteria or definitions, or sniffers, has shown promising results. Rule-based alerts for the detection of acute lung injury have demonstrated high sensitivity and specificity.[21,22] Real-time electronic alert algorithms for acute kidney injury (AKI) systems have the potential to increase AKI recognition, reduce the time to therapeutic interventions to prevent progression of AKI, and improve outcomes. These electronic alerts have been linked to intervention prompts and care bundles, and CDS has been shown to significantly reduce mortality and increase the proportion of AKI recognition, and investigations in hospitalized patients.[23] As most pediatric patients inherently have few of these risk factors, efforts in detecting children at risk for AKI have focused on the initiation of nephrotoxic medications. Nephrotoxic Injury Negated by Just-in-Time Action (NINJA) is an ongoing prospective quality improvement project to reduce nephrotoxic medication-associated AKI among noncritically ill hospitalized children.[24] It involves systematic EHR screening and a decision support process (trigger report). The trigger report is reviewed by pharmacists who recommend daily serum creatinine monitoring in patients who have the risk exposure. It was successful in reducing the number of AKI days.[25] EHR-based predictive models for AKI screening in hospitalized children have been developed and can be used to identify high-risk patients without serum creatinine data enabling targeted testing, early identification, and modification of care.

Legislative mandates and recommendations by the American College of Critical Care Medicine and the Surviving Sepsis Campaign require institutions to systematically screen for the early identification of patients with suspected septic shock and other sepsis-associated organ dysfunction. Automated systems for the early detection of sepsis are widely being used, especially in adult patients. There have been few published randomized controlled trials to evaluate whether automated systems for the early detection of sepsis improve outcomes. One systematic review showed that the trials were insufficient in showing the effects of automated systems on reducing the time to appropriate antibiotics and improving outcomes in the ICU.[26] Other systematic reviews on the impact of digital alerting systems on sepsis-related outcomes in hospitalized adults found that digital alerts considerably reduced hospital and ICU stay for patients with sepsis, but showed mixed results for outcome measures such as mortality and ICU transfer.[27] Process measures improvement (such as time to antibiotic administration, lactate measurement) were demonstrated across multiple types of hospital units, and evidence was most consistent for patients outside the ICU.[28] Development of trigger tools and automated alerts has been more challenging in children, especially for those admitted to the PICU. An ideal screening tool should be sensitive enough to detect sepsis, have a high positive predictive value to minimize false positive alerts and ensuing alarm fatigue and increase in clinician workload, and detect sepsis early in the course of the disease. Most automated sepsis alerts have a 2-step approach with a rule-based interruptive alert that prompts clinicians to huddle and assess the patient. One such computerized alert for identifying sepsis in the PICU relied on nurse assessment and had high sensitivity and a reasonable positive predictive value with minimal interruption to physician workflow.[29]

Early warning scores (EWS) were developed to aid clinicians in the early recognition of physiologic signs of deterioration, allowing timely intervention. The scores are based on routine measurements such as vital signs, clinical examination, and laboratory data, and are part of patient safety initiatives to improve situational awareness and avert adverse outcomes. A variety of pediatric early warning scores (PEWS) has been developed. Older PEWS systems were composed of rules applied to objective and subjective patient data and an associated actionable mitigation plan. Predictive analytical modeling using EHR-derived data has been successfully used to predict the early deterioration of hospitalized patients outside the PICU. In the PICU, CDS tools have been developed to detect patients at risk for deterioration. One such tool translated a paper tool to an automated CDS. Although it reduced the work of manual screening, there was a decrease in sensitivity and an increase in the number needed to screen, raising concerns about unstudied automated conversions of paper-tools.[30]

In contrast to CDS developed for the early detection of a single condition, platforms have been developed, mostly used for tele-critical care. These systems integrate real-time data from monitors and ventilators, which are incorporated into an integrated display, and feature a decision support surveillance system capable of detecting acute deterioration and other conditions.[31]

DATABASES AND REGISTRIES

Databases and registries serve several purposes, including quality improvement and operations. Registries from organizations such as the Virtual Pediatric Systems, LLC (VPS) and the Pediatric Cardiac Critical Care Consortium (PC4) collect granular data from PICUs and PCICUs in North America and around the world. Case-mix descriptions, resource utilization data, and risk-adjusted outcomes are included in reports to the participating hospitals. These registries have an important role in quality improvement and allow individual centers to benchmark their own outcomes and to learn from centers that have better outcomes. Data obtained from these registries have been used for research as well.

The Medical Information Mart for Intensive Care (MIMIC)-III and MIMIC-IV databases are unique as they can capture structured and granular data, including minute to minute changes in physiologic signals, time-stamped treatments, and medication dosage. The MIMIC-III database provides deidentified data for more than 40,000 patients admitted to ICUs at a single hospital. MIMIC-IV is an update to MIMIC-III. The eICU Collaborative Research Database is an additional large database with high granularity data from ICU patients monitored by the eICU Program, a telehealth system developed by Philips health care. These large databases are freely available and have spurred the development of ML algorithms, decision support tools, and clinical research.[32–35]

PATIENT PORTALS

A personal health record (PHR) is an electronic application through which individuals can access, manage, and share their health information, and that of others who are authorized, in a private, secure, and confidential environment.[36] Patient-centered care has become a core component of medical care. Patients were given the legal right to view and own their personal medical records in 1996. But it wasn't until the introduction of the EHR, and subsequently, EHR-tethered PHR electronic entry, or "patient portals," that patients could access their records easily. In addition to viewing information, some patient portals allow the patient to message their provider, schedule appointments, request prescription refills, update information, check benefits and coverage, download forms, and print educational material. Although patient portals are increasingly being used in the outpatient environment, use in the inpatient environment and specifically the ICU is challenging. Patient needs which determine the utility of patient portals are different for hospitalized patients. Acute care portals provide clinical data including information about the care team, clinical summaries and notes, results of laboratory and imaging and other tests, and a list of medications. This allows the patient to review the information at their convenience and correct errors such as missing medications or inconsistencies with verbal updates. Patient–provider communication regarding health concerns, needs and preferences, and clinical updates is an essential component. Patients should be able to review provider-generated content regarding daily schedule including events such as laboratory tests and imaging, daily goals and plan of care, expected hospital course, discharge criteria, and discharge planning needs, with the ability to provide feedback. Educational features have been included in the portals such as infobuttons linked to various educational sources closely linked to medications, diagnoses, or test results. Portals include safety-oriented content and allow reporting of safety concerns. While not directly affecting quality or safety, portals have built-in amenities that can enhance the patient experience. Availability of menus and food ordering, information for visitors such as maps, visiting hours, nearby accommodations, and entertainment to distract or prevent boredom are some of the amenities that have been incorporated into patient portals.[37]

Traditionally, patient portals are tethered to the EHR and accessed by users on their personal devices (or other laptop or desktop computers or smartphones). Innovative ways to engage parents in using patient portals include the use of tablet computers and monitors placed in patient rooms. In a study to assess parent use and perceptions of an inpatient portal application on a tablet computer that provided information about a child's stay on a medical/surgical unit at a tertiary children's hospital, parents were satisfied, reporting improved health care team communication and reduction of errors in care. The authors concluded that portals may engage parents in hospital care, facilitate parent recognition of medication errors, and improve perceptions of safety and quality.[38] A flat-panel touchscreen monitor placed in patient rooms displayed data from the EHR and allowed patients, parents, and professional staff access to patient data. Interviews of parents who used the system showed benefits such as increased parental situational awareness and potential error detection, and family empowerment and helping with care and advocacy. This technology altered communication, either aiding conversation with clinicians or obviating the need through the provision of information. In addition to concerns for privacy, the level of patient or family health literacy, lack of context and real-time explanations reduced the usefulness of the system and led to the potential for misinterpretation.[39] Close attention should be paid to the timing and content of information, without which, anxiety and stress can result while the patient or family member views the information. Other limitations to the use of patient portals include literacy, health literacy, and digital access.

ARTIFICIAL INTELLIGENCE, MACHINE LEARNING, AND DEEP LEARNING

Artificial intelligence (AI) can be described as a branch of computer science that studies computer technologies with the capacity to behave or function like human intelligence. ML is a subfield of AI that studies algorithms that learn from vast amounts of data and produce prediction or classification outputs; in other words, ML is an area of AI that uses computational algorithms and statistics to give computers the ability to learn without explicitly being programmed. Deep learning (DL) is a subtype of ML algorithms whereby algorithms are structured in multilayer nodes mimicking the neurons and synapses in the human brain.

The popularity of ML algorithms is due to 2 main factors; (1) availability of large amounts of data and (2) faster and cheaper computer processing power. In a data set, the relationship between the variables may already be known to humans. ML algorithms are designed to discover unknown and/or nonlinear and highly complex relationships, that humans cannot understand, among the variables in a data set. To discover those unknown relationships, ML algorithms need to "study" and "learn" from large amounts of data. The initial dataset used by an ML algorithm to train itself is called the *training dataset*. Once the ML algorithm trains itself, it must be tested on how well it performs in a separate dataset that is called the *test dataset*.

ML algorithms are used for 2 main tasks, *regression* and *classification*. In regression predictions, an ML algorithm is tasked to predict a continuous variable outcome, such as serum creatinine, whereas in classification predictions, the ML algorithm is designed to classify the data into different categories that are similar or different from each other; for example, a benign versus a malignant tumor.

ML algorithms can also be further divided into *supervised* and *unsupervised* learning types. In supervised learning, the dataset includes the variable defined by humans as the outcome variable that needs to be predicted. Humans inform an algorithm with the input variables and the output variable to be predicted, allowing the algorithm to find the relation between the input and output variables. In unsupervised learning, humans provide the whole data set without specifying the outcome variable to be predicted. The unsupervised learning ML model is tasked to discover unknown relations between the variables and make previously unknown classifications.

ML algorithms have been increasingly studied in pediatrics. DL algorithms called recurrent neural network and convolutional neural networks were used to predict real-time mortality in the PICU.[40–42] Sepsis in children has been evaluated using DL and other ML algorithms.[43–45] EWS and systems to predict the need for a hospitalized child to be transferred to the PICU has been studied for many years, but ML methods have been used only recently.[46,47] ML techniques have been used to predict clinical conditions at high risk of progressing to cardiac arrest among critically ill children admitted to the PICU,[48–50] early deterioration in those with parallel circulations,[51] and failure of high flow nasal cannula treatment within 24 hours of initiation.[52]

Despite the successful and very promising results of ML in medicine, there are concerns regarding ML methods, the most important of which is that ML algorithms are trained in biased datasets and real-life decisions are based on the resulting algorithm, that is biased. These biases can include race, sex, socioeconomic status, or others. All efforts should be made to minimize the bias in the dataset. Another concern in the medical community is that it is very difficult and sometimes impossible for humans to determine how the ML model (especially for DL algorithms) processed the data and produced the results. Therefore, some ML algorithms are considered as "black boxes." This perception decreases acceptance, trust, and use of ML algorithms in medicine by clinicians.[53] Although these developments are exciting, models using ML must be implemented as interventions that directly impact decision-making. So far, there is sparse evidence that the use of ML-based CDS is associated with improved clinician diagnostic performance.[54]

BIG DATA, CLINICAL INFORMATICS, AND THE LEARNING HEALTH SYSTEM

Big data are data "whose scale, diversity, and complexity require new architecture, techniques, algorithms, and analytics to manage it and extract value and hidden knowledge from it."[55] Processing of big data for clinical care, research, and administration generates knowledge. Thus, the role of clinical informatics is to provide the right tools to turn data into information, and information into knowledge. Informatics applications deliver this knowledge as CDS, transforming knowledge into action. The concept and processes to "close" the loop of the learning health cycle are shown schematically in **Fig. 2**.

CHALLENGES AND FUTURE DIRECTIONS

Health information systems play a vital role in providing high-quality care in the PICU. Despite technological advancements in health care, health care lags behind many other industries in the application of innovations. Some of the challenges stem from the nature of data (narrative data of clinical notes, physiologic waveforms), lack of standards in clinical terminology of data and metadata in health care, issues with connectivity and interoperability, and concerns regarding data privacy, confidentiality, and security. Implementation requires considerable resources and can cause unanticipated and undesirable consequences that can undermine provider acceptance, increase costs, sometimes lead to failed implementation, and result in harm to patients. Unintended consequences include increased clinician workload, changes in workflow, never-ending demands for system changes such as more sophisticated functionality and new features, altered communication patterns and practices, generation of new kinds of errors, and overdependence on technology. In 2011, the IOM Committee on Patient Safety and Health Information Technology released a report titled Health IT and Patient Safety: Building Safer Systems for Better Care.[56] The report outlined observations of potential health IT errors, concluding that several factors must be taken into consideration with implementation to prevent these errors from occurring. EHRs and CDS offer many benefits to clinicians and their patients, including better quality of care, improved patient safety, and greater efficiency. The involvement of end-users has been identified as fundamental to well-designed systems that are useable and useful in the context of busy workflows. Early engagement of the clinician in the design, development, implementation, and validation is crucial; this requires a great commitment of time and resources, knowledge, and interest. With the explosion of ML and predictive analytics, it is imperative for clinicians to be educated about the basics of these processes.

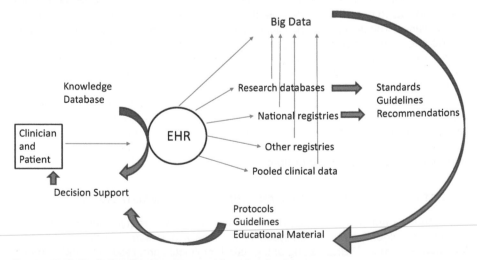

Fig. 2. Clinical informatics, big data, and learning health systems.

The recent SARS-CoV-2 pandemic has demonstrated that these barriers can be surmounted. Hospitals and health systems rapidly built multiple COVID-19 tools to meet evolving requirements to optimize care and maintain high-quality care and patient safety. These included CDS tools such as order sets and documentation to help nonintensivists care for critically ill patients. Dashboards and real-time analytics to screen, triage, and manage patients and allocate resources and manage operations were created. In addition, databases and registries to capture, store, manage and visualize population-level data, support research and determine clinical effectiveness, and widespread deployment of telemedicine for remote monitoring and management of patients were implemented. The health information technology-related changes have facilitated more effective patient care and resource management.[57,58]

Opportunities and challenges abound; clinician education and engagement are essential to ensure that the promises of clinical informatics and AI are realized.

CLINICS CARE POINTS

- Clinical informatics can support quality improvement and patient safety in the PICU.
- CDS, now an integral part of the workflow in the PICU, includes several tools and is increasingly leveraging artificial intelligence (AI).
- Understanding opportunities and challenges can improve engagement of clinicians with the design, validation, and implementation of CDS, and improve satisfaction, patient safety, care quality, and value.

DISCLOSURE

The authors have nothing to disclose.

REFERENCES

1. Institute of Medicine. Computer-based patient record: an essential technology for health care. Washington, DC: The National Academies Press; 1991. https://doi.org/10.17226/18459.
2. Institute of Medicine. In: Dick RS, Steen EB, Detmer DE, editors. The computer-based patient record: an essential technology for health care. Revised Edition. Washington, DC: National Academy Press; 1997.
3. Institute of Medicine. The learning healthcare system: Workshop summary. Washington, DC: The National Academies Press; 2007. https://doi.org/10.17226/11903.
4. The Office of the National Coordinator for Health Information Technology. https://www.healthit.gov/policy-researchers-implementers/clinical-decision-support-cds (accessed on 3/1/2022)
5. Buntin MB, Burke MF, Hoaglin MC, et al. The benefits of health information technology: a review of the recent literature shows predominantly positive results. Health Aff (Millwood) 2011;30(3):464–71.
6. Lau F, Kuziemsky C, Price M, et al. A review on systematic reviews of health information system studies. J Am Med Inform Assoc 2010;17(6):637–45.
7. Wright MC, Borbolla D, Waller RG, et al. Critical care information display approaches and design frameworks: A systematic review and meta-analysis. J Biomed Inform X 2019;3:100041.

8. Pickering BW, Herasevich V, Ahmed A, et al. Novel Representation of Clinical Information in the ICU: Developing User Interfaces which Reduce Information Overload. Appl Clin Inform 2010;1(2):116–31.

9. Khairat SS, Dukkipati A, Lauria HA, et al. The Impact of Visualization Dashboards on Quality of Care and Clinician Satisfaction: Integrative Literature Review. JMIR Hum Factors 2018;5(2):e22.

10. Dziadzko MA, Herasevich V, Sen A, et al. User perception and experience of the introduction of a novel critical care patient viewer in the ICU setting. Int J Med Inf 2016;88:86–91.

11. Ahmed A, Chandra S, Herasevich V, et al. The effect of two different electronic health record user interfaces on intensive care provider task load, errors of cognition, and performance. Crit Care Med 2011;39(7):1626–34.

12. Shaw SJ, Jacobs B, Stockwell DC, et al. Effect of a Real-Time Pediatric ICU Safety Bundle Dashboard on Quality Improvement Measures. Jt Comm J Qual Patient Saf 2015;41(9):414–20.

13. Reese TJ, Del Fiol G, Tonna JE, et al. Impact of integrated graphical display on expert and novice diagnostic performance in critical care. J Am Med Inform Assoc 2020;27(8):1287–92.

14. Ibrahim H, Sorrell S, Nair SC, et al. Rapid Development and Utilization of a Clinical Intelligence Dashboard for Frontline Clinicians to Optimize Critical Resources During Covid-19. Acta Inform Med 2020;28(3):209–13.

15. Pageler NM, Longhurst CA, Wood M, et al. Use of electronic medical record-enhanced checklist and electronic dashboard to decrease CLABSIs. Pediatrics 2014;133(3):e738–46.

16. Geva A, Albert BD, Hamilton S, et al. eSIMPLER: A Dynamic, Electronic Health Record-Integrated Checklist for Clinical Decision Support During PICU Daily Rounds. Pediatr Crit Care Med 2021;22(10):898–905.

17. Prgomet M, Li L, Niazkhanl Z, et al. Impact of commercial computerized provider order entry (CPOE) and clinical decision support systems (CDSSs) on medication errors, length of stay, and mortality in intensive care units: a systematic review and meta-analysis. J Am Med Inform Assoc 2017;24(2):413–22.

18. Kane-Gill SL, Dasta JF, Buckley MS, et al. Clinical Practice Guideline: Safe Medication Use in the ICU. Crit Care Med 2017;45(9):e877–915.

19. Chaturvedi RR, Etchegaray JM, Raaen L, et al. Technology Isn't the Half of It: Integrating Electronic Health Records and Infusion Pumps in a Large Hospital. Jt Comm J Qual Patient Saf 2019;45(10):649–61.

20. Ni Y, Lingren T, Huth H, et al. Integrating and Evaluating the Data Quality and Utility of Smart Pump Information in Detecting Medication Administration Errors: Evaluation Study. JMIR Med Inform 2020;8(9):e19774.

21. Azzam HC, Khalsa SS, Urbani R, et al. Validation study of an automated electronic acute lung injury screening tool. JAMIA 2009;16(4):503–8.

22. Koenig HC, Finkel BB, Khalsa SS, et al. Performance of an automated electronic acute lung injury screening system in intensive care unit patients. Crit Care Med 2011;39(1):98–104.

23. Zhao Y, Zheng X, Wang J, et al. Effect of clinical decision support systems on clinical outcome for acute kidney injury: a systematic review and meta-analysis. BMC Nephrol 2021;22(1):271.

24. Goldstein SL, Kirkendall E, Nguyen H, et al. Electronic health record identification of nephrotoxin exposure and associated acute kidney injury. Pediatrics 2013;132: e756–67.

25. Wang L, McGregor TL, Jones DP, et al. Electronic health record-based predictive models for acute kidney injury screening in pediatric inpatients. Pediatr Res 2017;82(3):465–73.
26. Warttig S, Alderson P, Evans DJ, et al. Automated monitoring compared to standard care for the early detection of sepsis in critically ill patients. Cochrane Database Syst Rev 2018;6(6).
27. Joshi M, Ashrafian H, Arora S, et al. Digital Alerting and Outcomes in Patients With Sepsis: Systematic Review and Meta-Analysis. J Med Internet Res 2019; 21(12):e15166.
28. Gale BM, Hall KK. The Use of Patient Monitoring Systems to Improve Sepsis Recognition and Outcomes: A Systematic Review. J Patient Saf 2020;16(3S Suppl 1):S8–11.
29. Dewan M, Vidrine R, Zackoff M, et al. Design, Implementation, and Validation of a Pediatric ICU Sepsis Prediction Tool as Clinical Decision Support. Appl Clin Inform 2020;11(2):218–25.
30. Dewan M, Muthu N, Shelov E, et al. Performance of a Clinical Decision Support Tool to Identify PICU Patients at High Risk for Clinical Deterioration. Pediatr Crit Care Med 2020;21(2):129–35.
31. Colquhoun DA, Davis RP, Tremper TT, et al. Design of a novel multifunction decision support/alerting system for in-patient acute care, ICU and floor (AlertWatch AC). BMC Anesthesiol 2021;21:196.
32. Johnson, Alistair, et al. "MIMIC-III Clinical Database" (version 1.4). PhysioNet (2016).
33. Johnson AEW, Pollard TJ, Shen L, et al. MIMIC-III, a freely accessible critical care database. Scientific Data 2016;3:160035.
34. Johnson, A., Bulgarelli, L., Pollard, T., Horng, S., Celi, L. A., & Mark, R. (2021). MIMIC IV (version 1.0). PhysioNet.
35. Pollard TJ, Johnson AEW, Raffa JD, et al. Scientific Data. 2018. Available at: https://www.nature.com/articles/sdata2018178.
36. Connecting for Health Personal Health Working Group. The personal health working Group: final report. Markle Foundation; 2003.
37. Grossman LV, Choi SW, Collins S, et al. Implementation of acute care patient portals: recommendations on utility and use from six early adopters. J Am Med Inform Assoc 2018;25(4):370–9.
38. Kelly MM, Hoonakker PL, Dean SM. Using an inpatient portal to engage families in pediatric hospital care. J Am Med Inform Assoc 2017;24(1):153–61.
39. Asan O, Scanlon MC, Crotty B, et al. Parental Perceptions of Displayed Patient Data in a PICU: An Example of Unintentional Empowerment. Pediatr Crit Care Med 2019;20(5):435–41.
40. Kim SY, Kim S, Cho J, et al. A deep learning model for real-time mortality prediction in critically ill children. Crit Care 2019;23:279.
41. Sanchez Fernandez I, Sansevere AJ, Gainza-Lein M, et al. Machine learning for outcome prediction in electroencephalograph (EEG)-monitored children in the intensive care unit. J Child Neurol 2018;33:546–53.
42. Aczon MD, Ledbetter DR, Laksana E, et al. Continuous Prediction of Mortality in the PICU: A Recurrent Neural Network Model in a Single-Center Dataset. Pediatr Crit Care Med 2021;22(6):519–29.
43. Kamaleswaran R, Akbilgic O, Hallman MA, et al. Applying artificial intelligence to identify Physiomarkers predicting severe sepsis in the PICU. Pediatr Crit Care Med 2018;19:e495–503.

44. Masino AJ, Harris MC, Forsyth D, et al. Machine learning models for early sepsis recognition in the neonatal intensive care unit using readily available electronic health record data. PLoS One 2019;14:e0212665.

45. Lamping F, Jack T, Rübsamen N, et al. Development and validation of a diagnostic model for early differentiation of sepsis and non-infectious SIRS in critically ill children – a data-driven approach using machine-learning algorithms. BMC Pediatr 2018;18:112.

46. Zhai H, Brady P, Li Q, et al. Developing and evaluating a machine learning based algorithm to predict the need of pediatric intensive care unit transfer for newly hospitalized children. Resuscitation 2014;85:1065–71.

47. Rubin J, Potes C, Xu-Wilson M, et al. An ensemble boosting model for predicting transfer to the pediatric intensive care unit. Int J Med Inf 2018;112:15–20.

48. Williams JB, Ghosh D, Wetzel RC. Applying machine learning to pediatric critical care data. Pediatr Crit Care Med 2018;19:599–608.

49. Kennedy CE, Aoki N, MariscalcoM Turley JP. Using time series analysis to predict cardiac arrest in a PICU. Pediatr Crit Caremed 2015;16:e332–9.

50. Bose SN, Verigan A, Hanson J, et al. Early identification of impending cardiac arrest in neonates and infants in the cardiovascular ICU: a statistical modelling approach using physiologic monitoring data. Cardiol Young 2019;29:1340–8.

51. Rusin CG, Acosta SI, Shekerdemian LS, et al. Prediction of imminent, severe deterioration of children with parallel circulations using real-time processing of physiologic data. J Thorac Cardiovasc Surg 2016;152(1):171–7.

52. Pappy G, Ledbetter D, Aczon M, et al. 1005: Early Prediction of HFNC Failure In the Pediatric ICU Using a Recurrent Neural Network. Crit Care Med 2021; 49(1):501.

53. Baloglu O, Latifi SQ. Nazha A What is machine learning? Arch Dis Child Educ Pract Ed 2021. edpract-2020-319415.

54. Vasey B, Ursprung S, Beddoe B, et al. Association of Clinician Diagnostic Performance With Machine Learning-Based Decision Support Systems: A Systematic Review. JAMA Netw Open 2021;4(3):e211276.

55. Harper E. Can big data transform electronic health records into learning health systems? Stud Health Technol Inform 2014;201:470–5.

56. Institute of Medicine. Health IT and patient safety: Building safer systems for better care. Washington, DC: The National Academies Press; 2012. https://doi.org/10.17226/13269.

57. Reeves JJ, Hollandsworth HM, Torriani FJ, et al. Rapid response to COVID-19: health informatics support for outbreak management in an academic health system. J Am Med Inform Assoc 2020;27(6):853–9.

58. Malden S, Heeney C, Bates DW, et al. Utilizing health information technology in the treatment and management of patients during the COVID-19 pandemic: Lessons from international case study sites. J Am Med Inform Assoc 2021;28(7):1555–63.

Mechanical Ventilation and Respiratory Support in the Pediatric Intensive Care Unit

Omar Alibrahim, MD[a,b], Kyle J. Rehder, MD, FCCM[a,b], Andrew G. Miller, MSc, RRT[c], Alexandre T. Rotta, MD, FCCM[a,b],*

KEYWORDS

- Mechanical ventilation • Noninvasive ventilation
- Continuous positive airway pressure • Bi-level positive airway pressure
- High-flow nasal cannula • Negative pressure ventilation • Children
- Pediatric intensive care

KEY POINTS

- Heated humidified high-flow nasal cannula support has gained increasing popularity in the management of children with respiratory distress due to its ease of use, portability, tolerability, and success in the treatment of patients across the pediatric age spectrum.
- Continuous positive airway pressure and bilevel positive airway pressure unload fatigued respiratory muscles, increase or maintain end-expiratory lung volume, prevent collapse of peripheral small airways during exhalation, and reduce work of breathing.
- The goal of invasive mechanical ventilation is not to normalize gas exchange but to achieve sufficient oxygenation and ventilation to ensure tissue viability until recovery of acceptable lung function while minimizing excessive work of breathing and complications.
- Patient–ventilator asynchrony increases work of breathing and patient discomfort and can aggravate lung injury.

INTRODUCTION

The need for respiratory support is one of the most common reasons children require critical care, and its use is ubiquitous to pediatric intensive care units (PICUs) throughout the world. It can be argued that no other treatment modality is more emblematic of pediatric critical care medicine as a specialty. Respiratory support comprises both noninvasive modalities (ie, heated humidified high-flow nasal cannula [HFNC], continuous positive airway pressure [CPAP], bilevel positive airway pressure

Funding Source: None.
[a] Division of Pediatric Critical Care Medicine, Duke University Medical Center, Durham, NC, USA; [b] Department of Pediatrics, Duke University School of Medicine, Durham, NC, USA; [c] Respiratory Care Services, Duke University Medical Center, Durham, NC, USA
* Corresponding author. Division of Pediatric Critical Care Medicine, 2301 Erwin Road, DUMC 3046, Durham, NC 27710, USA
E-mail address: alex.rotta@duke.edu

Pediatr Clin N Am 69 (2022) 587–605
https://doi.org/10.1016/j.pcl.2022.02.004
0031-3955/22/© 2022 Elsevier Inc. All rights reserved.

pediatric.theclinics.com

[BiPAP], negative pressure ventilation [NPV]) and invasive mechanical ventilation. In this article, we review the various essential elements and considerations involved in the planning and conduct of respiratory support used in the treatment of the critically ill child.

NONINVASIVE RESPIRATORY SUPPORT
Heated Humidified High-Flow Nasal Cannula

The use of HFNC for the treatment of children with respiratory distress or acute hypoxemic respiratory failure has increased significantly during the past decade, with nearly one-quarter of all patients admitted to the PICU now receiving this form of support.[1] The popularity of HFNC is likely related to its ease of use, portability, tolerability, and its success in the management of perinatal lung disease, acute viral bronchiolitis, and respiratory distress across the pediatric age spectrum.[2–5] Recent randomized controlled trials in children with critical bronchiolitis suggest that of HFNC may be superior to standard oxygen therapy[4,6] and equivalent to CPAP for meaningful outcomes, such as the need to escalate support to BiPAP or invasive mechanical ventilation.[7,8] HFNC has also been used to deliver continuous albuterol in patients with critical asthma, with outcomes comparable to aerosol face mask.[9,10]

Several mechanisms contribute to the clinical effect of HFNC. The bulk movement of gas delivered during HFNC therapy penetrates deeply into the hypopharynx and washes out CO_2, thus functionally reducing the anatomic dead space. In addition, the delivery of gas flow at high velocity into the nasal cavity helps offset inspiratory resistance through the nasal passages, thus effectively decreasing work of breathing. The high flow rates delivered into the nasopharynx also provide a low level of positive pressure that may overcome subtle upper airway obstruction, whereas the delivery of conditioned (heated and humidified) gas improves mucociliary clearance and reduces the metabolic work related to heating and humidifying the inspired air.[11,12]

All HFNC system must contain the following elements: (1) a blender for oxygen and air connected to pressurized sources, (2) a water reservoir attached to a heated humidifier, (3) a heated circuit that maintains gas temperature and humidity, and (4) a nonocclusive nasal cannula interface (**Fig. 1**). Aerosol treatment and specialty gases (eg, nitric oxide, helium–oxygen mixtures) can be delivered via HFNC. Medication deposition is affected by cannula size, location of the nebulizer within the circuit, type of system used, and flow, with lower flows resulting in higher aerosol deposition.[13]

On initiation of HFNC support, the clinician sets the gas temperature, the fraction of inspired oxygen (FiO_2), and the flow rate. For comfort, gas temperature is generally set 1°C to 2°C lower than body temperature, whereas FiO_2 should be chosen based on patient physiology and adjusted to target the desired peripheral capillary oxygen saturation (SpO_2). Although there is no consensus regarding the ideal initial gas flow rate, weight-based flow dosing is preferred, at least in infants.[8] Modest respiratory support is achieved with flow rates between 0.5 and 1 L/kg/min, whereas flows up to 2 L/kg/min further attenuate intrathoracic pressure swings associated with work of breathing and likely represent maximal support.[14] Flows in excess of 2 L/kg/min are unlikely to yield additional clinical benefit.[15]

Noninvasive Positive Pressure Ventilation

Noninvasive positive pressure ventilation (NIPPV) modalities, such as CPAP and BiPAP, have been used extensively in patients with extrathoracic airway obstruction, neuromuscular weakness, and in those with obstructive or restrictive lung disease (**Box 1**).[16–19] Of note, CPAP only delivers a continuous airway pressure; therefore,

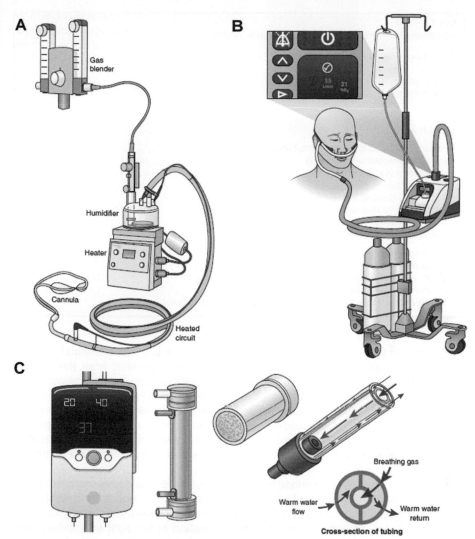

Fig. 1. Commonly used devices for delivery of heated humidified gas mixtures via HFNC. (*A*) HFNC system assembled using a blender, heater/humidifier, and heated wire circuit, (*B*) Airvo-2 HFNC system (Fisher & Paykel Healthcare), and (*C*) Precision Flow high-velocity nasal insufflation HFNC system (Vapotherm, Inc.). (*From* Alibrahim O, Slain KN. Noninvasive ventilation in the Pediatric Intensive Care Unit. In: Zimmerman JJ, Rotta AT, editors. Fuhrman & Zimmerman's Pediatric Critical Care, 6th edition. Philadelphia: Elsevier; 2022. P.646, with permission.)

by definition, it is not a true form of noninvasive ventilation because, unlike BiPAP, the minute volume during CPAP is generated exclusively by the patient, not by the device. CPAP and BiPAP unload fatigued respiratory muscles, increase or maintain end-expiratory lung volume, prevent collapse of peripheral small airways to allow for a more complete exhalation, and reduce work of breathing (**Box 2**).

During CPAP, the device provides constant positive pressure throughout the respiratory cycle while the patient breathes spontaneously. Flow may be variable or fixed,

---

Box 1
Indications for Noninvasive Positive Pressure Ventilation

Acute Lower Respiratory Tract Diseases
  Bronchiolitis
  Pneumonia
  Pulmonary edema
  Acute chest syndrome
  Atelectasis
  Asthma

Avoidance of Intubation or Reintubation
  Immunocompromised patients
  Neuromuscular disorders
  Cystic fibrosis
  Restrictive chest diseases
  Postoperative respiratory insufficiency
  Do-not-intubate status
  Postextubation respiratory insufficiency

Long-Term Use
  Sleep disordered breathing
  Chest wall deformities (eg, scoliosis)
  Neuromuscular diseases
  Chronic respiratory failure (eg, bronchopulmonary dysplasia)

---

depending on the device used. Although CPAP is generally well tolerated,[8,20] some children may need sedation to decrease anxiety or discomfort from the device–patient interface.[21] With BiPAP, the operator sets an expiratory positive airway pressure (EPAP), inspiratory positive airway pressure (IPAP), and FiO_2; when BiPAP modes with mandatory breaths are used, inspiratory time and mandatory respiratory rate must also be set. The IPAP assists with augmentation of tidal volume (V_T) during inspiration, whereas the EPAP maintains airway patency during expiration, prevents alveolar derecruitment, decreases intrathoracic pressure swings, and may improve triggering synchrony.

A well-fitted and sealed interface (eg, nasal or full-face mask) is essential for effective delivery of both CPAP and BiPAP. The occurrence of air leak around an ill-fitting interface may prevent maintenance of the desired airway pressures and be a source of discomfort to the patient. Conversely, the application of too tight an interface may cause skin breakdown and pressure ulcers, especially with prolonged use. Several patient interfaces are available for the delivery of CPAP or BiPAP (**Fig. 2**), including nasal

---

Box 2
Goals of Noninvasive Positive Pressure Ventilation

Short-Term Noninvasive Positive Pressure Ventilation
  Decrease work of breathing
  Improvement of gas exchange
  Avoidance of intubation

Long-Term Noninvasive Positive Pressure Ventilation
  Improve gas exchange
  Improve sleep duration and quality
  Prolong survival
  Improve quality of life

---

pillows, nasal masks, oro-nasal masks, full-face masks, helmets, and mouthpieces. Nasal, oro-nasal, and full-face masks are most commonly used in the PICU.

Hypoxemia and tachypnea that persist after 1 to 6 hours following initiation of NIPPV have been associated with treatment failure.[22–24] Therefore, intubation should be

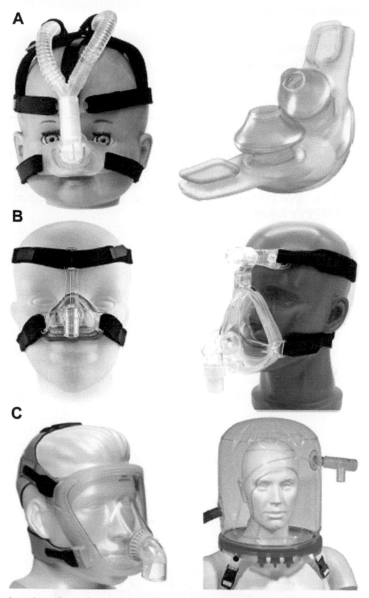

Fig. 2. Various interfaces for delivery of noninvasive ventilation support. (*A*) Nasal pillows (Medical Innovations PedFlow and Resmed Swift FX); and (*B*) Nasal (Sleepnet MiniMe 2) and oronasal (Respironics FitLife) and helmet (Arol NIV10301/X). Images courtesy of the manufacturers. (*From* Alibrahim O, Slain KN. Noninvasive ventilation in the Pediatric Intensive Care Unit. In: Zimmerman JJ, Rotta AT, editors. Fuhrman & Zimmerman's Pediatric Critical Care, 6th edition. Philadelphia: Elsevier; 2022. P.647, with permission.)

Box 3
Complications of Noninvasive Positive Pressure Ventilation

Inadequate gas exchange

Pulmonary aspiration

Gastric distention and perforation

Pressure skin injury (face, nose)

Eye injury and irritation/conjunctivitis

Air leak (pneumothorax, pneumomediastinum)

Agitation

Delay in intubation

---

considered if one is unable to decrease FiO_2 within a few hours from NIPPV initiation. NIPPV may mask progressive worsening of respiratory failure and lead to a delay in intubation, which increases the risk of associated complications, including death[25,26] (**Box 3**). Therefore, appropriate patient selection and a high index of suspicion for the recognition of NIPPVV failure are paramount.

Negative Pressure Ventilation

There has been renewed interest in recent years in the use of cuirass NPV in the management of pediatric acute respiratory failure.[27–29] The cuirass interface is a plastic shell that covers the anterior chest wall to deliver either continuous negative pressure (CNEP) or biphasic cuirass ventilation (BCV; **Fig. 3**). In CNEP mode, negative (subatmospheric) pressure is applied within the cuirass to the anterior chest wall and is maintained at a constant level throughout the respiratory cycle while the patient breathes spontaneously; this can be viewed as the negative equivalent of CPAP. During BCV, inspiratory and expiratory phases are fully controlled (control mode) by modifying the negativity of the air pressure applied to the chest wall during the respiratory cycle. Unlike restful spontaneous breathing, both inspiration and exhalation are active during BCV.

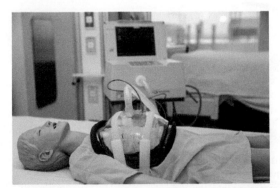

Fig. 3. Hayek RTX Cuirass ventilator. The chest cuirass is made of flexible plastic. This ventilator is capable of conventional NPV as well as high-frequency chest wall oscillations. (*From* Alibrahim O, Slain KN. Noninvasive ventilation in the Pediatric Intensive Care Unit. In: Zimmerman JJ, Rotta AT, editors. Fuhrman & Zimmerman's Pediatric Critical Care, 6th edition. Philadelphia: Elsevier; 2022. P.648, with permission.)

CNEP is usually chosen as the initial support mode, with a minimum support of negative 8 (−8) cm H_2O. This is then adjusted in decrements of 2 cm H_2O until work of breathing is noted to improve. A pressure of negative 14 (−14) cm H_2O generally is sufficient, but support can be escalated to more negative pressures (eg, −20 cm H_2O) as needed throughout the treatment course.

By lowering the intrathoracic pressure, NPV increases right ventricular (RV) preload and decreases RV afterload by facilitating venous return and decreasing pulmonary vascular resistance due to alveolar recruitment, respectively.[30]

INVASIVE MECHANICAL VENTILATION

The goal of invasive mechanical ventilation is not to normalize gas exchange but to achieve sufficient oxygenation and ventilation to ensure tissue viability until recovery of acceptable lung function while minimizing excessive work of breathing and complications. When precisely used, invasive mechanical ventilation is a life-saving intervention, yet care must be taken to avoid ventilator-induced lung injury (VILI).

Indications for Invasive Mechanical Ventilation

The decision to institute invasive mechanical ventilation is based primarily on the need to assist native pulmonary function in patients with acute respiratory failure. This could be from an inability to maintain adequate gas exchange or due to respiratory muscle fatigue or weakness. Although NIPPV is most commonly used earlier in the disease course, for mild or moderate respiratory insufficiency, or when endotracheal intubation is undesirable or contraindicated, invasive mechanical ventilation is indicated in the setting of more severe or rapidly evolving respiratory failure, refractory shock, neurologic impairment, muscle weakness, inability to maintain a patent airway, or any combination of the above. Additional indications for mechanical ventilation include the need to support performance of the left ventricle, to decrease metabolic demand, and to modulate pulmonary or cerebral blood flow in patients with pulmonary or intracranial hypertension, respectively.

There are no absolute criteria for derangement of gas exchange that mandate initiation of respiratory support. Blood gas analysis often is unnecessary to assist in the decision to initiate mechanical respiratory support and is no substitute for clinical assessment. Although some have used numeric cutoffs to define acute hypoxemic and hypercapnic respiratory failure (eg, PaO_2 <60 mm Hg while breathing >60% oxygen, $PaCO_2$ >60 mm Hg, and pH < 7.25) to assist with the decision to initiate invasive mechanical ventilation,[31] the basic tenet is that it should be initiated when clinical goals cannot be safely met using noninvasive methods. Similarly, if a patient's disease trajectory suggests rapid decline toward a need for invasive mechanical ventilation, clinical prudence dictates the early initiation of invasive mechanical ventilation before respiratory or cardiac arrest.

Basic Ventilator Function

The basics of ventilation begin with moving gas in and out of the lungs, usually maintained by an individual's diaphragm and other respiratory muscles. Forces that must be overcome to move air into the lungs include airway resistance and elastance of the respiratory system (ie, lungs and chest wall). When, either due to disease or poor respiratory muscle function, a patient needs assistance to move air in and out of the lungs, ventilators may provide either supportive or full pressure to generate the necessary tidal volume.

Phases of a Breath

The key components of a mechanical breath are trigger, flow pattern, limit, cycle, and inspiratory time (**Fig. 4**). The trigger parameter signals the ventilator to initiate a mechanical breath, whereas flow pattern describes how the air flows into the patient during inspiration. Individual breaths can be pressure or volume limited. During pressure ventilation, the breath is immediately pressurized to the set pressure, which persists until the cycle parameter is met. During volume limited ventilation, gas is delivered throughout the inspiratory phase until the set V_T is reached or the high-pressure alarm is activated. Although different ventilator modes may go by a host of names, the basics of trigger, flow pattern, limit, and cycle define the parameters of any mechanical breath.

Conventional ventilation modes include *control* modes, where the limit and inspiratory time are predetermined, *support* modes where only the limit is preselected, and mixed modes of these two breath types.[32] The mode's title will typically follow the limit parameter, that is, *volume control* for controlled breaths with a volume limit and *pressure support* for supported breaths with a pressure limit. Pure control modes (eg, assist control) will give each breath with a predetermined inspiratory time, whereas a mixed mode will provide a set number of control breaths (determined by the set ventilator rate) with additional opportunity for patient triggered breaths (supported breaths) above that set rate. In either of these modes, should the patient not initiate a spontaneous breath within a predetermined time, the ventilator will deliver a time-triggered control breath, such that the patient will receive at a minimum the set ventilator rate.

Inspiratory time is defined as the period from the start of flow into the patient to the start of exhalation. Expiratory time is defined as the period from the start of exhalation until the start of the next breath. Total cycle time is the sum of inspiratory and expiratory times (see **Fig. 4**).

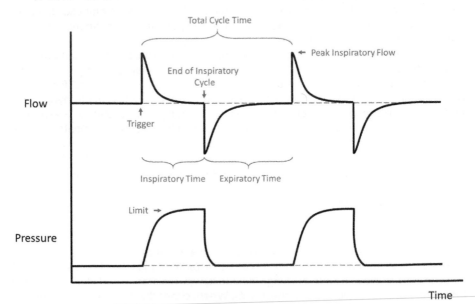

Fig. 4. Phases of a breath. (*Modified from* Rehder KJ, Cheifetz I. Mechanical ventilation and respiratory care. In: Zimmerman JJ, Rotta AT, editors. Fuhrman & Zimmerman's Pediatric Critical Care, 6th edition. Philadelphia: Elsevier; 2022. P.628, with permission.)

Initiating Breaths

Breaths can be initiated (triggered) by either the patient or the ventilator. Triggers include time, pressure, flow, minimum minute ventilation, apnea interval, and electrical signals (eg, electrical diaphragmatic activity). The most common triggers are time, flow, and pressure. All modern ventilators are capable of providing synchronized intermittent mandatory ventilation, in that when the patient is participatory, the ventilator uses a patient trigger to recognize the patient's desire for a breath and delivers either a mandatory machine breath or a pressure-supported breath. Flow or electrical triggers are typically the most sensitive and will allow for improved synchrony, particularly in infants or in patients with weak respiratory muscle effort.[33,34]

Flow Pattern

During inspiration, airway pressure and lung volume will increase until inspiratory flow is terminated. The most common flow patterns used are constant flow and decelerating flow. Constant flow can only be used during volume-limited ventilation. Constant flow will increase pressure and volume linearly, whereas decelerating flow will result in rapid pressure and volume increase at the beginning of a breath, which then slows toward the end of inspiration. Decelerating flow is most commonly used, as it more closely mimics natural breathing and is likely to meet patient flow demands; however, different flow patterns may be beneficial for specific disease processes.[32]

Limit

During assisted breathing, the ventilator will continue to deliver flow into the patient until a predetermined limit is reached. In volume-limited ventilation, the limit is a set volume of gas, and the peak inspiratory pressure (PIP) required to deliver that volume will be variable. Most modern ventilators will allow for more volume to be inspired than what is set, if so desired by the patient. In pressure-limited ventilation, the ventilator will provide flow until a set PIP is reached, resulting in variable tidal volumes. Delivered V_T is the integral of flow with respect to time for each of these breaths. Even when the set limit is reached and flow into the patient ceases, gas may not necessarily be allowed to leave the patient as the lungs are held in an inflated state until the beginning of expiration (cycling).

Adaptive modes allow the clinician to set a V_T or minute ventilation target, and the ventilator delivers pressure-limited breaths to meet that target based on lung compliance measured during test and subsequent breaths. These modes include pressure regulated volume control, average volume-assured pressure support, and adaptive support ventilation. Other adaptive modes of ventilation include proportional assist ventilation (PAV) and neurally adjusted ventilatory assist (NAVA). Each of these modes adjust the amount of support given breath to breath based on patient effort, either measured through flow-derived calculation of patient work (PAV) or through electrical measurement of diaphragm contraction (NAVA).

Exhalation

Ventilator cycling from inspiration to exhalation is most commonly signaled by time (ie, a set inspiratory time during a control breath) or flow (eg, 75%–80% reduction from peak inspiratory flow signaling the end of inspiration for a supported breath). When available, a preset threshold of diaphragmatic electrical signal may also be used as a cycling signal.

Exhalation is passive during almost all forms of invasive mechanical ventilation, with high-frequency oscillatory ventilation (HFOV) being the exception. At the determined end of inspiration during conventional mechanical ventilation, an expiratory valve opens and the chest wall and diaphragm recoil expels gas in an exponentially declining fashion determined by the mathematic product of lung compliance and airways resistance, or *time constant*. The expiratory time constant is the amount of time it takes for the lung to empty 63% of tidal volume, and therefore complete emptying of the lungs (greater than 98% emptying) takes at least 4 time constants. Time constants will be prolonged in states of high airway resistance and of high lung compliance. This is why longer expiratory times are necessary in small airways disease states such as asthma and bronchiolitis to allow complete exhalation and avoid gas trapping.

Initial Ventilator Settings

When initiating mechanical ventilation, it is imperative to understand the underlying pathophysiology: hypoxemic, hypercapnic, or neuromuscular respiratory failure. The ventilator itself will not cure the underlying disease, yet proper management—or mismanagement—can most certainly influence the course of lung disease; it can expedite recovery or worsen pulmonary function through the occurrence of VILI.

Because carbon dioxide rapidly equilibrates between the alveolar gas and the blood stream, carbon dioxide removal is primarily a function of alveolar minute ventilation. Minute ventilation, or the volume of gas moved in and out of the lungs per minute, is represented by the product of respiratory rate and tidal volume. Oxygenation, however, depends on a slower diffusion process and uses hemoglobin as a carrier molecule in the blood. As such, systemic oxygenation is not only dependent on moving oxygen into the alveoli, but on higher mean airway pressures to drive oxygen diffusion across the alveolar membrane, as well as optimizing ventilation perfusion (V/Q) ratio so that oxygen is able to bind to passing hemoglobin.

Appropriate setting and titration of the ventilator relies on an understanding of clinical goals and pathophysiology (ie, restrictive disease, obstructive disease, or a combination of the two).

Tidal Volume

Selecting the optimal V_T is largely dependent on the underlying disease process and should be indexed to predicted (ideal) body weight. For patients with *healthy lungs*, like those receiving mechanical ventilation for severe encephalopathy or neuromuscular failure, a V_T between 6 and 10 mL/kg is generally acceptable and should be easily achievable with modest PIPs. Patients with *restrictive lung disease*, like those with severe pneumonias or pediatric acute respiratory distress syndrome (PARDS) should be ventilated with V_T between 5 and 8 mL/kg as measured at the endotracheal tube.[35,36] Lower V_T in the range of 3 to 6 mL/kg should be used in patients with more severely decreased respiratory system compliance. To avoid VILI, the end-inspiratory alveolar pressure (ie, plateau pressure) should be targeted no higher than 28 cm H_2O (or 32 cm H_2O in patients with reduced chest wall compliance).[35,36] For patients with *obstructive disease*, like those with near-fatal asthma, large V_T (ie, 8–12 mL/kg) are often necessary to maintain an acceptable minute ventilation because these patients will also require a low respiratory rate to allow for full exhalation before a subsequent breath.[37] Due to the high airway resistance, this may necessitate very high PIP (as high as 50–60 cm H_2O). It must be underscored, however, that these high pressures are not directly transmitted to the alveoli because they are dynamic measurements taken during inspiratory flow and thus influenced by the high airway resistance. The plateau pressure, a static measurement obtained during an inspiratory hold in the absence of flow, is not influenced by airway resistance and is a better gauge of the forces being transmitted to the alveoli; it should be kept less than 30 cm H_2O to avoid barotrauma.

Ventilator Rate and Inspiratory Time

Ventilator rate is selected based on the age and ventilatory requirements of the patient and should subsequently be adjusted according to the $PaCO_2$ or end-tidal CO_2. Patients with *restrictive disease* generally require higher rates to achieve an acceptable minute ventilation due to the concomitant use of reduced V_T. Conversely, patients with *obstructive disease* will require lower rates to allow for complete exhalation before the next breath and prevent dynamic hyperinflation. Under normal circumstances, the inspiratory time for control breaths is selected to provide an inspiratory-to-expiratory time (I: E) ratio of at approximately 1:2, which approximates normal spontaneous breathing. Patients with restrictive disease usually have heterogeneous lung compliance with varying regional time constants, so a longer inspiratory time is necessary to allow for adequate gas distribution and avoid underventilation and underinflation. A long inspiratory time also increases the mean airway pressure, which is directly correlated with oxygenation and may be beneficial in restrictive processes such as acute respiratory distress syndrome (ARDS). Sufficient expiratory time must be provided to allow for complete exhalation, which is particularly important in patients with obstructive disease. If inspiration starts before the prior exhalation is completed, gas trapping will result. In mechanically ventilated children with asthma, the expiratory time must be lengthened to avoid gas trapping (**Fig. 5**). This is best accomplished by decreasing the respiratory rate rather than by shortening the inspiratory time, because the latter could result in insufficient time for the delivery of the desired V_T when airway resistance is high.

Continuous positive airway pressure, positive end expiratory pressure, and FiO_2

CPAP denotes the maintenance of positive airway pressure throughout the respiratory cycle with no positive pressure breaths delivered, whereas positive end expiratory pressure (PEEP) refers to the maintenance of airway pressure more than the atmospheric pressure between breaths; for the remainder of this article, we will use PEEP as a uniform term for both these pressures when applied to the intubated patient

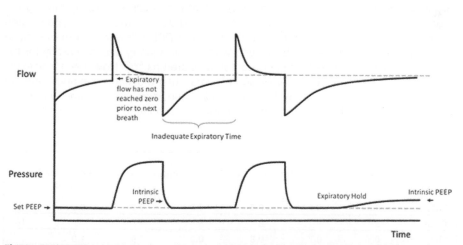

Fig. 5. Scalars demonstrating gas trapping in a patient with obstructive small airways disease. (*Modified from* Rehder KJ, Cheifetz I. Mechanical ventilation and respiratory care. In: Zimmerman JJ, Rotta AT, editors. Fuhrman & Zimmerman's Pediatric Critical Care, 6th edition. Philadelphia: Elsevier; 2022. P.631, with permission.)

undergoing invasive mechanical ventilation. We reserved the term CPAP for the application of CPAP via a tight-fitting interface for the nonintubated patient, as previously discussed.

Atelectasis is common in lung diseases characterized by nonuniform or heterogeneous parenchymal involvement. Recruitment of collapsed alveoli requires higher airway pressures than those needed to sustain inflation once the alveoli are open, and the reopening of these alveoli may cause shear injury to the alveolar epithelium, a process known as atelectrauma. PEEP is an essential element of an open lung ventilation strategy that, when properly set, (1) increases end-expiratory lung volume above closing volume to prevent cyclic alveolar collapse, (2) maintains stability of alveolar segments, (3) increases oxygenation by improving V/Q matching, and (4) reduces work of breathing by unloading the diaphragm.

The optimal PEEP is the level at which there is an acceptable balance between the desired clinical goals and undesired adverse effects. Clinicians should target PEEP to optimal lung expansion and to maintain adequate oxygenation with a "nontoxic" inspired oxygen concentration.[35,36] Arbitrary limits cannot be placed on the level of PEEP required to maintain adequate gas exchange, which are highly variable among disease processes or even for the same patient at different time points. For patients with normal lungs, low levels of PEEP in the range of 4 to 5 cm H_2O are generally sufficient to maintain adequate oxygenation and prevent atelectasis. Patients with *restrictive disease* and poor lung compliance, such as those with ARDS, will require higher PEEP to prevent alveolar collapse during expiration. A helpful guideline is to titrate PEEP based on a PEEP/FiO_2 table [**Table 1**], where patients with a high oxygen requirement receive higher PEEP and patients with low oxygen requirement receive lower PEEP.[38] Recent data suggest that clinicians underutilize PEEP in the setting of ARDS, and that the application of PEEP lower than indicated is associated with increased mortality.[39] Restrictive syndromes caused by obesity, anasarca, or increased abdominal pressure will also benefit from higher PEEP to stabilize the alveoli at end-expiration, which can be best titrated using esophageal manometry.

In obstructive lung disease of the small airways (eg, asthma), the target level of PEEP can be controversial. The application of PEEP may benefit patients with expiratory flow limitation from dynamic compression of the small airways by moving the equal pressure point down the airway and enabling decompression of hyperinflated upstream alveoli.[40] The application of low levels of PEEP (lower than the intrinsic-PEEP) may relieve dyspnea by facilitating ventilator triggering and synchrony for the intubated patient capable of drawing spontaneous breaths.[40,41] However, for patients with severe airflow obstruction receiving neuromuscular blockade, the application of PEEP is uniformly associated with hyperinflation and increased intrathoracic pressures that could result in hemodynamic compromise. In these patients, our practice

Table 1						
PEEP/FiO_2 combinations based on the ARDS clinical trials network lower PEEP/Higher FiO_2 protocol[a]						
FiO_2	0.3	0.4	0.4	0.5	0.5	0.6	0.7
PEEP	5	5	8	8	10	10	10
FiO_2	0.7	0.7	0.8	0.9	0.9	1.0	
PEEP	12	14	14	16	18	18–24	

FiO_2, fraction of inspired oxygen; PEEP, positive end-expiratory pressure.
  [a] Data from reference[33].

is to use zero PEEP while under neuromuscular blockade and apply a low level of PEEP (lower than the intrinsic-PEEP and generally not greater than 8 cm H_2O) to facilitate ventilator synchrony in patients contributing with spontaneous breaths.

In conjunction with PEEP, FiO_2 is adjusted to achieve adequate oxygenation. High concentrations of oxygen can contribute to lung injury through development of reactive oxygen species and should be avoided. The exact threshold that increases the risk of oxygen-associated lung injury is not clear, but a $FiO_2 \leq 0.5$ is generally considered safe. With evidence of adequate oxygen delivery, a permissive hypoxemia strategy may be safely applied to permit the application of lower FiO_2.[35]

Patient-Ventilator Asynchrony

A primary goal of mechanical ventilation is the coordination of the patient's natural breathing pattern with mechanical breaths. The patient should be able to receive a breath when attempting to inspire, just as they should be able to effortlessly exhale when ready. Patient–ventilator asynchrony increases work of breathing and patient discomfort and can aggravate lung injury. Patients exhibiting asynchrony during mechanical ventilation often demonstrate improved oxygenation and ventilation after neuromuscular blockade; however, adjustments to ventilator settings can often avoid the need for neuromuscular blockade and are preferred.

Triggering Asynchrony

Asynchrony associated with breath triggering is common and can be classified into (1) missed triggering, (2) delayed triggering, (3) autotriggering, (4) double triggering, and (5) reverse triggering.[42] The first two forms of asynchrony cause air hunger by not providing a supported breath when the patient desires a breath, whereas the remaining forms provide mechanical breaths when the patient should not be receiving a breath.

Missed triggering: Missed triggering refers to a patient's effort that fails to trigger the ventilator, such that effort is not accompanied by a supported mechanical breath (**Fig. 6**). Most commonly, poor patient effort (often secondary to muscle weakness) results in a breath that is insufficient to reach the trigger threshold. A trigger threshold that is set inappropriately high may lead to missed triggering even when the patient can generate a normal effort. The missing (ineffective) triggering presents as either a pressure or flow deflection along with visualized patient effort that is not followed by a ventilator breath. Missed triggers can also be detected using waveform capnography.

Delayed triggering: Delayed triggering is defined as a lag from sensing the trigger to delivering the mechanical breath (see **Fig. 6**), usually intrinsic to the trigger sensitivity and electronic response of the ventilator.

Autotriggering: Autotriggering occurs when mechanical breaths are delivered neither in response to patient effort nor a timed breath (see **Fig. 6**). Factors commonly associated with autotriggering include an inadequately low triggering threshold, circuit leak, water in the circuit, and ventilator sensing of patient cardiac oscillations.

Double triggering: Double triggering occurs when two consecutive inspirations happen within an interval of less than half of the mean inspiratory time (see **Fig. 6**). A common reason for double triggering is when the patient's native inspiratory time exceeds the set inspiratory time, usually due to high patient demand or coughing. As the second breath is triggered while the patient is still inhaling, a higher V_T may be inadvertently delivered with subsequent increase in alveolar pressure.

Reverse triggering: Reverse triggering occurs when the ventilator delivers a breath not triggered by the patient (usually a time-triggered breath), and the distension of the

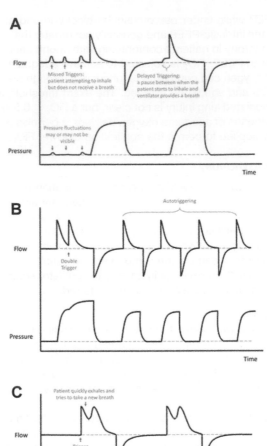

Fig. 6. Scalars representing different types of patient–ventilator asynchrony. (*A*) The trigger sensitivity is initially set such that the patient is unable to trigger a breath; a flow deflection signals attempted inhalation without an associated breath. Subsequently, the trigger is set such that the patient attempts to inhale, and there is a delay before the ventilator responds with a breath. (*B*) The patient initially experiences a double trigger event, with a second breath triggered before beginning exhalation, resulting in additional tidal volume delivered with an increase in pressure. The patient then begins to experience autotriggering, with repeated breaths given immediately following exhalation. The latter may be easily mistaken for tachypnea, but examination of the patient will reveal no respiratory effort. (*C*) This patient is experiencing flow asynchrony in the form of inadequate flow demand. The patient begins to inhale but in unable to draw enough flow to meet his needs, slightly exhales, then once again inhales. The pressure waveform has a scooped appearance as the patient "sucks" flow from the circuit. (*From* Rehder KJ, Cheifetz I. Mechanical ventilation and respiratory care. In: Zimmerman JJ, Rotta AT, editors. Fuhrman & Zimmerman's Pediatric Critical Care, 6th edition. Philadelphia: Elsevier; 2022. P.636, with permission.)

lungs causes the diaphragm to contract, thus triggering a spontaneous breath. The combination of the mechanical breath and late diaphragm contraction may result in larger than intended V_T, along with a prematurely terminated breath while the patient is still trying to inhale.

Flow Asynchrony

Flow asynchrony occurs during inspiration, most commonly when the patient's demand exceeds the delivered flow.[42,43] The pressure scalar can be useful in assessing flow asynchrony. A commonly witnessed pattern for inadequate flow is an "M-shaped" flow pattern as the patient maximizes the available flow, slightly exhales, and then inhales again to the maximal available flow (see **Fig. 6**). Less common is a delivered flow that is in excess of the patient's needs, resulting in an early peak in airway pressure and potential for larger tidal volumes.

Cycling Asynchrony

Patients can experience notable discomfort when their neural inspiratory time and ventilator cycling criteria are mismatched.[42,43] Premature cycling refers to the ventilator terminating inspiration while the patient is still maintaining an inspiratory effort, often in the presence of a leak in the ventilator circuit or around the endotracheal tube. Delayed cycling refers to the prolongation of inspiration beyond the start of the patient's expiration. In addition to high PIP as the patient attempts to exhale against a closed expiratory valve, a shortened expiratory time may result in gas trapping.[43]

Nontraditional Ventilator Modes

The most commonly used nontraditional mode of ventilation is high frequency ventilation, defined by supraphysiologic breath rates (greater than 150 breaths/min) and very small tidal volumes that approximate—or are lower than—the anatomic dead space.[44] The three main types of high frequency ventilation used in clinical practice are HFOV, high frequency jet ventilation (HFJV), and high-frequency percussive ventilation. Due to their very low V_T, these modes of ventilation are theorized to be lung-protective, yet definitive evidence of their role in the treatment of pediatric ARDS are lacking. Oxygenation may be supported by a high baseline mean airway pressure, whereas ventilation occurs via a mix of gas exchange principles including flow streaming, asymmetric velocity profiles, augmented dispersion, cardiogenic mixing, diffusion, convection, and Pendelluft ventilation.[45]

Airway pressure release ventilation (APRV), also called bilevel ventilation, is a nontraditional mode of ventilation primarily used for hypoxemic respiratory failure in the patient capable of maintaining a spontaneous breathing effort. APRV uses prolonged sustained lung inflation with unrestricted spontaneous breathing to maintain a high mean airway pressure to support oxygenation. Ventilation occurs through spontaneous small breaths (generated by the patient) which occur above that sustained inflation, coupled with intermittent brief release breaths, with rapid exhalation and reinflation to augment CO_2 clearance.[46] A recent randomized controlled trial demonstrated APRV to be associated with increased mortality in pediatric ARDS.[47]

Each of these modes has theoretic advantages and, when applied correctly, can often improve short-term gas exchange. Despite these reported short-term improvements in physiologic outcomes, convincing evidence demonstrating that these modes improve meaningful clinical outcomes is lacking. In addition, inexpert management of any of these modes carries a high potential for iatrogenic lung injury. These unique forms of ventilation are most commonly used as rescue when conventional modes cannot meet clinical goals, but may also be used early as part of a comprehensive lung protective strategy for certain disease processes, including air leak syndromes and inhalational injury.

SUMMARY

In the setting of respiratory failure or respiratory insufficiency, mechanical ventilation serves to augment the patient's native respiratory effort, either noninvasively or invasively. The application of continuous positive pressure also helps maintain optimal V/Q matching in the setting of restrictive or heterogeneous lung disease. Ventilator management should focus on lung protection to avoid VILI and allow for best chance for lung recovery. Specific strategies will also need to be adjusted based on underlying lung and cardiovascular pathophysiology. Finally, titrating settings for optimal patient–ventilator synchrony will improve gas exchange and comfort while also helping minimize VILI.

CLINICS CARE POINTS

- Close monitoring of patient response is paramount following initiation NIPPV because hypoxemia and tachypnea that persist after 1 to 6 hours following initiation of NIPPV have been associated with treatment failure.
- Blood gas analysis often is unnecessary to assist in the decision to initiate mechanical respiratory support and is no substitute for clinical assessment.
- Patients with restrictive lung disease (eg, severe pneumonias, PARDS) should be ventilated with V_T between 5 and 8 mL/kg. Lower V_T in the range of 3 to 6 mL/kg should be used in patients with more severely decreased respiratory system compliance.
- Patients with obstructive lung disease (eg, near-fatal asthma) often require large V_T (ie, 8–12 mL/kg) and low respiratory rates to allow for complete exhalation before the start of the next breath and prevent dynamic hyperinflation.
- Clinicians should target PEEP to optimal lung expansion and to maintain adequate oxygenation with a "nontoxic" inspired oxygen concentration.
- Nontraditional ventilator modes (eg, HFOV, HFJV) are most commonly used as rescue when conventional modes cannot meet clinical goals but may also be used early as part of a comprehensive lung protective strategy for certain disease processes.

CONFLICT OF INTEREST STATEMENT

A.T. Rotta received honoraria from Breas US and Vapotherm Inc for consulting, development of educational materials, and lecturing. The remaining authors do not have any potential conflicts to disclose.

REFERENCES

1. Morris JV, Kapetanstrataki M, Parslow RC, et al. Patterns of Use of Heated Humidified High-Flow Nasal Cannula Therapy in PICUs in the United Kingdom and Republic of Ireland. Pediatr Crit Care Med 2019;20(3):223–32.
2. Wilkinson D, Andersen C, O'Donnell CP, et al. High flow nasal cannula for respiratory support in preterm infants. Cochrane Database Syst Rev 2016;2: CD006405.
3. Franklin D, Babl FE, Schibler A. High-Flow Oxygen Therapy in Infants with Bronchiolitis. N Engl J Med 2018;378(25):2446–7.
4. Franklin D, Babl FE, Schlapbach LJ, et al. A Randomized Trial of High-Flow Oxygen Therapy in Infants with Bronchiolitis. N Engl J Med 2018;378(12):1121–31.

5. Ward JJ. High-flow oxygen administration by nasal cannula for adult and perinatal patients. Respir Care 2013;58(1):98–122.

6. Kepreotes E, Whitehead B, Attia J, et al. High-flow warm humidified oxygen versus standard low-flow nasal cannula oxygen for moderate bronchiolitis (HFWHO RCT): an open, phase 4, randomised controlled trial. Lancet 2017; 389(10072):930–9.

7. Cesar RG, Bispo BRP, Felix P, et al. High-Flow Nasal Cannula versus Continuous Positive Airway Pressure in Critical Bronchiolitis: A Randomized Controlled Pilot. J Pediatr Intensive Care 2020;9(4):248–55.

8. Milesi C, Essouri S, Pouyau R, et al. High flow nasal cannula (HFNC) versus nasal continuous positive airway pressure (nCPAP) for the initial respiratory management of acute viral bronchiolitis in young infants: a multicenter randomized controlled trial (TRAMONTANE study). Intensive Care Med 2017;43(2):209–16.

9. Gates RM, Haynes KE, Rehder KJ, et al. High-Flow Nasal Cannula in Pediatric Critical Asthma. Respir Care 2021;66(8):1240–6.

10. Gauto Benitez R, Morilla Sanabria LP, Pavlicich V, et al. High flow nasal cannula oxygen therapy in patients with asthmatic crisis in the pediatric emergency department. Rev Chil Pediatr 2019;90(6):642–8.

11. Hasani A, Chapman TH, McCool D, et al. Domiciliary humidification improves lung mucociliary clearance in patients with bronchiectasis. Chron Respir Dis 2008;5(2):81–6.

12. Dysart K, Miller TL, Wolfson MR, et al. Research in high flow therapy: mechanisms of action. Respir Med 2009;103(10):1400–5.

13. Li J, Fink JB, MacLoughlin R, et al. A narrative review on trans-nasal pulmonary aerosol delivery. Crit Care 2020;24(1):506.

14. Weiler T, Kamerkar A, Hotz J, et al. The Relationship between High Flow Nasal Cannula Flow Rate and Effort of Breathing in Children. J Pediatr 2017;189: 66–71 e63.

15. Milesi C, Pierre AF, Deho A, et al. A multicenter randomized controlled trial of a 3-L/kg/min versus 2-L/kg/min high-flow nasal cannula flow rate in young infants with severe viral bronchiolitis (TRAMONTANE 2). Intensive Care Med 2018;44(11): 1870–8.

16. Luo F, Annane D, Orlikowski D, et al. Invasive versus non-invasive ventilation for acute respiratory failure in neuromuscular disease and chest wall disorders. Cochrane Database Syst Rev 2017;12:CD008380.

17. Jat KR, Mathew JL. Continuous positive airway pressure (CPAP) for acute bronchiolitis in children. Cochrane Database Syst Rev 2019;1:CD010473.

18. Korang SK, Feinberg J, Wetterslev J, et al. Non-invasive positive pressure ventilation for acute asthma in children. Cochrane Database Syst Rev 2016;9: CD012067.

19. Morley SL. Non-invasive ventilation in paediatric critical care. Paediatr Respir Rev 2016;20:24–31.

20. Yanez LJ, Yunge M, Emilfork M, et al. A prospective, randomized, controlled trial of noninvasive ventilation in pediatric acute respiratory failure. Pediatr Crit Care Med 2008;9(5):484–9.

21. Abadesso C, Nunes P, Silvestre C, et al. Non-invasive ventilation in acute respiratory failure in children. Pediatr Rep 2012;4(2):e16.

22. Mayordomo-Colunga J, Medina A, Rey C, et al. Predictive factors of non invasive ventilation failure in critically ill children: a prospective epidemiological study. Intensive Care Med 2009;35(3):527–36.

23. James CS, Hallewell CP, James DP, et al. Predicting the success of non-invasive ventilation in preventing intubation and re-intubation in the paediatric intensive care unit. Intensive Care Med 2011;37(12):1994–2001.

24. Mayordomo-Colunga J, Pons M, Lopez Y, et al. Predicting non-invasive ventilation failure in children from the SpO(2)/FiO(2) (SF) ratio. Intensive Care Med 2013;39(6):1095–103.

25. Mosier JM, Sakles JC, Whitmore SP, et al. Failed noninvasive positive-pressure ventilation is associated with an increased risk of intubation-related complications. Ann Intensive Care 2015;5:4.

26. Demoule A, Girou E, Richard JC, et al. Benefits and risks of success or failure of noninvasive ventilation. Intensive Care Med 2006;32(11):1756–65.

27. Hassinger AB, Breuer RK, Nutty K, et al. Negative-Pressure Ventilation in Pediatric Acute Respiratory Failure. Respir Care 2017;62(12):1540–9.

28. Moffitt CA, Deakins K, Cheifetz I, et al. Use of Negative Pressure Ventilation in Pediatric Critical Care: Experience in 56 PICUs in the Virtual Pediatric Systems Database (2009-2019). Pediatr Crit Care Med 2021;22(6):e363–8.

29. Rotta AT. Randomized Controlled Trial of Negative Pressure Ventilation: We First Need a National Patient Registry. Pediatr Crit Care Med 2021;22(6):e369–70.

30. Shekerdemian LS, Bush A, Shore DF, et al. Cardiorespiratory responses to negative pressure ventilation after tetralogy of fallot repair: a hemodynamic tool for patients with a low-output state. J Am Coll Cardiol 1999;33(2):549–55.

31. Sarnaik AP, Clark JA, Heidemann SM. Respiratory Distress and Failure. In: Kliegman RM, St Geme JW III, editors. Nelson Textbook of pediatrics. 21 ed. Philadelphia: Elsevier; 2020. p. 583–601.

32. Mireles-Cabodevila E, Hatipoglu U, Chatburn RL. A rational framework for selecting modes of ventilation. Respir Care 2013;58(2):348–66.

33. Murias G, Villagra A, Blanch L. Patient-ventilator dyssynchrony during assisted invasive mechanical ventilation. Minerva Anestesiol 2013;79(4):434–44.

34. Stein H, Firestone K, Rimensberger PC. Synchronized mechanical ventilation using electrical activity of the diaphragm in neonates. Clin Perinatol 2012;39(3):525–42.

35. Pediatric Acute Lung Injury Consensus Conference G. Pediatric acute respiratory distress syndrome: consensus recommendations from the Pediatric Acute Lung Injury Consensus Conference. Pediatr Crit Care Med 2015;16(5):428–39.

36. Rimensberger PC, Cheifetz IM. Pediatric Acute Lung Injury Consensus Conference G. Ventilatory support in children with pediatric acute respiratory distress syndrome: proceedings from the Pediatric Acute Lung Injury Consensus Conference. Pediatr Crit Care Med 2015;16(5 Suppl 1):S51–60.

37. Darioli R, Perret C. Mechanical controlled hypoventilation in status asthmaticus. Am Rev Respir Dis 1984;129(3):385–7.

38. Brower RG, Lanken PN, MacIntyre N, et al. Higher versus lower positive end-expiratory pressures in patients with the acute respiratory distress syndrome. N Engl J Med 2004;351(4):327–36.

39. Khemani RG, Parvathaneni K, Yehya N, et al. Positive End-Expiratory Pressure Lower Than the ARDS Network Protocol Is Associated with Higher Pediatric Acute Respiratory Distress Syndrome Mortality. Am J Respir Crit Care Med 2018;198(1):77–89.

40. Marini JJ. Should PEEP be used in airflow obstruction? Am Rev Respir Dis 1989;140(1):1–3.

41. Stewart TE, Slutsky AS. Occult, occult auto-PEEP in status asthmaticus. Crit Care Med 1996;24(3):379–80.

42. Gilstrap D, MacIntyre N. Patient-ventilator interactions. Implications for clinical management. Am J Respir Crit Care Med 2013;188(9):1058–68.
43. Gilstrap D, Davies J. Patient-Ventilator Interactions. Clin Chest Med 2016;37(4): 669–81.
44. Miller AG, Bartle RM, Rehder KJ. High-Frequency Jet Ventilation in Neonatal and Pediatric Subjects: A Narrative Review. Respir Care 2021;66(5):845–56.
45. Hupp SR, Turner DA, Rehder KJ. Is there still a role for high-frequency oscillatory ventilation in neonates, children and adults? Expert Rev Respir Med 2015;9(5): 603–18.
46. Turner DA, Rehder KJ, Cheifetz IM. Nontraditional modes of mechanical ventilation: progress or distraction? Expert Rev Respir Med 2012;6(3):277–84.
47. Lalgudi Ganesan S, Jayashree M, Chandra Singhi S, et al. Airway Pressure Release Ventilation in Pediatric Acute Respiratory Distress Syndrome. A Randomized Controlled Trial. Am J Respir Crit Care Med 2018;198(9):1199–207.

Research in Pediatric Intensive Care

Andrew Prout, MD[a,b,*], Kathleen L. Meert, MD[b,c,d]

KEYWORDS

- Research agenda • Core outcome sets • Precision medicine • Clinical trials
- Pediatric intensive care unit • Infants • Children

KEY POINTS

- Research agendas guide the investment of time and resources and are usually based on review of the medical literature and expert opinion.
- Core outcome sets are an agreed on set of outcomes to be measured in all clinical trials of a specific disease or disorder and make it easier to compare, contrast, and combine results across individual trials.
- Precision medicine refers to the goal of identifying biologically similar groups of patients within a specific disease or syndrome that have different responses to therapy.
- Recent and planned clinical trials focus on disease and treatment heterogeneity and the use of core outcomes sets, which include patient- and family centered outcomes.

INTRODUCTION

Clinical research in pediatric intensive care has increased in quantity and quality over the past several decades.[1] National and international research networks, large electronic registries, sophisticated statistical software, innovative trial designs, shifts in funding priorities toward pragmatic clinical trials, and other advancements have contributed to this growing body of research. Yet, many important clinical questions remain unanswered due to the lack of high-quality evidence. To address this gap, some have suggested that research in pediatric intensive care units (PICUs) should be incorporated into clinical work as a "standard of care" much the same way as children with cancer are enrolled into iterative clinical trials where the treatment arm consists of small modifications to standard care.[2] Resources for research in PICUs

[a] Division of Pediatric Critical Care Medicine, Discipline of Pediatrics, Children's Hospital of Michigan, Floor Carls Building, 3901 Beaubien Boulevard, Detroit, MI, 48201, USA; [b] Central Michigan University, Mt. Pleasant, MI, USA; [c] Discipline of Pediatrics, Children's Hospital of Michigan, Detroit, MI, USA; [d] Children's Hospital of Michigan, Suite H-07, 3901 Beaubien Boulevard, Detroit, MI 48201, USA
* Corresponding author. Pediatric Critical Care Medicine, Children's Hospital of Michigan, 4th Floor Carl's Building,3901 Beaubien Boulevard, Detroit, MI 48201.
E-mail address: prout2a@cmich.edu

Pediatr Clin N Am 69 (2022) 607–620
https://doi.org/10.1016/j.pcl.2022.01.015
0031-3955/22/© 2022 Elsevier Inc. All rights reserved.

include multidisciplinary care teams, continuous physiologic monitoring, electronic health records (EHR), access to biological samples from invasive devices, and abundance of laboratory and radiologic data. However, challenges to conducting research in PICUs also exist, such as heterogeneity in patient age and diagnoses, high rates of underlying comorbidities, rare diseases, lack of equipoise for important research questions, need for timely informed consent, family stress, and high clinical demands on intensivists, leaving little time for investigative pursuits. Although the topic of "Research in PICUs" is extremely broad, this review focuses on a few common themes receiving increased attention in the literature, including research agendas, core outcome sets, precision medicine, and novel clinical trial strategies.

DISCUSSION
Research Agendas

Research agendas are developed to guide the investment of time and resources toward areas deemed most in need of advancement. Funding agencies, professional societies, and research networks are examples of organizations that create and disseminate research agendas. Although often based on literature reviews, conference proceedings, and professional guidelines, most research agendas rely heavily on expert opinion.

In 2016, the *Eunice Kennedy Shriver* National Institute of Child Health and Human Development Pediatric Trauma and Critical Illness Branch (PTCIB) identified 3 research priorities for pediatric intensive care to which funding would be directed.[3] These included (1) mechanisms of trauma and critical illness and therapies to improve outcomes, (2) multisystem organ dysfunction syndrome (MODS) as a cause or consequence of critical illness, and (3) co-occurrence of physical and psychological trauma and prevention and treatment of injury and its sequelae. Collaborations among multidisciplinary teams were deemed essential to address the gaps in understanding of mechanisms of critical illness and to optimize strategies for prevention and treatment. Priorities of the PTCIB were informed by recommendations from leading researchers and clinicians in critical care.

A global clinical research agenda for pediatric intensive care was put forth in 2017 by Peters and colleagues after seeking the input of PICU investigators from 5 continents.[1] After considering recent advances, the international group of experts identified 10 research themes considered to directly influence patient care. These included ventilation techniques and interfaces; fluid, transfusion, and feeding strategies; optimal targets for vital signs; MODS definitions, mechanisms and treatments; trauma prevention and treatment; improving safety; comfort of the patient and family; appropriate care in the face of medical complexity; defining post-PICU outcomes; and improving knowledge generation and adoption with novel trial designs and implementation strategies. The importance of clinical research in low- and middle-income countries, as well as highly resourced PICUs was highlighted.

Several disease-focused research agendas have been put forth by specialty societies. These agendas often emerge during development of guidelines aimed at managing specific conditions. Experts using various predefined methods for creation of evidence-based treatment guidelines uncover gaps in knowledge through the process; these gaps become the basis for future research recommendations. Examples include research recommendations for pediatric traumatic brain injury,[4] sepsis,[5] acute respiratory distress syndrome (ARDS),[6] cardiac arrest,[7] cardiac intensive care,[8] and critical complications of oncologic disorders.[9] The Society of Critical Care Medicine and European Society of Intensive Care Medicine Surviving Sepsis Campaign identified 29 pathophysiologic questions and proposed 23 randomized controlled trials during the process of developing international guidelines for the management of septic shock and sepsis-associated organ dysfunction in children.[5] Some common research priorities described across guidelines include greater knowledge and understanding of pathophysiology, new treatments, integration of treatments, biomarkers and identification of subpopulations, common data elements, supportive therapies, deescalation of care, nonmortality outcomes, and the role of unit structure and process improvement on outcomes.

Although most research agendas are based on the literature and expert opinion, experts may have insufficient information or bias toward specific issues resulting in agendas that may not have the biggest impact on patient outcomes. To inform a research agenda that could maximally reduce morbidity and mortality in PICUs, the Collaborative Pediatric Critical Care Research Network (CPCCRN) identified pathophysiologies responsible for new morbidities and mortality after critical illness and potential therapeutic advances that could reduce or prevent these adverse outcomes.[10,11] Data were collected by a multicenter structured chart review. A significant new morbidity was defined as a worsening of functional status compared with preillness baseline based on Functional Status Scale scores. The most common pathophysiologies leading to adverse outcomes were low cardiac output and cardiac arrest, inflammation-related organ failure, and central nervous system trauma. Chronic illness frequently contributed to adverse outcomes. Necessary therapeutic advances included drug therapies, cell regeneration, and improved immune and inflammatory modulation. Patient-level data that identify pathophysiologies driving morbidity and mortality in PICUs may be useful in informing a research agenda that is ultimately intended to reduce these adverse outcomes.

Research agendas for PICU nursing care have also been developed.[12] In a recent review of nursing research priorities, themes for pediatric intensive care included resuscitation, nurse-led interventions, pressure-related tissue damage, ventilation, outcome measures, technology, transfer, and discharge.

Core Outcome Sets

The number of children in a single PICU who are eligible for a particular clinical trial is relatively small compared with the number of children needed to gain clinically and statistically significant trial results. Therefore, multicenter networks with the ability to combine data across centers are important for conducting rigorous clinical trials. In addition, to synthesize the results of individual clinical trials in systematic reviews and meta-analyses, comparable outcomes across studies must be used.

The Core Outcome Measures in Effectiveness Trials (COMET) initiative was started in 2010 to help foster the development of *core outcome sets* (COS) in medicine.[13] A COS is "an agreed-upon standardized set of outcomes that should be measured and reported, as a minimum, in all clinical trials in specific areas of health or health care."[13] Use of a COS does not restrict a trial to only the outcomes included in the COS; other outcomes relevant to the research question can and should be added. However, including the COS developed for a specific health condition will make it easier to compare, contrast, and combine the results of individual trials when appropriate. COMET promotes the use of evidence-based review of outcomes along with clinician, researcher, patient, and family participation in development of COS. Including stakeholders in the development process helps to ensure that clinically meaningful patient- and family centered outcomes are identified.

PICU mortality rates approximate 2% to 4% in high-resource settings. As more children are surviving critical illness, the presence of new morbidities and long-term child and family dysfunction have become evident. Thus, evaluation of outcomes beyond hospital discharge that capture broader aspects of child and family life are important.[14]

To address this need, Fink and colleagues in collaboration with the Pediatric Acute Lung Injury and Sepsis Investigators (PALISI) network and the CPCCRN developed an evidence-based, stakeholder-informed PICU COS.[15] Stakeholders included clinicians, researchers, and family advocates from 6 continents. First, a scoping review of PICU-related studies was carried out to identify potential core outcome domains and instruments to evaluate the domains.[16,17] Outcomes of interest were those pertaining to PICU survivors and families of children who experienced critical illness. To supplement the scoping review, semistructured interviews were conducted with PICU survivors and caregivers to gain their perspectives on meaningful outcomes. These steps were followed by a 2-round modified Delphi electronic survey with stakeholders to finalize the PICU COS and recommended instruments.

The final PICU COS ultimately included 4 global domains (overall, cognitive, physical, emotional) and 4 specific outcomes (child quality of life, survival, pain, communication). To include additional outcomes valued by families that did not reach preset inclusion criteria through the Delphi process, a PICU COS-extended was also reported. Final steps include reporting of feasible instruments to evaluate the global domains and specific outcomes included in the PICU COS and dissemination to end users for implementation. It has been recommended that the PICU COS be reviewed and updated in 5 to 10 years to keep it consistent with new knowledge that develops and relevant as health care outcomes change.[15]

Other specialties related to pediatric intensive care are also in various stages of developing a COS, including pediatric anesthesiology[18] and neonatology.[19] COS for specific pediatric diseases or conditions (eg, epilepsy,[20] appendicitis,[21] gastroschisis[22]) and specific health care settings (eg, low- and middle-income countries[23]) are also in process.

Precision Medicine in the Pediatric Intensive Care Unit

Precision medicine generally refers to the goal of identifying biologically similar groups of patients within a previously understood disease or syndrome who require different treatments. Recent advances in breast cancer[24] and asthma[25] treatment have led to subclassification of patients with these diseases into biological subgroups that have dramatically different responses to therapy. These findings have led to similar efforts to develop precision therapeutics in many fields of medicine, including pediatric intensive care.

Most novel therapeutics for common PICU syndromes (eg, sepsis and ARDS) have failed to improve patient outcomes in clinical trials.[26] One reason for failure is that these syndromes have heterogeneous courses, outcomes, and responsiveness to therapy, with some patients being helped by a particular therapy and others being harmed, leading to an overall lack of detectable benefit.[27] This *heterogeneity of treatment effect* is one driving force in the recent proliferation of approaches to classify pediatric and adult patients with sepsis or ARDS into subgroups.[28–33]

These classification methodologies use clinical data,[34] biomarkers,[31] genomic and metabolomic data,[35] or a combination[29] to categorize patients with a given syndrome into groups. The goal of these groupings may be to define patients who are biologically similar, who have a similar likelihood of response to a given therapy, or who have a different risk of adverse outcome. In general, a *phenotype* of a syndrome can be understood as a set of clinical features used in definition of a subgroup, often with enrollment in a clinical trial based on this presentation.[27] This methodology is distinct from classification by *endotypes*, which is most commonly used to describe patients with a similar observed presentation but different subclinical characteristics.[25] Importantly, classification into an endotype implies that the subclinical features identified are part of the causal structure of the clinical presentation.[27] This distinction highlights the different goals of different approaches to subclassification in precision medicine in the PICU. Phenotypes may be more useful for predicting responsiveness to a given therapy, whereas endotypes may be more predictive of trajectory or outcome.

Some approaches use multiple data sources to classify patients, including clinical and laboratory data as well as integrated genomic or metabolomic data.[29] Whatever the data source, a key step in developing subclasses is the choice of *agnostic or knowledge-based approaches*.[36] In general, agnostic approaches use advanced modeling to define subgroups based on all available data (especially with high-dimensional genomic or metabolomic data). In contrast, knowledge-based approaches use previous knowledge of underlying pathophysiologic derangements to define subgroups that may benefit from a specific intervention.

Challenges in the development of precision medicine in the pediatric intensive care unit

A common challenge for the development of precision medicine is the volume of data. Many precision medicine approaches rely on high-volume multiomic data; this can include genomic, metabolomic, proteomic, and transcriptomic data, which can be sampled from many patients at multiple time points. Integrating these data to form clinically relevant subclasses requires novel data analytical strategies and is computationally challenging. Researchers must also consider the behavior of identified subclasses over time, given the rapidly changing pathophysiology of critically ill patients, as well as the background health status of the patient.

Precision medicine in sepsis

Multiple research groups have derived and validated classification strategies for children with sepsis (**Table 1** for a summary of the approaches). One approach used genome-wide expression profiling[28] to define subclasses of children with septic shock with differential gene expression. These patients had different risk of mortality based on cluster classification with different clinical phenotypes and a higher risk of mortality with steroid administration in one subgroup. This approach has been further refined to develop a biomarker-based risk model based on the underlying differential gene expression.[37] Another approach used prior knowledge to define subgroups with dysregulated immunity among pediatric patients with sepsis and MODS.[31,38] A retrospective analysis of a previously completed randomized controlled trial of anakinra found a substantial mortality benefit in adult patients with one of these subgroups.[39] A multicenter interventional trial is currently in progress for one of these subgroups,[40] and an adaptive randomized trial to study targeted immune therapy based on subgroup membership has been funded and will begin enrollment soon.[41]

Several investigators have used clinical data to group patients with similar characteristic patterns of organ failure, abnormal vital signs, and differential mortality. One research group[34] identified pediatric patients with MODS and used machine learning to identify 4 subgroups of MODS with distinct clinical characteristics and differential mortality. These researchers also evaluated the trajectory of MODS during the first 3 days of each patient encounter and described a heterogeneous treatment effect of hydrocortisone based on subgroup membership.

In adults with sepsis, genome-wide expression profiles have revealed subgroups of patients with pathogenically altered immunity.[42] These patients displayed differential

Table 1
Comparison of reviewed precision medicine strategies for identification of subgroups in sepsis

Classification Characteristics	Wong et al,[28] 2009; Wong et al,[35] 2015	Carcillo et al,[38] 2019	Sanchez-Pinto et al,[34] 2020	Scicluna et al,[42] 2017	Seymour et al,[29] 2019
Level of classification					
Genomic	x	—	—	x	x
Metabolomic	x	—	—	—	—
Molecular	x	x	—	x	—
Clinical	—	—	x	—	x
Classification strategy					
Agnostic	x	—	x	x	x
Knowledge-based	—	x	—	—	—
Statistical methodology					
Hierarchical clustering	x	—	—	—	—
K means clustering	—	—	—	x	x
Other machine learning	—	—	x	—	—
Time course					
Static	x	x	—	x	x
Temporal	—	—	x	—	—
Target					
Planned therapeutic trial	—	x	—	—	—
Mechanistic clarification	x	---		x	x
Risk for poor outcome	—	—	x	—	—

activation of pathways associated with immune suppression, hyperinflammation, increased immune activity, and increased pattern recognition and mobility signaling. The subgroups had substantially different acute organ failure severity and mortality. Using clinical data, another group of investigators[29] also defined 4 subgroups in adults with sepsis that had differential patterns of acute organ failure and mortality. These subgroups were also identified in patients enrolled in previously completed randomized controlled trials, and different subgroups had significantly different response rates to the interventions studied in these trials.

Precision medicine in acute respiratory distress syndrome

Researchers have undertaken similar efforts to derive and validate clinically relevant subgroups of ARDS in children and adults. Using peripheral blood RNA transcriptomics, a single-center study defined 3 subgroups characterized by different patterns of immune activation, complement activity, and inflammatory cytokines.[33] These groups had differing duration of mechanical ventilation and mortality. Latent class analysis in adults with ARDS using clinical and biological data revealed 2 subgroups with distinct mortality and inflammatory profiles.[30] Membership in these groups was associated with heterogeneous responses to fluid management,[43] positive end-expiratory pressure,[30] and simvastatin[44] in secondary analyses of prior clinical trials.

Common themes and future directions

Precision medicine enables appropriately targeted therapies based on underlying pathophysiology and may lead to better outcomes by delivering the optimal treatment to patients most likely to benefit. Understanding the potential clinical applicability of any method of subclassifying patients within a heterogeneous syndrome requires understanding the goal of the classification system (eg, prognostic, predictive of response to therapy, understanding the underlying pathophysiology, or a combination). Many of these subgroups have strong clinical and biological plausibility with differential gene expression, outcomes, and responsiveness to therapies in secondary analyses of previous clinical trials. Despite substantial advances in the field, the complexity of rapidly changing pathophysiology, multiple simultaneous interventions, high-dimensional data, and the role of preexisting conditions make development of clinically relevant and actionable subgroups challenging. As the field of precision medicine in the PICU advances, researchers and clinicians should remain aware of these challenges and continue to refine our efforts to focus on clinically meaningful understanding of the complex syndromes in the children we treat.

Clinical Trial Strategies

There are substantial challenges to the development and implementation of high-quality, practice-changing research in critically ill children. Novel clinical trial designs and evidence-based modifications of existing strategies may help to address the significant gaps in evidence for managing critically ill children.[4,45,46] Recent and planned clinical trials are focusing on disease and treatment heterogeneity[41] and assessing patient- and family centered outcomes.[47–49]

Heterogeneity and precision medicine implications

One goal of precision medicine, as discussed earlier, is to define subgroups that predict responsiveness to treatment. One clear application is the use of an identified subgroup to direct administration of the intervention; this relies on the relevance of the subgroup to the intervention being studied (such as impaired innate immunity as a precursor for granulocyte-macrophage colony-stimulating factor administration in children with sepsis).[40] Further support for directing randomization based on clinical phenotype is based on retrospective secondary analyses of existing trials showing benefit or harm in specific subgroups.[29,35,39,44] These analyses suggest that a prospective trial that randomizes patients based on subgroup identification will show a benefit of the therapy in the selected subgroup. This strategy is known as *predictive enrichment* and is recommended by the Food and Drug Administration (FDA) for use in clinical trials of therapeutic interventions.[50] The FDA also recommends consideration of *prognostic enrichment*, which involves inclusion of high-risk patients who are most likely to benefit from an intervention. A combination of prognostic and predictive enrichment was beneficial for identification of children likely to benefit from corticosteroids in septic shock in a retrospective secondary analysis.[51] These enrichment strategies may assist in identifying effective interventions for carefully selected subgroups of patients.

Adaptive randomization refers to making changes in the allocation of patients to a treatment arm of a trial based on interim evaluation.[52] *Platform trials* enroll patients with a similar disease into multiple potential interventional arms to test multiple hypothesized interventions. Adaptive randomization modifies the likelihood of new patients enrolled in a trial being randomized to receive a specific treatment based on interim analysis (**Fig. 1** displays a hypothetical adaptive randomization platform trial). Randomization to a specific interventional arm is based on the likelihood of the intervention being beneficial for the newly enrolled patient based on data from previous similar patients in the trial. The REMAP-CAP trial is an ongoing adaptive randomization platform trial to investigate the benefit of multiple treatment strategies for adults with community-acquired pneumonia. It was initiated before the SARS-CoV-2 pandemic but transitioned to enroll patients with COVID-19 pneumonia.[53] The REMAP-CAP trial has tested multiple domains of treatment on each enrolled patient, resulting in early evidence supporting the use of steroids in patients with COVID-19 pneumonia,[54] among other significant findings. Using platform trials to test multiple interventions in the same patient and in the same trial promotes more efficient use of resources and accelerates research.

Novel trial designs

Although innovative approaches to randomized controlled trials are likely to improve knowledge generated from these trials, other investigators have used novel trial designs to generate evidence more efficiently for real-world practice. Randomized controlled trials can be challenging to conduct and interpret in the PICU. Selection using precision medicine techniques or specific selection criteria challenges generalizability. Critically ill patients, by definition, have rapidly changing disease and often

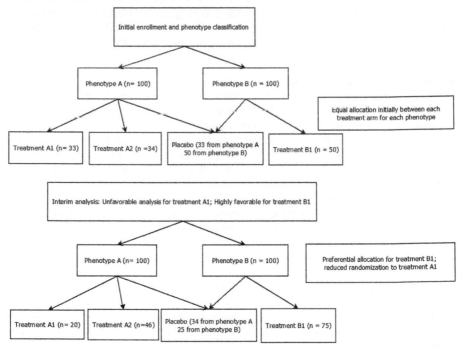

Fig. 1. Hypothetical platform response-adaptive randomization trial. Patients are stratified into 2 phenotypes (A, B) that receive different treatments. Phenotype A receives one of two potential therapies and phenotype B receives one. After interim analysis, patients with phenotype B are preferentially randomized to receive treatment (over placebo) due to substantial probability of benefit. Patients with phenotype A are preferentially allocated to receive treatment A2 but remain allocated to placebo in the same 1:1:1 ratio. If these trends persist in the second interim analysis, treatment A1 may be dropped from the trial, and another treatment arm may be added for patients with phenotype A.

receive multiple simultaneous interventions. Discerning the effect of a single treatment, even when patients are randomized, can be challenging.

One approach to address these challenges is *comparative effectiveness research* (CER). CER "is the generation and synthesis of evidence that compares the benefits and harms of alternative methods to prevent, diagnose, treat, and monitor or improve the delivery of care."[55] The choice of study designs used in CER can vary. The Approaches and Decisions for Acute Pediatric Traumatic Brain Injury (ADAPT)[56] trial is a comparative effectiveness trial that uses an observational design and propensity scoring to control for potential confounders. ADAPT assesses the relative benefit of multiple therapeutic strategies in children with traumatic brain injury. CERs with observational designs, such as ADAPT, are especially useful in disease processes where patients receive multiple interventions, care is highly variable, and evidence for best practices is limited.

An alternative approach to enrollment of all patients with a certain disease process is assessment of the best strategy to provide supportive care across a variety of disease states. There remains wide variation in practice with a lack of adequate evidence about the best strategy to provide sedation for children with respiratory failure requiring mechanical ventilation, mode and delivery of nutrition, and the effect and implementation of early rehabilitation, among many other questions that affect our daily practice. These supportive therapies are provided to patients across a variety of disease states, and trials are planned,[57] underway,[58] or have been completed[59] to build the evidence base for appropriate supportive care across the spectrum of pediatric critical illness.

Structural innovations

Because of the relative rarity of many pediatric critical illnesses, successful clinical research in the PICU requires multicenter trials for generalized applicability. One approach is to develop and initiate a *de novo* infrastructure focused on a single disease among centers with dedicated researchers that can act as local site investigators. However, this approach is costly and labor-intensive. An alternative strategy is to form a research network that can perform multiple trials across a sustained time period. Two of the largest pediatric intensive care research networks are the CPCCRN and PALISI. These networks have produced high-quality research that has had a direct impact on clinical practice.[59–62] A major advantage of these and similar multicenter networks is the development of personnel with familiarity in procedures for multicenter research and infrastructure that does not have to be rebuilt with each trial; this allows for adaptation to multiple simultaneous or sequential trials. The existing research infrastructure was leveraged by a PALISI group of investigators to rapidly advance our understanding of the multisystem inflammatory syndrome in children associated with SARS-CoV-2 in real time during the COVID pandemic (MIS-C),[63] highlighting the flexibility and power of preexisting collaborative networks.

Another approach to increasing the size and granularity of observational trials is to enroll patients using clinical data directly imported from EHR. EHR include a substantial amount of high-dimensional data, especially in patients who require intensive care. These granular data can be used to classify patients into subgroups using precision medicine approaches,[29,34] perform CER,[64] analyze longitudinal characteristics predictive of decompensation,[65] and develop novel risk classification scores,[66] among other potential applications. There are, however, challenges in performing research using EHR data. Adequate deidentification and data security require significant investment in data security and storage. Most "multicenter" trials have been performed in multiple hospitals within a single health care system because of differences in EHR implementation; this leads to substantial challenges in merging data from multiple centers.[64] The multiple formats of clinical data, highly variable missing data, and data volume also make adequate data preparation and interpretation difficult. Despite these challenges, the development of observational cohorts using EHR may allow characterization of previously undetected predictive factors, effects, and outcomes across the range of critical illnesses.

SUMMARY

Significant progress has been made in the practice of pediatric intensive care because of new research methodologies and priorities, and significant progress is on the horizon. Dr Robert C. Tasker, editor-in-chief of *Pediatric Critical Care Medicine*, discussed the direction of our specialty's primary journal in a recent interview.[67] Dr Tasker highlighted pioneers in the field who have described clinically meaningful patient-centered outcomes, observational cohorts of physiology-based data and large multicenter high-dimensional databases, as well as multicenter trials with granular and meaningful individual patient data. Research in pediatric critical care medicine is moving away from low-fidelity administrative data and single-center studies and toward high-quality large studies that reveal important information about pathophysiology and treatment responsiveness.

Increasing recognition of the importance of disease and treatment-response heterogeneity by precision medicine techniques increases the chance that specific patients will benefit from a targeted therapy. Novel platform trial designs, testing multiple interventions, and observational research identifying the effect of natural practice variations may address the rapidly changing pathophysiology and multiple simultaneous interventions for patients in the PICU. Multicenter research and the use of high-dimensional EHR data increase the generalizability and clinical relevance of research findings. Focusing on outcomes beyond mortality that are important to patients and families increases the potential applicability and uptake of clinical research. In short, identifying the right treatment of the right patient that delivers the right outcome should be the focus of our endeavors. Careful implementation of novel methodology and rigorous scientific practice will advance the state of our field and improve the morbidity and mortality caused by critical illness in children.

CLINICS CARE POINTS

- Research agendas guide the investment of time and resources toward areas most in need of new or advanced knowledge.

- Core outcome sets are an agreed on set of outcomes that should be evaluated in all clinical trials of a specific disease or disorder. Core outcomes facilitate the combining of data from multiple trials for systematic reviews and meta-analyses.

- Precision medicine refers to defining specific subgroups within a disease or syndrome that predict responsiveness to treatment, risk of adverse outcome, or different underlying pathophysiology.

- Platform trials increase efficiency by testing multiple interventions in study patients with a single disease process.

- Adaptive randomization improves the likelihood of finding a beneficial treatment by preferentially assigning patients to treatments that have a high probability of being beneficial based on interim analysis.

- Comparative effectiveness research compares the benefits and harms of alternative methods to prevent, diagnose, treat, and monitor or improve delivery of care using various study designs.
- Research networks that are flexible, efficient, and productive can perform multiple sequential or simultaneous clinical trials in critically ill children.
- Research using EHR faces significant barriers but represents a promising source of granular clinical data for observational cohorts.

DISCLOSURE

The authors have nothing to disclose.

REFERENCES

1. Peters MJ, Argent A, Festa M, et al. The intensive care medicine clinical research agenda in paediatrics. Intensive Care Med 2017;43(9):1210–24.
2. Zimmerman JJ, Anand KJS, Meert KL, et al. Research as a standard of care in the PICU. Pediatr Crit Care Med 2016;17(1):e13–21.
3. Maholmes V, Tamburro RF, Jenkins TL. Toward a research agenda on pediatric trauma and critical illness. JAMA Pediatr 2016;170(1):7–8.
4. Kochanek PM, Tasker RC, Carney N, et al. Guidelines for the management of pediatric severe traumatic brain injury, third edition: Update of the brain trauma foundation guidelines. Pediatr Crit Care Med 2019;20(3):S1–82.
5. Weiss SL, Peters MJ, Alhazzani W, et al. Surviving sepsis campaign international guidelines for the management of septic shock and sepsis-associated organ dysfunction in children. Pediatr Crit Care Med 2020;E52–106.
6. Jouvet P, Thomas NJ, Willson DF, et al. Pediatric Acute Respiratory Distress Syndrome: Consensus Recommendations from the Pediatric Acute Lung Injury Consensus Conference. Pediatr Crit Care Med 2015;16(5):428–39.
7. Maconochie IK, Aickin R, Hazinski MF, et al. Pediatric life support 2020 international consensus on cardiopulmonary resuscitation and emergency cardiovascular care science with treatment recommendations. Pediatrics 2021;147(1):S1–47.
8. Reddy S, Polito A, Staveski S, et al. A process for academic societies to develop scientific statements and white papers: Experience of the Pediatric Cardiac Intensive Care Society. Cardiol Young 2019;29(2):174–7.
9. Critical complications in pediatric oncology and hematopoietic cell transplant | frontiers research topic. Available at: https://www.frontiersin.org/research-topics/11226/critical-complications-in-pediatric-oncology-and-hematopoietic-cell-transplant. Accessed August 26, 2021.
10. Pollack MM, Banks R, Holubkov R, et al. Morbidity and mortality in critically ill children. i. pathophysiologies and potential therapeutic solutions. Crit Care Med 2020;48(6):790–8.
11. Meert KL, Banks R, Holubkov R, et al. Morbidity and mortality in critically ill children. II. A qualitative patient-level analysis of pathophysiologies and potential therapeutic solutions*. Crit Care Med 2020;48(6):799–807.
12. Mörelius E, Foster M, Gill FJ. A scoping review of nursing research priorities in pediatric care. J Pediatr Nurs 2020;52:e57–69.
13. COMET Initiative | Home. Available at: https://www.comet-initiative.org/. Accessed October 21, 2021.

14. Dalton HJ, Pollack MM. Mortality is passé: the importance of morbidity as an outcome. Pediatr Crit Care Med 2018;19(7):683–4.

15. Fink EL, Maddux AB, Pinto N, et al. A core outcome set for pediatric critical care. Crit Care Med 2020;48(12):1819–28.

16. Maddux A, Pinto N, Fink E, et al. Postdischarge outcome domains in pediatric critical care and the instruments used to evaluate them: a scoping review. Crit Care Med 2020;48(12):e1313–21.

17. Fink EL, Jarvis JM, Maddux AB, et al. Development of a core outcome set for pediatric critical care outcomes research. Contemp Clin Trials 2020;91(November 2019):105968.

18. Razavi C, Walker SM, Moonesinghe SR, et al. Pediatric perioperative outcomes: Protocol for a systematic literature review and identification of a core outcome set for infants, children, and young people requiring anesthesia and surgery. Paediatr Anaesth 2020;30(4):392–400.

19. Webbe JWH, Duffy JMN, Afonso E, et al. Core outcomes in neonatology: development of a core outcome set for neonatal research. Arch Dis Child Fetal Neonatal Ed 2020;105(4):425–31.

20. Crudgington H, Rogers M, Bray L, et al. Core Health Outcomes in Childhood Epilepsy (CHOICE): Development of a core outcome set using systematic review methods and a Delphi survey consensus. Epilepsia 2019;60(5):857–71.

21. Knaapen M, Hall NJ, Moulin D, et al. International core outcome set for acute simple appendicitis in children: results of A systematic review, Delphi study, and focus groups with young people. Annals of Surgery 2020.

22. Allin B, Hall N, Ross A, et al. Development of a gastroschisis core outcome set. Arch Dis Child Fetal neonatal edition 2019;104(1):F76–82.

23. Wooldridge G, Murthy S, Kissoon N. Core outcome set in paediatric sepsis in low- and middle-income countries: a study protocol. BMJ open 2020;10(4).

24. Barker A, Sigman C, Kelloff G, et al. I-SPY 2: an adaptive breast cancer trial design in the setting of neoadjuvant chemotherapy. Clin Pharmacol Ther 2009; 86(1):97–100.

25. Lötvall J, Akdis CA, Bacharier LB, et al. Asthma endotypes: a new approach to classification of disease entities within the asthma syndrome. J Allergy Clin Immunol 2011;127(2):355–60.

26. Marshall JC. Why have clinical trials in sepsis failed? Trends Mol Med 2014;20(4): 195–203.

27. Seymour CW, Gomez H, Chang C-CH, et al. Precision medicine for all? Challenges and opportunities for a precision medicine approach to critical illness. Crit Care (London, England) 2017;21(1):257.

28. Wong HR, Cvijanovich N, Lin R, et al. Identification of pediatric septic shock subclasses based on genome-wide expression profiling. BMC Med 2009;7:34.

29. Seymour CW, Kennedy JN, Wang S, et al. Derivation, validation, and potential treatment implications of novel clinical phenotypes for sepsis. JAMA 2019;321: 2003–17.

30. Calfee CS, Delucchi K, Parsons PE, et al. Subphenotypes in acute respiratory distress syndrome: Latent class analysis of data from two randomised controlled trials. Lancet Respir Med 2014;2(8):611–20.

31. Carcillo JA, Halstead ES, Hall MW, et al. Three hypothetical inflammation pathobiology phenotypes and pediatric sepsis-induced multiple organ failure outcome. Pediatr Crit Care Med 2017;18(6):513–23.

32. Knox DB, Lanspa MJ, Kuttler KG, et al. Phenotypic clusters within sepsis-associated multiple organ dysfunction syndrome. Intensive Care Med 2015; 41(5):814–22.
33. Yehya N, Varisco B, Thomas N, et al. Peripheral blood transcriptomic sub-phenotypes of pediatric acute respiratory distress syndrome. Crit Care (London, England) 2020;24(1).
34. Sanchez-Pinto LN, Stroup EK, Pendergrast T, et al. Derivation and validation of novel phenotypes of multiple organ dysfunction syndrome in critically ill children. JAMA Netw Open 2020;3(8):e209271.
35. Wong HR, Cvijanovich NZ, Anas N, et al. Developing a clinically feasible person-alized medicine approach to pediatric septic shock. Am J Respir Crit Care Med 2015;191(3):309–15.
36. Jacobs L, Wong HR. Sepsis subclasses: be careful of what you wish for. Pediatr Crit Care Med 2017;18(6):591–2.
37. Wong HR, Salisbury S, Xiao Q, et al. The pediatric sepsis biomarker risk model. Crit Care 2012;16(5):R174.
38. Carcillo JA, Berg RA, Wessel D, et al. A multicenter network assessment of three inflammation phenotypes in pediatric sepsis-induced multiple organ failure. Pediatr Crit Care Med 2019;20(12):1137–46.
39. Shakoory B, Carcillo JA, Chatham WW, et al. Interleukin-1 receptor blockade is associated with reduced mortality in sepsis patients with features of macrophage activation syndrome: reanalysis of a prior phase iii trial. Crit Care Med 2016;44(2): 275–81.
40. Hall M. GM-CSF for Reversal of immunopAralysis in pediatriC sEpsis-induced MODS Study - Full Text View - ClinicalTrials.gov. Available at: https://clinicaltrials.gov/ct2/show/NCT03769844. Accessed September 22, 2021.
41. Award Information | HHS TAGGS. Available at: https://taggs.hhs.gov/Detail/AwardDetail?arg_AwardNum=PL1HD105462&arg_ProgOfficeCode=50.   Accessed September 22, 2021.
42. Scicluna BP, van Vught LA, Zwinderman AH, et al. Classification of patients with sepsis according to blood genomic endotype: a prospective cohort study. Lancet Respir Med 2017;5(10):816–26.
43. Famous KR, Delucchi K, Ware LB, et al. ARDS subphenotypes respond differ-ently to randomized fluid management strategy. Am J Respir Crit Care Med 2016;195(3):331–8.
44. Calfee CS, Delucchi KL, Sinha P, et al. Acute respiratory distress syndrome sub-phenotypes and differential response to simvastatin: secondary analysis of a randomised controlled trial. Lancet Respir Med 2018;6(9):691–8.
45. Topjian AA, Raymond TT, Atkins D, et al. Part 4: Pediatric Basic and Advanced Life Support: 2020 American Heart Association Guidelines for Cardiopulmonary Resuscitation and Emergency Cardiovascular Care. Circulation 2020;142(16 2): S469–523.
46. Weiss SL, Peters MJ, Alhazzani W, et al. Surviving sepsis campaign international guidelines for the management of septic shock and sepsis-associated organ dysfunction in children. Pediatr Crit Care Med 2020;21(2):e52–106.
47. Watson RS, Asaro LA, Hutchins L, et al. Risk factors for functional decline and impaired quality of life after pediatric respiratory failure. Am J Respir Crit Care Med 2019;200(7):900–9.
48. Choong K, Fraser D, Al-Harbi S, et al. Functional Recovery in Critically Ill Chil-dren, the "WeeCover" Multicenter Study. Pediatr Crit Care Med 2018;19(2): 145–54.

49. Zimmerman JJ, Banks R, Berg RA, et al. Trajectory of mortality and health-related quality of life morbidity following community-acquired pediatric septic shock. Crit Care Med 2020;48(3):329–37.
50. FDA. Enrichment strategies for clinical trials to support determination of effectiveness of human drugs and biological products. Guidance for Industry 2019;(March):1–41.
51. Wong HR, Atkinson SJ, Cvijanovich NZ, et al. Combining prognostic and predictive enrichment strategies to identify children with septic shock responsive to corticosteroids 2016;44(10):e1000–3.
52. Lin J, Lin LA, Sankoh S. A general overview of adaptive randomization design for clinical trials. J Biometrics Biostatistics 2016;07(02).
53. REMAP-CAP Trial. Available at: https://www.remapcap.org/. Accessed September 24, 2021.
54. Angus DC, Derde L, Al-Beidh F, et al. Effect of hydrocortisone on mortality and organ support in patients with severe COVID-19: The REMAP-CAP COVID-19 Corticosteroid domain randomized clinical trial. JAMA 2020;324(13):1317–29.
55. Institute of Medicine (U.S.). Committee on Comparative Effective Research Prioritization. Initial national priorities for comparative effectiveness research. Published online 2009:227.
56. ADAPT | Approaches and Decisions in Acute Pediatric TBI Trial. Available at: https://www.adapttrial.org/. Accessed September 30, 2021.
57. Clinical Effectiveness of the "PICU Up!" Multifaceted Early Mobility Intervention for Critically III Children - Full Text View - ClinicalTrials.gov. Available at: https://clinicaltrials.gov/ct2/show/NCT04989790. Accessed September 30, 2021.
58. Early Versus Late Parenteral Nutrition in the Pediatric Intensive Care Unit - Full Text View - ClinicalTrials.gov. Available at: https://clinicaltrials.gov/ct2/show/NCT01536275. Accessed September 30, 2021.
59. Watson RS, Asaro LA, Hertzog JH, et al. Long-term outcomes after protocolized sedation versus usual care in ventilated pediatric patients. Am J Respir Crit Care Med 2018;197(11):1457.
60. Agus MSD, Wypij D, Hirshberg EL, et al. Tight glycemic control in critically ill children. N Engl J Med 2017;376(8):729–41.
61. Moler FW, Silverstein FS, Holubkov R, et al. Therapeutic hypothermia after in-hospital cardiac arrest in children. N Engl J Med 2017;376(4):318–29.
62. Publications | CPCCRN. Available at: https://www.cpccrn.org/publications/. Accessed October 1, 2021.
63. Feldstein LR, Rose EB, Horwitz SM, et al. Multisystem inflammatory syndrome in u.s. children and adolescents. N Engl J Med 2020;383(4):334–46.
64. Narus SP, Srivastava R, Gouripeddi R, et al. Federating clinical data from six pediatric hospitals: process and initial results from the PHIS+ Consortium. AMIA Annu Symp Proc 2011;2011:994.
65. Kausch SL, Lobo JM, Spaeder MC, et al. Dynamic transitions of pediatric sepsis: a markov chain analysis. Front Pediatr 2021;0:1060.
66. Wellner B, Grand J, Canzone E, et al. Predicting unplanned transfers to the intensive care unit: a machine learning approach leveraging diverse clinical elements. JMIR 2017;5(4):e45.
67. Tasker RC, Wolbrink T. Emerging Trends in Research: Clinical Research Concepts by Dr Robert Tasker for OPENPediatrics. Open Pediatrics. 2021. Available at: https://soundcloud.com/openpediatrics/emerging-trends-in-research-clinical-research-concepts-by-dr-robert-tasker-for-openpediatrics. Accessed August 29, 2021.

Education in the Pediatric Intensive Care Unit

Jeff A. Clark, MD

KEYWORDS

• Medical education • Pediatric intensive care unit • Adult learning

KEY POINTS

- In addition to imparting knowledge, teaching the ability to make rapid, error-free medical decisions are key to allow clinicians to function optimally in the PICU environment
- Use of newer methods of education such as simulation and electronic methods have increasing roles in PICU education
- Traditional methods such as bedside teaching remain vital in the education of clinicians

INTRODUCTION

Effective practice in the pediatric intensive care unit (PICU) requires a broad skill set. As physicians, our primary responsibilities include providing safe, effective, and compassionate care for our patients and teaching others to do the same. To accomplish this, knowledge is essential, but by itself is insufficient to ensure quality patient care. The ability to use knowledge for medical decision making is fundamental to the practice of medicine, and the ability to make decisions rapidly and accurately is a critical skill in PICU. In addition to clinical decision making, technical skills, an ethical framework, leadership and a commitment to safety and quality and the ability to provide emotional support to families and other staff are essential skills for intensivists. All these skills need to be taught and learned.

Although challenges exist, the broad range of pathology and the high acuity in the PICU is an excellent place for education. The high acuity and fast pace often lead to interruptions in teaching and limit teaching time. High clinical loads and constraints of a multidisciplinary team also decrease opportunities to teach. The transition to faculty-led care over the last few decades has likely improved patient care but has decreased valuable learning opportunities for trainees. These issues and others have contributed to the teaching challenges that currently exist for critical care trainees.

Pediatric Critical Care Medicine, Ascension St. John Children's Hospital, 22101 Moross Road, Detroit, MI 48236, USA
E-mail address: Jeff.clark2@ascension.org

Pediatr Clin N Am 69 (2022) 621–631
https://doi.org/10.1016/j.pcl.2022.01.016
0031-3955/22/© 2022 Elsevier Inc. All rights reserved.

Most physicians have benefitted immeasurably from faculty who are gifted at teaching, guiding us through training while both pushing and inspiring us. Although we often recognize effective teaching when we experience it, quantifying what makes an effective teacher is difficult. Those faculty members who are skilled often appear to have an innate understanding of when to teach, how best to impart knowledge and skills, when to push students to find answers and when to lead students to answers. Teaching and promoting these skills in a challenging environment have led to novel approaches to teaching in critical care, and re-emphasis of effective and time-honored teaching activities. In addition, the science of how we make decisions is beginning to influence medical education and may prove helpful in improving PICU education and subsequent clinical care.

Decision Making

Medical decision making is the most important skill physicians need. The decisions we make have a profound impact on our patient's daily care, and ultimately their health. Faulty decision making is thought to be the primary cause of medical errors.[1,2] An understanding of how physicians make decisions is critical to improving patient care and should influence how we teach our trainees.

In a busy clinical setting such as the PICU, we can sometimes take medical decision making for granted. Medical decisions are made dozens of times a day and often under the stress of time constraints, patient instability, and high emotions. We make decisions based on data and experience and most of the time these decisions are appropriate. However, when medical errors occur, faulty decision making is most often to blame. Although we make decisions on all aspects of patient care, including testing, admission location, and treatment, almost all are predicated on an accurate diagnosis. If diagnosis is in error, most other clinical decisions are affected. Faulty diagnoses lead to significant morbidity, mortality, and increased length of stay. It is estimated that 75% of all malpractice activity in the United States involves diagnostic errors.[3] Diagnostic errors result from failures in knowledge or system flaws, but most often are due to cognitive error. Cognitive errors can result from lack of knowledge, but more frequently they are a result of failure of proper application of knowledge for clinical decision making. Therefore, the way we process information and make decisions is key to our ability to practice medicine and should therefore be central to the way we teach learners. Our understanding of human decision has increased significantly over the last 2 decades, yet little of this knowledge has influenced medical education.

The human decision-making process occurs in 2 ways.[4] We make decisions hundreds of times a day, and most decisions occur automatically without significant thought. This type of decision making does not require reasoning and is referred to as intuitive reasoning. These decisions are reflexive and are either "hardwired" or learned by repetitive experiences over time. They are often referred to in cognitive sciences as type I thinking. We get through our day making most decisions this way. What to eat for breakfast, when to cross the street, and what we say to greet others are all examples of intuitive decisions. They rely primarily on pattern recognition. For example, we recognize street signs, traffic patterns, and cross the street. These decisions require little effort or conscious deliberation. In medicine, we often make decisions similarly, especially when there are time constraints. A 3-year-old with wheezing and respiratory distress is likely having an asthma flare and receives albuterol before a full examination of all diagnostic data. Most of the time we are correct in this provisional diagnosis and the treatment is appropriate. But not always.

Other decisions we make are not intuitive and require active thought and reasoning. These decisions are often referred to as "analytical," or type II thinking, and require a more structured thought process and effort. In the same example where a child presents with wheezing and may have asthma, there are other causes of wheezing at this age. The consideration of additional diagnostic data such as heart rate, respiratory rate, perfusion, or chest radiograph may affect our interpretation of wheezing in this child and its likely causes. Creating a problem list and using it to arrive at a list of differential diagnoses is an example of analytical reasoning. This activity requires a structured thought process using knowledge and logic along with patient-specific data to arrive at a conclusion. Because this is an active process that relies on a conscious, deliberate evaluation of known data, it is often more reliable and less prone to error. However, it occurs at the expense of time and effort, and is therefore impractical for most medical decisions. We typically reserve this type of thinking for situations that do not fit expected patterns. As time (and possibly energy) become limited, such as in a busy PICU, it is easy to understand how this type of thinking may become less common, and lead to the possibility of increased diagnostic error. If we can appropriately apply both forms of decision making to patient care, this would allow us to maximize our clinical accuracy and efficiency. It may seem superfluous to make some decisions without much thought while giving considerable thought to others. However, these are not simply the same processes given different amounts of conscious thought. They are fundamentally different processes, occurring in separate areas of the brain and require different neural pathways.[4] Therefore, our ability to understand how we make decisions and when each type of decision making is appropriate may allow us to minimize errors.

Intuitive or reflexive decisions allow us to move through our day with relative ease and get things accomplished. However, this form of decision making is much more prone to error and therefore potentially problematic in medicine. It is particularly vulnerable to biases and can more frequently lead to medical errors. Cognitive biases are faulty patterns of thought that lead to erroneous conclusions.[5] In the PICU, we are especially vulnerable when we are under pressure to arrive at conclusions and make decisions. Many types of cognitive biases have been described and some are particularly common in the setting of medical decision making. An example of a clinical scenario in which decision making may fall victim to biases is as follows: A 3-year-old is admitted to the PICU from the emergency department with wheezing and respiratory distress. The child has been given the provisional diagnosis of bronchiolitis with bronchospasm and placed on high-flow nasal cannula support. In the PICU, the child is given a nebulized beta-agonist medication, and toward the end of the treatment, develops ventricular tachycardia and pulselessness. Further investigation reveals the patient has acute heart failure and administration of beta-agonist therapy likely precipitated the arrhythmia. Multiple types of biases may have contributed to the erroneous diagnosis and treatment decisions for this child. Examples include *availability bias*, in which common diagnoses, because of their frequency, preclude consideration of alternate diagnoses. *Anchoring bias* leads to fixation on a prominent diagnostic feature (eg, wheezing) and allowing this feature to drive subsequent decision making without thorough examination of other features. In addition, d*iagnostic momentum* commonly leads to errors where a label is attached to a patient and remains unchallenged. These are a few examples of biases that prevent accurate thinking and accurate conclusions. Although learning and remembering all biases that can cloud our judgment would be onerous, understanding the common biases that exist and that can influence our thinking is the first step in mitigating their effects and preventing faulty conclusions. Understanding and teaching proper methods for debiasing may have a significant role in medical education as a way of improving critical thinking and preventing errors.

Adult Learning

Adult learning occurs along a spectrum, much like childhood developmental progression.[6] Skills acquired at one level are built upon to achieve the next level of proficiency. At a novice level, learners rely primarily on rules (pattern recognition) to guide decision making and are therefore particularly prone to biases. An example of novice learning in medicine is illustrated in the scenario of the 3-year-old with wheezing. A trainee may have learned that all patients over the age of 2 years who are wheezing should receive a trial of albuterol nebulization. Knowledge is limited, little discriminatory reasoning is used, and errors are more common. As knowledge and skills progress, learners can identify features of a clinical scenario that are unusual or atypical. They can use prior experience and reasoning along with increased knowledge to more accurately assess and arrive at conclusions. With enough experience and knowledge, outliers become more readily identifiable and identifying them can become "intuitive." With progression toward more advanced learning, biases become less problematic, as the ability to predict their effect on decision making improves. Although understanding that errors in judgment can be made and knowing the common scenarios under which they occur is inherent to medical education, the explicit discussion of how they occur, and a thorough understanding of their type and influence are uncommon. Although little data exist regarding the effect of minimizing bias in medical decision making, several strategies have been proposed.

Explicit teaching of critical thinking is one strategy.[5] Critical thinking is a necessary and vital skill in the PICU. Critical thinking is not a method of decision making per se, but rather, a way of thinking about thinking. It has been described as "the ability to engage in purposeful, self-regulatory judgment."[4] It requires one to be critical of their own thought process and identify biases in attempts to prevent errors in judgment. It is the understanding that a dual decision-making process exists and is prone to biases. This is a skill that is particularly difficult to master. It has been shown in medicine that clinicians with the least knowledge and skill are more likely to overestimate their skills, underestimate the skills of others, and are less aware of the potential for errors.[7] This is true both for technical skills and behavioral and humanistic skills such as leadership and empathy. In fact, proficiency with behavioral and humanistic skills appears to be essential for subsequent mastery of technical skills.[8] These nontechnical skills are particularly important in PICU practice. Intensivists use these skills every day to improve teamwork and support family and staff and ultimately improve outcomes. Our ability to teach these skills is therefore essential.

STRATEGIES TO IMPROVE DIAGNOSTIC ACCURACY AND CLINICAL DECISION MAKING
Critical Thinking

With the importance of diagnostic accuracy and clinical decision making in medicine, multiple strategies have been proposed to improve teaching of these skills. Although data to support their implementation are scarce, these strategies are based on understanding of the effect of biases on medical decision making. In 2017, Hayes and colleagues proposed 5 steps educators can use to improve the teaching of critical thinking in the ICU (Table 1). The first is to make the thinking process explicit. Discussion of "how" and "why" a trainee may have arrived at a decision is essential to the learning process as it forces them to begin to evaluate their own thought process and recognize biases that may affect their thought process. The second is to explicitly discuss biases, including how to recognize them and prevent them from affecting decision making. The third step involves modeling and teaching inductive reasoning.

Table 1 Strategies to improve critical thinking	
Strategies	**Description**
Make the thinking process explicit	Probe the thought process used to arrive at a conclusion
Discuss cognitive biases as strategies to eliminate bias	
Model and teach inductive reasoning	Results in a more inclusive problem list and leads to broader differential diagnoses list
Use questions to stimulate critical thinking	Use questions aimed at identifying the thought process not knowledge
Assess critical thinking	Give feedback as milestones from novice to advanced

Adapted from Hayes et. al [5]

Clinicians often use deductive reason to arrive at a conclusion, taking one or a few facts to reach a provisional diagnosis, which is supported or refuted with additional patient data. This process begins with a narrower focus based on assumptions of likelihood that can interfere with arrival at the actual diagnosis and is more prone to biases. Inductive reasoning uses all available data to generate a differential diagnosis. The clear analogy of this is to begin with an accurate and inclusive problem list and allow that to drive the creation of a list of differential diagnoses. Priorities can then be created for the diagnoses and decisions regarding additional tests or data can be decided, until a provisional or more definitive diagnosis can be determined. The fourth step is to use questions to stimulate critical thinking. Asking a trainee to describe why they think a patient is wheezing may stimulate discussions on the underlying understanding of the basis of disease and reveal biases that may prevent accurate decision making. Lastly, the trainee's critical thinking skills must be assessed to allow additional training focused on achieving proficiency.

Reflective Learning

As part of their 50th anniversary review series, the Society of Critical Care Medicine published a review of education in the ICU in 2021.[8] Along with the acquisition of knowledge and skills, it emphasized the importance of reflective learning. "Reflective learning is an experiential process of personal insight development, in which one's own and others' experiences are used to change attitudes and behaviors to promote optimal patient care and staff wellbeing. Reflective learning underpins all learned behaviors, but the capacity for reflection is itself a skill that varies between individuals." Reflective learning reviews past events to evaluate what went well and what did not to develop strategies to improve performance in future situations. The ability to accurately self-reflect and improve can be learned, and evidence indicates that those who lack these skills are less likely to progress in their education. This suggests that the skills of self-evaluation are required before the acquisition of more complex skills such as critical thinking or technical ability. The earlier these skills are taught and acquired, the more rapidly proficiency at more complex skills can be acquired.

Self-reflection is a critical skill for ICU physicians, where openness to self-reflection is a key component. As an example, morbidity and mortality conference is a time-honored tradition in medicine, but it is likely that few trainees ever look forward to participating in this activity because of the presentation of objective facts (usually errors or deficiencies) and traditional focus on blame. Although information critical to quality improvement can and has come from these types of activities, studies suggest that mandated self-reflection activities may not be as beneficial and potentially have negative effects on the future ability to self-reflect.[9] Group self-reflection activities can be intimidating for trainees or less experienced clinicians. But data suggest that self-reflection practiced as a group event instead of in isolation may be more effective.[8] Effective self-reflection should look dispassionately but critically at events and the development of strategies to continue to emphasize and encourage good practices and avoid errors and undesirable practices. Group self-reflection exercises, such as debriefing sessions or Schwartz rounds[10] have significant benefits for personal self-growth and education, and team functioning. Numerous studies support the concept of effective self-reflection and strategies to implement these in ICU practice.

Bedside Teaching

Sir William Osler said "Medicine is learned at the bedside, not in a classroom."[11] Bedside teaching has always been considered the gold standard for education in PICU. It is at the bedside that trainees learn the skills of history taking and physical examination, and many other essential skills for PICU practitioners. Lack of these skills is at the root of most medical errors. Lack of physical examination skills has been directly linked to increased diagnostic errors.[12] In addition to preventing errors, improvement in these clinical skills may lessen the reliance on ancillary tests and help reduce health care costs. The patient's bedside provides excellent opportunities for faculty members to demonstrate and model humanistic skills such as empathy, integrity, compassion, and leadership skills that are fundamental in critical care.

Most PICU clinicians have likely benefitted immensely from skillful bedside education. By many accounts, however, reliance on bedside teaching is declining. Although the reason for this is not clearly defined, numerous factors likely are responsible, including multiple demands on faculty time, heavy clinical load, duty hour restrictions, and possibly a decreased confidence of faculty members in their ability to perform bedside teaching. In addition, reliance on alternate forms of teaching such as electronic methods and simulation likely play a role. In the face of these demands and emphasis on alternate methods of education, a re-emphasis on bedside teaching is needed. One way to accomplish this may be to increase the comfort of younger clinicians to teach at the bedside. This can be accomplished by observation and group "practice" with mentors.

Just as with other skills, bedside teaching is something that can be taught and learned. Quantifying the effectiveness of bedside teaching is difficult. However, in a recent study based on feedback from a wide range of physicians at varying points in their training, Ten Cate and colleagues[11] reported numerous desirable bedside teaching traits. The themes identified included well-prepared teachers who provided a safe teaching environment, teaching geared toward the learner's level of expertise, and stressed both the uniqueness of the personalized care for each patient and focusing on patient satisfaction and outcomes. The authors concluded that few clinicians have formal education in these skills and suggested the development of an Entrustable Professional Activity (EPA) for bedside teaching to improve the education of both teachers and learners.

OTHER TOOLS FOR TEACHING IN THE ICU

Adult learners are in general self-motivated and have a desire to be self-directed. However, not all trainees benefit from the same teaching techniques. For example, some learners require near-complete knowledge of a subject before attempting to apply this knowledge for problem solving, whereas others assimilate information better while attempting to utilize it, even when knowledge is incomplete. To be effective as educators and maximize learning, we must recognize that differences exist. This may require alternative methods of knowledge and skill acquisition be available to learners, and a willingness to support these alternatives.

Many different types of education occur in the PICU. Nonpatient facing educational activities such as case discussions, journal article reviews, didactic discussions, morbidity and mortality discussions have all been mainstays of teaching on inpatient units, including ICUs and all have utility in the education process. Alternative educational activities have more recently become popular as they are more easily incorporated into the current ICU environment and the limited number of hours for teaching and learning. Electronic forms of education and conferencing are becoming increasingly common in training programs, especially with younger learners who are more facile with electronic media.

Electronic Learning

Electronic formats for learning in medicine have been increasing in number and type for decades, and medical school curricula are now largely electronic based. However, these formats have been slow to be adopted in postgraduate training. Residency programs in anesthesiology have a well-described online curriculum[13,14] and radiology programs commonly use electronic learning for residents,[15] but most other specialties primarily rely on in-person educational activities. These methods may be effective for transfer of knowledge, but likely insufficient for learning other skills such as teamwork, collaboration, technical skills, and other skills that benefit from clinical, interpersonal, or multidisciplinary environments.

Multiple types of e-learning activities are used in postgraduate education and include Internet-based tutorials (eg, lectures), virtual patients, interactive videoconferences, and discussion groups. More recently, podcasts and chat groups have become common. Electronic learning has been shown to be equally effective compared to nonelectronic learning in terms of satisfaction and knowledge acquisition.[16] Additional benefits also exist and may continue to encourage transition of certain activities to e-learning. These include the flexibility in allowing learners to view information and participate in learning at times that are convenient for their schedule. This makes these activities desirable for both learners and educators and allows faculty to effect teaching and knowledge acquisition without taking time away from patient care responsibilities. Other benefits include the ability to tailor educational activities to a learners' ability and style, which is not always possible in a traditional lecture setting with multiple learner types.

The adoption of electronic learning for postgraduate training began to change more rapidly in 2020 with the onset of the COVID-19 pandemic and the need for social distancing. Training programs were forced to rapidly develop online teaching activities for both trainees and continuing medical education. Many of these activities have been converted back to in-person learning, but a number have been well received and learners may continue to benefit from an electronic format of learning.[17] Mock codes, which have traditionally been an in-person activity, have been conducted in a virtual format. In addition, virtual teaching rounds have also been reported. Satisfaction with these activities has been reported to be acceptable, but possibly only because no in-person alternative existed. It is unclear if these or other virtual activities improve teaching outcomes and will continue to have a heightened role in PICU education or whether the convenience of these sessions outweighs the lack of interactive discussions that would otherwise occur during in-person activities.

Simulation

Medical simulation remains an important part of PICU education as it allows acquisition of skills without the potential of patient harm. Although simulators in health care have existed in some fashion since the 1960s, their use did not become widespread until the last 20 years. This may partly be due to an improvement in equipment and increased availability, but also likely due to the more widespread acceptance of the benefits of simulation. Simulation encompasses a wide range of educational activities. Common types include simulated patients, task trainers, and high-fidelity mannequin-based simulation. Simulation has a particular benefit for PICU training as it allows trainees to practice critical high-risk skills without putting patients at risk. In addition to skill acquisition, it allows for multidisciplinary and team training and feedback that is vital to optimum PICU functioning.

Simulation has become standard in certain training programs such as surgery and anesthesiology. This is likely due to its effectiveness in task training as well as its effectiveness at crisis situation training. Data support its effectiveness for improving knowledge, procedural skills, and team functioning.[18–21] The improvement in patient care and outcomes is less well-defined. Most pediatric critical care fellowship programs use some form of simulation. This includes use of task trainers such as intubation and central venous cannulation trainers, in situ mock codes, and high-fidelity mannequins for teaching clinical skills as well as team training. Fellowship program directors agree that simulation is a necessary part of their training program and fellows, in general, agree that simulation improves their skills and abilities.[22] The degree to which simulation is effective in resident or student PICU education is not known.

The efficacy of simulation-based task training has been demonstrated in multiple specialties, including critical care.[23–25] Task-based trainers for intubation and central venous cannulation are common, and their use has been associated with improved outcomes for intubation success and decreased central line–associated bloodstream infection.[26] The use of task trainers allows practice and mastery of manual skills without risk to patients, development of repetitive maneuver dexterity and memory, and learning and streamlining of sequential processes to avoid unnecessary and potentially harmful steps in a procedure and improve success. The ability of trainees to practice tasks on trainers has received overwhelmingly positive reviews from participants.[27–29]

Along with task simulators, patient simulation has increased in popularity among training programs. Patient simulation can mimic the experience of providing care for critically ill children and is usually accomplished with the use of high-fidelity patient mannequins. These mannequins mimic many critical organ and tissue functions thereby increasing the realism of the simulation and ultimately, the utility of learning sessions. Mannequin-based simulation supports discussion of physiology and pathophysiology, diagnostic accuracy, treatment, and team function. In addition, nontechnical skills such as professionalism, ethical behavior and decision-making, empathy, and giving bad news to families can be modeled and practiced using mannequin-based simulation.

Realism is an important part of simulation because it allows for greater suspension of disbelief and therefore greater stress. The ability to model stress and evaluate its effect on performance is one of the most powerful teaching aspects of medical simulation. In situ simulation involves medical simulation that takes place in the ICU setting where the trainees work. This type of simulation has the benefits of placing learners in a realistic environment that resembles the one in which they routinely function. Understanding how trainees function in this type of environment is critical to their ability to function adequately in the PICU. Feedback from in situ sessions can significantly improve identification of personal skills that may either excel or suffer under stress, to modify behavior and to further tailor educational activities for individual learners. In addition, in situ simulation provides situations to identify location-specific problems that may be unique to a particular clinical setting such as malfunctioning equipment, space limitations, or other factors that may affect team function and patient outcome. By simulation of actual emergencies with the physicians, nurses, therapists, technicians, and other staff who provide care, team training and quality of care can be significantly improved.

As much as simulation has become a vital part of PICU training, barriers exist. The primary barrier is cost, as simulation equipment and space to house and perform simulation are both costly and scarce. In addition, simulation requires staff who have the knowledge to organize, program, carry out, and maintain simulation equipment and space. An additional barrier is the lack of data. Despite simulation becoming part and parcel of many training programs, data supporting its effectiveness in improving education in ICUs are sparse. There is even less data on the effects on patient care. Hopefully, as more studies show the utility of simulation to train physicians and improve patient care and outcomes, funding will increase and allow all trainees and patients to benefit from this educational modality.

SUMMARY

Many novel teaching techniques are available to educators for enhancing PICU training. However, traditional teaching methods still hold a vital place in continuing to educate our trainees. A better understanding of how to use these techniques along with an understanding of how we make decisions in medicine should continue to influence how we educate our trainees in attempts to not only optimize education but patient care and outcomes.

CLINICS CARE POINTS

- Diagnostic errors are common in medicine and lead to significant morbidity and mortality.
- Teaching students to recognize and manage inherent biases can lead to improved diagnositc ability and decreased errors.
- Promotion of critical thinking and reflective learning are additional tools that may help prevent errors.
- Electronic learning modalities and simulation are becoming more common and sought after by trainees.

DISCLOSURE

The author has nothing to disclose.

REFERENCES

1. Saber Tehrani AS, Lee H, Mathews SC, et al. 25-Year summary of US malpractice claims for diagnostic errors 1986-2010: an analysis from the National Practitioner Data Bank. BMJ Qual Saf 2013;22(8):672–80.

2. Cifra CL, Custer JW, Singh H, et al. Diagnostic Errors in Pediatric Critical Care: A Systematic Review. Pediatr Crit Care Med 2021;22(8):701–12.
3. Graber ML, Franklin N, Gordon R. Diagnostic error in internal medicine. Arch Intern Med 2005;165(13):1493–9.
4. Croskerry P. From mindless to mindful practice–cognitive bias and clinical decision making. N Engl J Med 2013;368(26):2445–8.
5. Hayes MM, Chatterjee S, Schwartzstein RM. Critical Thinking in Critical Care: Five Strategies to Improve Teaching and Learning in the Intensive Care Unit. Ann Am Thorac Soc 2017;14(4):569–75.
6. Carraccio CL, Benson BJ, Nixon LJ, et al. From the educational bench to the clinical bedside: translating the Dreyfus developmental model to the learning of clinical skills. Acad Med 2008;83(8):761–7.
7. Kruger J, Dunning D. Unskilled and unaware–but why? A reply to Krueger and Mueller (2002). J Pers Soc Psychol 2002;82(2):189–92.
8. Bion J, Brown C, Gomersall C, et al. Society of Critical Care Medicine 50th Anniversary Review Series: Critical Care Education. Crit Care Med 2021;49(8):1241–53.
9. Curtis P, Taylor G, Riley R, et al. Written reflection in assessment and appraisal: GP and GP trainee views. Educ Prim Care 2017;28(3):141–9.
10. Hughes J, Duff AJ, Puntis JWL. Using Schwartz Center Rounds to promote compassionate care in a children's hospital. Arch Dis Child 2018;103(1):11–2.
11. van Dam M, Ramani S, Ten Cate O. An EPA for better Bedside Teaching. Clin Teach 2021;18(4):398–403.
12. Clark BW, Derakhshan A, Desai SV. Diagnostic Errors and the Bedside Clinical Examination. Med Clin North Am 2018;102(3):453–64.
13. Marchalot A, Dureuil B, Veber B, et al. Effectiveness of a blended learning course and flipped classroom in first year anaesthesia training. Anaesth Crit Care Pain Med 2018;37(5):411–5.
14. Chu LF, Ngai LK, Young CA, et al. Preparing Interns for Anesthesiology Residency Training: Development and Assessment of the Successful Transition to Anesthesia Residency Training (START) E-Learning Curriculum. J Grad Med Educ 2013;5(1):125–9.
15. Sivarajah RT, Curci NE, Johnson EM, et al. A Review of Innovative Teaching Methods. Acad Radiol 2019;26(1):101–13.
16. Cook DA, Levinson AJ, Garside S, et al. Internet-based learning in the health professions: a meta-analysis. JAMA 2008;300(10):1181–96.
17. Pitt MB, Li ST, Klein M. Novel Educational Responses to COVID-19: What is Here to Stay? Acad Pediatr 2020;20(6):733–4.
18. Bullard MJ, Leuck JA, Howley LD. Unifying interdisciplinary education: designing and implementing an intern simulation educational curriculum to increase confidence in critical care from PGY1 to PGY2. BMC Res Notes 2017;10(1):563.
19. Johnson EM, Hamilton MF, Watson RS, et al. An Intensive, Simulation-Based Communication Course for Pediatric Critical Care Medicine Fellows. Pediatr Crit Care Med 2017;18(8):e348–55.
20. Khobrani A, Patel NH, George RL, et al. Pediatric Trauma Boot Camp: A Simulation Curriculum and Pilot Study. Emerg Med Int 2018;2018:7982315. https://doi.org/10.1155/2018/7982315.
21. Green M, Tariq R, Green P. Improving Patient Safety through Simulation Training in Anesthesiology: Where Are We? Anesthesiol Res Pract 2016;2016:4237523. https://doi.org/10.1155/2016/4237523.

22. Henricksen JW, Troy L, Siefkes H. Pediatric Critical Care Medicine Fellowship Simulation Use Survey. Pediatr Crit Care Med 2020;21(10):e908–14.
23. Bresler L, Perez M, Hubert J, et al. Residency training in robotic surgery: The role of simulation. J Visc Surg 2020;157(3 Suppl 2):S123–9.
24. Lorello GR, Cook DA, Johnson RL, et al. Simulation-based training in anaesthesiology: a systematic review and meta-analysis. Br J Anaesth 2014;112(2):231–45.
25. L'Her E, Geeraerts T, Desclefs JP, et al. Simulation-based teaching in critical care, anaesthesia and emergency medicine. Anaesth Crit Care Pain Med 2020;39(2): 311–26.
26. Steiner M, Langgartner M, Cardona F, et al. Significant Reduction of Catheter-associated Blood Stream Infections in Preterm Neonates After Implementation of a Care Bundle Focusing on Simulation Training of Central Line Insertion. Pediatr Infect Dis J 2015;34(11):1193–6.
27. Robinson AR, Gravenstein N, Cooper LA, et al. A mixed-reality part-task trainer for subclavian venous access. Simul Healthc 2014;9(1):56–64.
28. Zendejas B, Brydges R, Hamstra SJ, et al. State of the evidence on simulation-based training for laparoscopic surgery: a systematic review. Ann Surg 2013; 257(4):586–93.
29. Latif RK, Bautista AF, Memon SB, et al. Teaching aseptic technique for central venous access under ultrasound guidance: a randomized trial comparing didactic training alone to didactic plus simulation-based training. Anesth Analg 2012; 114(3):626–33.

Moving?

Make sure your subscription moves with you!

To notify us of your new address, find your **Clinics Account Number** (located on your mailing label above your name), and contact customer service at:

Email: journalscustomerservice-usa@elsevier.com

800-654-2452 (subscribers in the U.S. & Canada)
314-447-8871 (subscribers outside of the U.S. & Canada)

Fax number: 314-447-8029

Elsevier Health Sciences Division
Subscription Customer Service
3251 Riverport Lane
Maryland Heights, MO 63043

*To ensure uninterrupted delivery of your subscription, please notify us at least 4 weeks in advance of move.

Printed and bound by CPI Group (UK) Ltd, Croydon, CR0 4YY

03/10/2024

01040468-0011